Intellectual Disability and Dementia

of related interest

Understanding Learning Disability and Dementia
Developing Effective Interventions
Diana Kerr
ISBN 978 1 84310 442 1
eISBN 978 1 84642 675 9

Caring for the Physical and Mental Health of
People with Learning Disabilities
David Perry, Louise Hammond, Geoff Marston, Sherryl Gaskell and James Eva
ISBN 978 1 84905 131 6
eISBN 978 0 85700 225 9

How to Break Bad News to People with Intellectual Disabilities
A Guide for Carers and Professionals
Irene Tuffrey-Wijne
Foreword by Professor Baroness Sheila Hollins
ISBN 978 1 84905 280 1
eISBN 978 0 85700 583 0

Personalisation and Dementia
A Guide for Person-Centred Practice
Helen Sanderson and Gill Bailey
ISBN 978 1 84905 379 2
eISBN 978 0 85700 734 6

Enriched Care Planning for People with Dementia
A Good Practice Guide to Delivering Person-Centred Care
Hazel May, Paul Edwards and Dawn Brooker
ISBN 978 1 84310 405 6
eISBN 978 1 84642 960 6

Risk Assessment and Management for Living Well with Dementia
Charlotte L. Clarke, Heather Wilkinson, John Keady and Catherine E. Gibb
Foreword by Professor Murna Downs
Bradford Dementia Group Good Practice Guides series
ISBN 978 1 84905 005 0
eISBN 978 0 85700 519 9

Intellectual Disability *and* Dementia

Research into Practice

Edited by Karen Watchman

Foreword by Diana Kerr

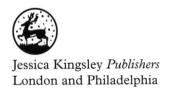

Jessica Kingsley *Publishers*
London and Philadelphia

Figures 10.1–10.4 on page 166 reproduced with permission from the Foundation for People with Learning Disabilities

First published in 2014
by Jessica Kingsley Publishers
73 Collier Street
London N1 9BE, UK
and
400 Market Street, Suite 400
Philadelphia, PA 19106, USA

www.jkp.com

Library of Congress Cataloging in Publication Data
A CIP catalog record for this book is available from the Library of Congress

British Library Cataloguing in Publication Data
A CIP catalogue record for thi book is available from the British Library

ISBN 978 1 84905 422 5
eISBN 978 0 85700 796 4

Printed and bound in Great Britain

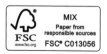

Contents

Figures

Tables

Foreword

Diana Kerr

Since the work of Wolfensberger and John O'Brien, amongst others, in the 1980s, services have been challenged to provide support and services that enable people with an intellectual disability to have meaningful, fulfilling lives. This has presented services with the need to become person-centred and so cater for the individual rather than the group. 'See the person not the disability' has become an often-heard mantra.

Wonderfully, people with an intellectual disability are, like the rest of the population, living longer and often into old age. This longevity inevitably brings with it the conditions of older age, one of which is dementia. The worry and indeed the reality in many cases is that with the onset of dementia many of the gains made over the years will be lost. People with an intellectual disability and dementia are at risk of again being defined by their diagnosis and increasingly marginalised or returned to inappropriate settings. To avoid this, people with an intellectual disability who develop dementia need to have a sure, coherent, consistent, adequately funded and resourced service based on informed, and evidence-based research and practice.

There are some good and even excellent examples of person-centred, sensitive provision, as this book demonstrates. This provision is, however, scattered and often the result of organisations and individuals pushing for their service to respond appropriately to the changing needs of people. They are, as a consequence, often limited to a specific locality and vulnerable to changing funding and social policies.

Much literature and practice in the past has concentrated on diagnosis and the early stage of dementia and as a consequence mid- and later-stage experiences and needs have been neglected. The lack of a suitable palliative care approach or pathway being an example of this lack of forward planning.

The range of chapters in this book provide a wealth of information that can and should inform provision throughout the whole course of the condition. There is well-researched and evidenced information about good practice and the way forward in relation to assessment, diagnosis, training, care pathways, service design and the experience of families, carers and peers. There is also welcome attention paid to the philosophy of care and support that must underpin all our interventions.

In 2007, in the final paragraph of *Understanding Learning Disability and Dementia* I wrote:

> Much that is written about in this book is not complicated; it is not expensive. In fact much is free or cheap to implement. It should not, therefore, be beyond the capacity of those who fund and provide services to people with a intellectual disability to maintain all the gains made for people with a intellectual disability since the 1980s as they enter old age and develop dementia.

Not everything included in this book is free or cheap, but it does already exist somewhere. If it can be implemented somewhere then why not everywhere, particularly as part of a longer-term strategic approach?

Seven years on from my original plea it is time that all who are involved with the provision of support and care of people with an intellectual disability who have dementia grasp the nettle and, having read this book, take the best and aim to implement it. There remains a need for more research beyond the scope of this book, but what is in here will inform and guide good practice from diagnosis to death.

Introduction

Karen Watchman

Background

There is increasing realisation that whilst people with an intellectual disability now enjoy a longer life expectancy, this brings with it an increased risk of dementia particularly for those with Down syndrome. There are growing bodies of research that include people with dementia and people with an intellectual disability. However, this is in stark contrast to the limited amount of research that is inclusive of people with both an intellectual disability and dementia. Those with an intellectual disability already face marginalisation at an individual and cultural level, due to society's perception of their disability. This book will show how the potential for further marginalisation increases due to the lack of accurate figures about the number of people with an intellectual disability who have dementia, the lack of adapted communication as dementia increases, a lack of specialist knowledge of intellectual disability and dementia and the impact of not sharing information about the diagnosis with the person.

The growing number of people with an intellectual disability living with dementia undoubtedly presents significant challenges to the individuals themselves, their families, health and social care services and the staff who provide support. The incidence and prevalence of dementia in people with an intellecutal disability is not decreasing. On the contrary, the issue will increase internationally as this population continues to enjoy a longer life expectancy, and develops later life conditions. This also applies to countries underrepresented among the contributors to this book, notably those in eastern Europe faced with their first-ever cohort of people ageing with an intellectual disability, and those countries where institutionalisation in long-stay hospitals remains the norm. The plea is to appreciate the importance of knowledge exchange on a wider scale, in a way that avoids countries and individuals working in isolation.

The origins of this book lie in my own background, having worked with people with an intellectual disability for many years. Whilst attitudes in some areas have changed significantly, the same cannot be said for approaches to supporting people with an intellectual disability who also have dementia. When developing a postgraduate course on intellectual disability and dementia, I was struck by the lack of a contemporary edited text in this area to augment the comprehensive work in 1999 (Janicki and Dalton, 1999) and 2000 (Janicki and Ansello, 2000). Practical and constructive examples have since been published highlighting issues and challenges in care settings such as Kerr (2007), where definitions of dementia and of intellectual disability and an explanation of the different realities of people with dementia can also be found. In addition to offering a resource for academic studies, I am mindful that although researchers and students have access to academic articles through their university, practitioners do not. Consequently, this book is for those developing, delivering or studying an education or training programme about an issue that impacts on people with an intellectual disability and dementia. It is also for those planning and developing services for people ageing with an intellectual disability, or supporting a person with an intellectual disability and dementia, their family or peers.

Emerging themes

In bringing together research, individual experience and evidence from practice covering a range of different topics and perspectives, a number of common themes have emerged:

- Recognition of the difference in clinical presentation and progression of dementia in people with Down syndrome.

- The lack of a clear evidence base for pharmacological interventions, with a reliance on anecdotal information.

- Awareness that existing dementia diagnosis tools and assessment methods are not suitable for most people with an intellectual disability.

- Recognition of the increased risk of dementia being misdiagnosed due to other treatable, but often undetected, conditions associated with ageing in people with an intellectual disability.

- Lack of recognition of the role that friends and families of those with an intellectual disability and dementia have, in addition to being able to provide a crucial source of information.

- The importance of talking about dementia to people with an intellectual disability, their family and peers.

- The need to know more about the first-hand experiences and preferences of people with an intellectual disability who have dementia.

- Awareness that co-production, at an individual, service or system level, is currently not happening with people who have an intellectual disability and dementia.

- A call for the development of specialist training, in addition to upskilling of staff in generic intellectual disability services and dementia services.

- Redevelopment of existing support services to accommodate changing physical, social and environmental needs, on a 24-hour basis.

- The emergence of in place progression dementia specific care settings for people with intellectual disabilities and dementia to complement ageing in place provision.

- The importance of a palliative approach from the point of diagnosis, with a recognised pathway needed that begins earlier in the course of dementia, rather than only at end of life.

Whilst each chapter can be read as standalone, the book has been developed in three sequential parts and asks a simple, yet crucial, question of the reader at each stage:

- What do we know?

- How do we know it?

- What are we going to do about it?

Part 1 – What do we know?

Whilst general population screening for dementia is not recommended in the UK, the screening of those known to be at risk will help with earlier detection. This enables a person's baseline functioning to be recorded whilst they are still healthy, with the likelihood that any significant changes would be investigated sooner. Part 1 of this book begins by looking at the association between Down syndrome and dementia. Amanda Sinai, Trevor Chan and Andre Strydom explain the prevalence and incidence rates of dementia among people with Down syndrome and among those with other types of intellectual disability. Liam Reese Wilson, Tiina Annus, Shahid Zaman and Anthony Holland take us through the clinical links, highlighting differences in the course and presentation of dementia as it affects people with Down syndrome. They introduce the growing body of evidence for frontotemporal (frontal lobe) symptoms as a pre-clinical manifestation of Alzheimer's disease among those with Down syndrome.

Antonia Coppus informs of how the issue of diagnosis is addressed at a Down syndrome outpatient clinic in the Netherlands. The clinic does not only screen for dementia, but also other conditions which, if untreated, may mask or mimic early signs of dementia leading to misdiagnosis. For example 30 per cent of those attending the clinic did not have the correct prescription for their glasses and 70 per cent had undetected hearing loss. Whilst there are at least 15 clinics in the UK for children with Down syndrome, services for adults are scarce (Marder and Dennis, 2013). The Fife model in Scotland (Jones *et al.*, 2010) is one of only a few developed in response to the known different health needs of people with Down syndrome, and the lack of specific training among primary care practitioners and secondary care professionals. Findings in Fife are similar to those in the Netherlands, with 66 per cent of people with Down syndrome attending having at least one new health need which was identified by the clinic, and 12 per cent having between five and eight new health needs identified. Some chapters, such as these first three, focus specifically on Down syndrome, because of the known association, whilst others focus on people with an intellectual disability more generally.

Ken Courtenay and Nicole Eady give a comprehensive overview of the purpose of anti-dementia medication and its application among people with intellectual disabilities. Whilst anecdotally, medication may slow down progression in the early stages of dementia, this is likely to be short-lived with the potential for increased susceptibility to side effects as tolerance to the medication increases. The extreme sensitivity to neuroleptic (anti-psychotic) medication, when the person has Lewy body dementia in particular should be noted. The lack of an evidence base in pharmacological approaches with people who have an intellectual disability leads to growing interest in non-pharmacological interventions. Nancy Jokinen discusses the challenges raised for organisations and individual carers due to the lack of evidence for non-pharmacological interventions with people who have an intellectual disability and dementia. This results in learning and practice being drawn from both sectors, particularly general dementia care, despite the known differences between both populations in age and where people typically live. Developed from the limited research on the subjective experiences of people with an intellectual disability and dementia, Sunny Kalsy-Lillico discusses how psychological experiences can be enhanced by those who provide support. She highlights the focus in literature of early signs and diagnosis of dementia, rather than interventions post-diagnosis for the person and their family. Sunny discusses the importance of social relationships of the individual, their physical environment and cultural understandings of, and tolerance for, confusion and frailty. Both Nancy and Sunny stress the importance of providing support in an individualised way that encourages a focus on the person, rather than 'the intellectual disability' or 'the dementia'.

Part 2 – How do we know?

Intentionally situated at the centre of the book, and a noticeably shorter section, are the experiences and personal accounts of people with an intellectual disability and their families. By asking the question 'How do we know?' this section brings together a mixture of evidence from research and practice, including individual experiences. In doing so, it becomes apparent that the answer is that we know very little from the perspective of the person with an intellectual disability and dementia. Consent has been given to reproduce individual stories and case studies either from the person with an intellectual disability, as part of the research process, or from their carer. Names have been changed throughout unless indicated otherwise.

Noelle Blackman and David Thompson share reflections from people with intellectual disabilities in the UK-based GOLD group

(Growing Older with Learning Disabilities). This explores issues raised when a family member or a friend has dementia. It reinforces the reciprocity of caring that often exists, although is not always recognised, between an adult with an intellectual disability and their friend, in addition to a sibling or ageing parent.

I introduce the first of the case examples in the book, based on a longitudinal research project. The experiences shared in this chapter highlight how staff are often ill-equipped to identify and support individuals with an intellectual disability and dementia. This can apply to staff in intellectual disability services in addition to those providing dementia care, although for different reasons. The importance of relearning practice in intellectual disability services is highlighted, where staff typically focus on independent living and supporting the development of new skills. Approaches should still be person-centred and value based, but will need to focus on maintaining and consolidating existing skills, with a greater crossover needed whereby intellectual disability services and dementia services learn from each other. I reflect on the three different care settings that the research participants called 'home', identifying the least satisfactory option as being a generic older people's service, where people with Down syndrome in particular are significantly younger than other residents.

The vulnerability of ageing parents of people with an intellectual disability is underreported, particularly in relation to their caring role over a prolonged period of time (Cairns *et al.*, 2013). Yet, increasing care needs will arise, with the onset of dementia. Rachel Carling-Jenkins, Christine Bigby and Teresa Iacono give insight into the experiences of diagnosis and post-diagnostic support for families in Australia. Their research shows consistency with the situation in the UK and Canada over the lack of a policy framework for younger people with intellectual disability, who find themselves lost in both the aged care system and the intellectual disability system. The importance of planning for any resulting transition to avoid a crisis situation is discussed. Christine Towers gives an example of how this may work in practice, based on a project at the Foundation for People with Learning Disabilities, UK. The project has developed resources that support families to plan ahead with their son or daughter who has an intellectual disability, and to address issues that will arise after a diagnosis of dementia. Christine presents strategies for a partnership approach that includes, but is not coordinated by, the family to ensure that longer-term needs are recognised and discussed after a diagnosis of dementia, in addition to immediate needs relating to the condition.

Part 3 – What are we going to do?

The shift required from supporting people with an intellectual disability to live as independently as possible, through to supporting their maintenance of skills and eventual decline is a thread that runs throughout the book. Social care staff are currently recruited and trained to provide a different form of support; different to the reality of what is required in the mid and end stages of dementia. The examples provided in Part 3 demonstrate the need for a redesign of current provision. This highlights the importance of services having a protocol for future development, which includes a redesign of staff training, residential provision and day programmes. By addressing the question 'What are we going to do?' contributors have considered how we can expand on the limited evidence base, with suggestions for how this can be developed to inform practice. Irene Tuffrey-Wijne and I respond first to the challenge by addressing the lack of consistent practice when talking to people with an intellectual disability about their diagnosis of dementia. This means that the person themselves is often unaware of why they are experiencing changes, which makes it harder to plan meaningfully together for their future. It restricts what can be told to friends, who may be in a position to play a supportive role, particularly in shared accommodation. The responsibility to explain, or communicate, the reasons for the changes in a consistent manner lies with those who do not have dementia, based on the experience and understanding of the person.

The importance of staff training is discussed by Karen Dodd, not just to impart knowledge, but to bring about a shift in attitude and practice. In addition to traditional didactic means of teaching and training, non-traditional methods should also be considered. This includes online or cascade approaches for knowledge exchange, and to maximise the potential audience internationally. Leslie Udell continues Part 3 of the book with an honest reflection on 20 years of dementia specific service provision for people with an intellectual disability at Winniserv non-profit organisation in Canada, and of lessons learned along the way. Leslie has observed the misdiagnosis of dementia on a number of occasions when in reality a treatable condition was the cause, often one that was not detected until significantly later. Leslie's experience at Winniserv recognises the need for adopting a palliative approach from the point of diagnosis, rather than only at the end of life stage, and her insight paves the way for today's service providers and commissioners to learn from their extensive experience. Many intellectual disability services in the UK and internationally are considering, or are already supporting, people in a dementia specific small group home or single person accommodation. Whilst recognising the role of ageing in place where appropriate, this also reflects a move towards an in place progression model (Janicki, 2011). Here, specialised training and adapted dementia specific environments continue to accommodate those with an intellectual disability as dementia progresses. Mary McCarron, Philip McCallion, Evelyn Reilly and Niamh Mulryan acknowledge the challenge to traditional intellectual disability service approaches and philosophies, and explain the response of an intellectual disability service in Ireland. This has included adapting more than one care setting to accommodate people with intellectual disabilities as they progress through different stages of dementia.

Susan Benbow, Moni Grizell and Andrew Griffiths also consider the service context, this time within the field of intellectual disability and older people psychiatry, where again a lack of clarity has been observed over which service can best meet individual need. A warning is issued about care being duplicated, or not provided at all, with a need for the person and their family to be given information at all stages. Good practice examples are shared, showing the importance of a locally agreed joint pathway and a care plan that identifies the required input from each service, in addition to the person and their family. In order to understand how far strategies and service delivery are achieving their aim of supporting people with an intellectual disability to live well with dementia, we need to be able to measure the outcomes of the care and support received. Karen Dodd concludes this section with a call to clarify what we are trying to achieve in services for people with intellectual disabilities and dementia. She introduces a new staged outcome measure designed to prevent deterioration in care as dementia progresses and to plan ahead for effective and meaningful support. Using 17 domains that accompany the person through the early, mid and late stages of dementia, the intention is to ensure quality outcomes for each person throughout the course of the condition.

It is evident that content of this book is from the economically developed countries of UK, Ireland, USA, Canada, Netherlands and Australia. Data is lacking from other parts of the world, reflecting the need for research and the development of a practice base in other areas. Also missing are the experiences of people with an intellectual disability from minority ethnic groups, and research evidence or examples of the use of assistive technology, telecare and telehealth with this population. All three parts of the book are consistent in the need to build a greater evidence base about dementia in people with an intellectual disability. The breadth of material included, whether informed by clinical or psychosocial evidence, user perspective, or practice, collectively call for existing knowledge to be shared. My hope is that the examples given, and experiences shared, open the door that informs future research, policy, practice and service development, both nationally and internationally. Until then, the one voice that needs to be heard will continue to remain silent – that of the person with an intellectual disability who has dementia.

A note on terminology

The terms 'intellectual disability' and 'Down syndrome' are used throughout consistent with international terminology. In the UK people with intellectual disabilities are commonly referred to as people with learning disabilities and this is reflected in some of the references.

References

Cairns, D., Brown, J., Tolson, D. and Darbyshire, C. (2013) Caring for a child with learning disabilities over a prolonged period of time: an exploratory survey on the experiences and health of older parent carers living in Scotland. *Journal of Applied Research in Intellectual Disability*. doi: 10.1111/jar.12071.

Janicki, M. (2011) Quality outcomes in group home dementia care for adults with intellectual disabilities. *Journal of Intellectual Disability Research* 55, 8, 763–776.

Janicki, MP. and Ansello, EF. (2000) *Community Supports for Aging Adults with Lifelong Disabilities*. Baltimore: Paul Brooks Publishing.

Janicki, MP. and Dalton, A. (1999) *Dementia, Aging and Intellectual Disabilities: A Handbook*. Philadelphia, PA: Brummer/Mazel.

Jones, J., Hathaway, D., Gilhooley, M., Leech, A. and MacLeod, S. (2010) Down's's syndrome health screening – the Fife model. *British Journal of Learning Disabilities* 38, 1, 5–9.

Kerr, D. (2007) *Understanding Learning Disability and Dementia*. London: Jessica Kingsley Publishers.

Marder, L. and Dennis, J. (2013) *Healthcare Services and Support for People with Down's's Syndrome in the UK: Down's Syndrome Medical Interest Group*. Available at www.dsmig.org.uk/library/articles/uk-healthcare.html, accessed on 4 December 2013.

PART 1

The Association between Intellectual Disabilities and Dementia

What Do We Know?

The Epidemiology of Dementia in People with Intellectual Disabilities

Amanda Sinai, Trevor Chan, Andre Strydom

The ageing population of people with intellectual disabilities

Significant improvements in health and social care for people with an intellectual disability have led to a dramatic increase in the life expectancy of this population over the past 50 years. The improvements in life expectancy have been particularly striking within the population of people with Down syndrome. It has been estimated that the survival of babies with Down syndrome and congenital birth defects increased from 0 to around 18 years or more in the early 1990s in the USA (Yang *et al.*, 2002) and the number of people with Down syndrome surviving to over 40 years old has been estimated to have doubled in Northern European countries since 1990 (de Graaf *et al.*, 2011). It can therefore be deduced that, at least in the developed world, there is now a much larger proportion of people with intellectual disability living into older adulthood, with associated increased rates of age-related conditions, including dementia. Dementia is now a common factor contributing to death in people with Down syndrome in the UK, and has been found to be a factor in the death in 30 per cent of older people with Down syndrome in Sweden (Englund *et al.*, 2013).

What is dementia?

Dementia is essentially a clinical syndrome which has been defined by various classification systems such as International Classification of Diseases, ICD-10 (World Health Organization, 1993) and the

Diagnostic and Statistical Manual of Mental Disorders, DSM-IV (American Psychiatric Association, 2000). Both ICD-10 and DSM-IV require development of a decline in memory and other cognitive functions to make a diagnosis of dementia. ICD-10 requires that symptoms are present for at least six months (World Health Organization, 1993). An updated version of DSM has been published in 2013, called DSM-5 (American Psychiatric Association, 2013). It remains to be seen how the fifth edition of DSM, known as DSM-5, will affect epidemiological research in this field. Diagnostic Criteria for Psychiatric Disorders for Use with Adults with Learning Disabilities (DC-LD) is a diagnostic classification system based on ICD-10, designed for use in adults with moderate to profound intellectual disability (Cooper et al., 2003).

There are several different types of dementia, such as Alzheimer's disease, vascular, Lewy body and frontotemporal dementias, with different aetiologies and different incidence and prevalence rates. In the general population, Alzheimer's disease is the most common subtype of dementia, followed by vascular dementia.

Factors affecting population estimates of dementia rates in the population of people with intellectual disabilities

The commonest epidemiological parameters of disorders are prevalence and incidence rates. Prevalence refers to the proportion of a population found to have a condition at a given time. Incidence is the number of new cases of the condition found in a defined population in a given period. Accurate epidemiological estimates of dementia in the intellectual disability population can be influenced by many factors, including diagnostic issues, assessment methods, criteria used, population studied, and type of dementia included. Some of these issues will briefly be considered before a summary of what is known about the epidemiological profile of dementia in the population of people with an intellectual disability.

Diagnostic issues and assessment tools

There are inherent difficulties in assessing for, and diagnosing, dementia in the population of people with an intellectual disability that can affect the estimation of prevalence and incidence rates. First, most adults with an intellectual disability have pre-existing cognitive deficits, including loss of short-term memory, and it can be quite difficult to establish a decline in cognition or function, particularly in those with limited speech abilities and low functional abilities. Second, most of the neuropsychological screening and assessment tools used in the general population are not suitable for adults with an intellectual disability. Although there are some tools that have been specifically developed for use in the population of people with intellectual disabilities, there are no established assessment batteries with satisfactory psychometric properties that can be used across the ability spectrum. Clinicians may therefore need to rely on informants' report of symptoms (Jamieson-Craig *et al.*, 2010), which may not always be accurate.

The diagnostic stability of dementia diagnoses in those with an intellectual disability, who did not have Down syndrome, has been explored by Strydom *et al.* (2013a). They established that diagnostic instability may be more common in the intellectual disability population due to additional challenges in diagnosing dementia. These additional challenges may include variable quality of informant reports, difficulties in the assessment of those with moderate and severe intellectual disability or sensory impairments, difficulties in detecting protracted periods of plateau in vascular dementia and the 'floor effect' in advanced dementia in the absence of longitudinal information.

Definitions of dementia used

As a result of the differences between criteria, estimates of population rates may vary according to the definition of dementia used. For example, the ICD-10 criteria often result in a more restrictive diagnosis and subsequent lower estimates of population rates. Estimates may also vary according to which subtypes of dementia are included; many epidemiological surveys tend to focus on Alzheimer's disease, and may miss cases of other dementias such as frontotemporal dementia, as these have a different presentation and age of onset. Study designs therefore require specific consideration to ensure inclusion of rarer types of dementia.

It is well established that there are much higher rates of Alzheimer's disease in people with Down syndrome as compared to the general population, and compared to other people with an intellectual disability. It is therefore important to be clear about whether adults with Down syndrome are included or excluded from epidemiological studies of dementia in those with an intellectual disability, and it is easier to interpret rates if those with Down syndrome and those without Down syndrome are reported separately.

The age thresholds used in epidemiological studies of dementia may also affect prevalence and incidence estimates. Dementia often occurs at a younger age than expected, particularly in people with Down syndrome, and rates may be underestimated if relevant age groups are excluded. Finally, living arrangements may also be important, as those living in institutions, which remain prevalent in some parts of the world, may differ in many ways from community-dwelling older adults with an intellectual disability, which could affect their likelihood of survival and of subsequently developing dementia.

The impact of these issues upon dementia estimates in the intellectual disability population can be demonstrated by the available literature. In a postal survey of known dementia cases amongst adults using intellectual disability services in New York State, USA, Janicki and Dalton (2000) found an overall prevalence rate of 6.1 per cent in those aged 60 and older. This figure was comparable to that in the general population, although rates were much higher in the Down syndrome population than in those who did not have Down syndrome. However, the survey may have underestimated dementia rates as it relied upon identification of those with known diagnoses, rather than screening for unidentified cases. In contrast, Shooshtari *et al.* (2011) used data from administrative provincial databases in Canada and a matched case-control design, and found a prevalence for dementia of 13.8 per cent for adults with intellectual disabilities aged 55 and older when compared to the matched comparison group.

Prevalence of dementia in people with intellectual disabilities

Dementia prevalence in people with Down syndrome

A number of studies have confirmed that dementia is common in older adults with Down syndrome, and that the prevalence increases sharply between ages 40 and 60. In a large study of people with

Down syndrome aged 45 years and older in the Netherlands, it was found that up to the age of 60 the prevalence of dementia doubled with each five-year interval up to the age of 49 – the prevalence was 8.9 per cent. Between the ages of 50 and 54, it was 17.7 per cent and between 55 and 59, it was estimated at 32.1 per cent (Coppus *et al.*, 2006). A study in the UK found that prevalence rates using CAMDEX (Cambridge Mental Disorders of the Elderly Examination) criteria for Alzheimer's disease increased from 3.4 per cent, to 10.3 per cent, to 40 per cent among 30–39, 40–49 and 50–59 age groups, respectively (Holland *et al.*, 1998). An Irish study, using modified DSM-IV (Diagnostic and Statistical Manual of Mental Disorders) criteria, found age-specific prevalence rates of 1.4 per cent for those under age 40, 5.7 per cent for those aged 40–49 and 30.4 per cent for those aged 50–59 (Tyrrell *et al.*, 2001).

Studies have varied in their estimates of prevalence of dementia beyond the age of 60. Tyrrell *et al.* (2001) have described a rate of 41.7 per cent among those aged 60 and over, and 50 per cent among those aged 70 or older. One study from the Netherlands, based on an institutional sample, described a 100 per cent prevalence rate in adults with Down syndrome aged 70 and older (Visser *et al.*, 1997). However, also in the Netherlands, Coppus *et al.* (2006) described a decrease in prevalence to 25.6 per cent at ages 60 and over, which was due to an increase in mortality rate in those with dementia.

No gender differences have been found for dementia rates in older adults with Down syndrome (Coppus *et al.*, 2006; Tyrrell *et al.*, 2001). However, the average age of menopause of women with Down syndrome has been found to be younger than in the general population (Schupf *et al.*, 1997), and women with Down syndrome who experience early onset of menopause have been shown to also have earlier onset and increased risk for developing Alzheimer's disease when compared to those who had a later onset of menopause (Schupf *et al.*, 2003). Also, the age at menopause for women with Down syndrome has been shown to be correlated with the age at dementia (Coppus *et al.*, 2010; Cosgrave *et al.*, 1999).

Dementia prevalence in people with intellectual disabilities other than Down syndrome

Cooper (1997) conducted a population-based study of 134 older people with an intellectual disability aged 65 and over (five of whom had Down syndrome) in the UK. Dementia was diagnosed in 21.6 per cent, which was found to be substantially higher than general population rates. Strydom *et al.* (2007) established a sample of 222 adults with an intellectual disability aged 60 and older in London, UK. The overall dementia prevalence was found to be 13.1 per cent among those aged 60 and older, and 18.3 per cent among those aged 65 and older. Alzheimer's disease was found to be the most common type of dementia, and had a prevalence of 12 per cent among those aged 65 and older, three times greater than comparable general older adult population rates. Lewy body and frontotemporal dementias were also relatively common.

Zigman *et al.* (2004) identified ten cases with possible, definite or complicated Alzheimer's disease (prevalence rate 9% for those aged 65 and older; 12% for those 75 years and older), in a USA-based longitudinal study of 126 adults with an intellectual disability without Down syndrome over the age of 65. These rates were within the range of rates for older adults in the USA without an intellectual disability (Zigman *et al.*, 2004).

Incidence of dementia in people with intellectual disabilities

When looking at dementia incidence studies, it is important to consider the rigour with which dementia cases at entry are excluded, the age distribution of the cohort, the length of follow-up and the diagnostic methods and criteria used.

Dementia incidence in people with Down syndrome

Visser *et al.* (1997) studied dementia incidence over a six-year period among 307 institutionalised participants in the Netherlands. The incidence rate over six years was 36 per cent among those aged 40 years and above at entry to the study. Coppus *et al.* (2006) found that incidence increased with increasing age, and did not appear to taper off in those aged 60 and over. The decreased prevalence in adults with Down syndrome aged 60 and older noted in this cohort therefore seems to be due to an increase in mortality rates of those with dementia.

In an institutional sample of adults with Down syndrome, Margallo-Lana *et al.* (2007) found that the survival period from onset of dementia until death of those who had died was 3.5 years for incident cases, while the mean age at death was 59.3 years. In this study, the incidence rate of dementia was found to be 25 per cent over 15 years, which seems to be low compared to other studies, possibly due to the difficulties in diagnosing dementia in those with a more profound or complex intellectual disability.

Dementia incidence in people with intellectual disabilities without Down syndrome

Zigman *et al.* (2004) also reported incidence rates from their longitudinal study of adults with an intellectual disability without Down syndrome over the age of 65, although the sample size reduced with each subsequent wave of data collection. The incidence rate for Alzheimer's disease was found to be eight cases over three years in a cohort of an estimated 100 participants (aged 65–84), with a cumulative incidence rate of 0.31.

In the UK, incidence of dementia was found to be higher in the population with intellectual disabilities not associated with Down syndrome as compared to the age-matched general population (Strydom *et al.*, 2013b). The overall dementia incidence rates for those aged 60 and older was found to be 54.6. For those aged 65 and older the overall dementia incidence rate was 60.8. Incidence rates in the non-Down syndrome intellectual disability population peaked at ages 70–74, dropping off after 75, particularly amongst men with intellectual disabilities, in contrast to a steady increase in the general population (Corrada *et al.*, 2010). This pattern may be due to high mortality rates in older adults with intellectual disabilities, giving rise to a healthy survivor effect, which may affect men more than women.

Impact on services and families

The increase in life expectancy of older adults with intellectual disabilities and higher incidence and prevalence rates of dementia in these individuals mean that dementia is, and will continue to be, a significant condition in the intellectual disability population. This implies that the care demands on families, paid carers and services are set to increase as people with intellectual disability live longer. The need to identify those at risk, offer diagnostic assessments to those with emerging symptoms, and provide appropriate treatment and environmental and care adjustments for those affected will continue to increase. This means a corresponding increase in resource allocation is required, along with ensuring that carers are provided with appropriate training.

Development of specialist residential, day and health services may be worthwhile as well as the up skilling of generic services. There are merits for both development of specialist dementia clinics for those with an intellectual disability, as well as increasing the skills for generic memory clinics to be able to provide appropriate and timely diagnostic, treatment and intervention services to these individuals.

Guidance in the UK does not support population level dementia screening (National Institute for Health and Care Excellence, 2006). However, screening may be useful in the intellectual disability population given the high incidence, particularly if more effective treatments become available. Further research is required to develop suitable screening strategies, and to identify the underlying aetiology and risk factors for dementia. Early and accurate diagnosis of dementia can lead to appropriate health and social intervention in a timely and effective manner.

Conclusion

In summary, the prevalence of dementia in people with Down syndrome increases from under 10 per cent in individuals in their 40s to more than 30 per cent for those in their 50s, with some studies reporting rates in excess of 50 per cent for those aged 60 and over (Strydom *et al.*, 2010). Dementia may also be three to four times more common in older people with an intellectual disability who do not have Down syndrome than in the general population. Despite the diagnostic issues, there is a need to offer suitable diagnostic services and treatment, and to consider the support and care needs of the increasing number of adults with an intellectual disability and dementia.

References

American Psychiatric Association (2000) *Diagnostic and Statistical Manual of Mental Disorders.* 4th edition. Arlington, VA: American Psychiatric Association.
American Psychiatric Association (2013) *Diagnostic and Statistical Manual of Mental Disorders.* 5th edition. Arlington, VA: American Psychiatric Association.

Cooper, S. (1997) High prevalence of dementia among people with learning disabilities not attributable to Down's's syndrome. *Psychological Medicine 27*, 3, 609–616.

Cooper, SA., Melville, C. and Einfeld, S. (2003) Psychiatric diagnosis, intellectual disabilities and diagnostic criteria for psychiatric disorders for use with adults with learning disabilities/mental retardation (DC-LD). *Journal of Intellectual Disability Research 47*, 1, 3–15.

Coppus, A., Evenhuis, H., Verberne, GJ. *et al.* (2006) Dementia and mortality in persons with Down's's syndrome. *Journal of Intellectual Disability Research 50*, 10, 768–777.

Coppus, AMW., Evenhuis, HM., Verberne, GJ. *et al.* (2010) Early age at menopause is associated with increased risk of dementia and mortality in women with Down's syndrome. *Journal of Alzheimer's Disease 19*, 2, 545–550.

Corrada, MM., Brookmeyer, R., Paganini-Hill, A., Berlau, D. and Kawas, CH. (2010) Dementia incidence continues to increase with age in the oldest old: The 90+ study. *Annals of Neurology 67*, 1, 114–121.

Cosgrave, M., Tyrrell, J., McCarron, M., Gill, M. and Lawlor, BA. (1999) Age at onset of dementia and age of menopause in women with Down's syndrome. *Journal of Intellectual Disability Research 43*, 6, 461–465.

de Graff, G., Vis, JC., Haveman, M. *et al.* (2011) Assessment of prevalence of persons with Down's syndrome: A theory-based demographic model. *Journal of Applied Research in Intellectual Disabilities 24*, 3, 247–262.

Englund, A., Jonsson, B., Zander, CS., Gustafsson, J. and Anneren, G. (2013) Changes in mortality and causes of death in the Swedish Down's syndrome population. *American Journal of Medical Genetics Part A, 161A*, 642–649.

Holland, A., Hon, J., Huppert, FA., Stevens, F. and Watson, P. (1998) Population-based study of the prevalence and presentation of dementia in adults with Down's syndrome. *British Journal of Psychiatry 172*, 6, 493–498.

Jamieson-Craig, R., Scior, K., Chan, T., Fenton, C. and Strydom, A. (2010) Reliance on carer reports of early symptoms of dementia among adults with intellectual disabilities. *Journal of Policy and Practice in Intellectual Disabilities 7*, 1, 34–41.

Janicki, MP. and Dalton, AJ. (2000) Prevalence of dementia and impact on intellectual disability services. *Mental Retardation 38*, 3, 276–288.

Margallo-Lana, ML., Moore, PB., Kay, DWK. *et al.* (2007) Fifteen year follow-up of 92 hospitalized adults with Down's syndrome: Incidence of cognitive decline, its relationship to age and neuropathology. *Journal of Intellectual Disability Research 51*, 6, 463–477.

National Institute for Health and Care Excellence (2006, last modified October 2012) *Dementia – Supporting People with Dementia and their Carers in Health and Social Care.* National Institute for Health and Care Excellence.

Schupf, N., Zigman, W., Kapell, D., Lee, JH., Kline, J. and Levin, B. (1997) Early menopause in women with Down's syndrome. *Journal of Intellectual Disability Research 41*, 3, 264–267.

Schupf, N., Pang, D. and Patel, BN. *et al.* (2003) Onset of dementia is associated with age at menopause in women with Down's syndrome. *Annals of Neurology 54*, 4, 433–438.

Shooshtari, S., Martens, PJ., Burchill, CA., Dik, N. and Naghipur, S. (2011) Prevalence of depression and dementia among adults with developmental disabilities in Manitoba, Canada. *International Journal of Family Medicine. Article ID 319574.* doi:10.1155/2011/319574.

Strydom, A., Livingston, G., King, M. and Hassiotis, A. (2007) Prevalence of dementia in intellectual disability using different diagnostic criteria. *British Journal of Psychiatry 191*, 150–157.

Strydom, A., Chan, T., Fenton, C., Craig, R., Livingston, G. and Hassiotis, A. (2013a) Validity of criteria for dementia in older people with intellectual disability. *American Journal of Geriatric Psychiatry 21*, 3, 279–288.

Strydom, A., Chan, T., King, M., Hassiotis, A. and Livingston, G. (2013b) Incidence of dementia in older adults with intellectual disabilities. *Research in Developmental Disabilities 34*, 6, 1881–1885.

Strydom, A, Shooshtari, S., Lee, L. *et al.* (2010) Dementia in older adults with intellectual disabilities-epidemiology, presentation and diagnosis. *Journal of Policy and Practice in Intellectual Disabilities 7*, 2, 96–110.

Tyrrell, J., Cosgrave, M., McCarron, M. *et al.* (2001) Dementia in people with Down's syndrome. *International Journal of Geriatric Psychiatry 16*, 12, 1168–1174.

Visser, FE., Aldenkamp, AP., van Huffelen, AC. and Kuilman, M. (1997) Prospective study of the prevalence of Alzheimer-type dementia in institutionalized individuals with Down's syndrome. *American Journal on Mental Retardation 101*, 4, 412.

World Health Organization (1993) *The ICD-10 Classification of Mental and Behavioural Disorders – Diagnostic Criteria for Research.* World Health Organization: Geneva.

Yang, Q., Rasmussen, SA. and Friedman, JM. (2002) Mortality associated with Down's syndrome in the USA from 1983 to 1997: A population based-study. *Lancet 359*, 9311, 1019–1025.

Zigman, W., Schupf, N., Devenny, D. *et al.* (2004) Incidence and prevalence of dementia in elderly adults with mental retardation without Down's syndrome. *American Journal on Mental Retardation 109*, 2, 126–141.

2

Understanding the Process

Links between Down Syndrome and Dementia

Liam Reese Wilson, Tiina Annus,
Shahid H. Zaman, Anthony J. Holland

Introduction

The past three decades have seen significant improvements in the life expectancy of people with Down syndrome living in economically advanced countries. Because of this many people with Down syndrome are now living to an age when the risk of developing Alzheimer's disease increases significantly. That this represents a significant health concern for people with Down syndrome is indisputable, especially given the absence, at present, of an effective preventative treatment. For this reason, a deeper understanding by clinicians of the brain processes that lead to Alzheimer's disease developing in people with Down syndrome in later life, and the problems involved in diagnosis, is necessary and will benefit people with Down syndrome, as it may lead to a more informed, accurate and timely diagnosis. First, it is necessary to understand the link between these two disorders – one present from conception (Down syndrome) and the other developing in later life (Alzheimer's disease). In doing so we will consider the strong genetic, molecular and clinical links between the two. Second, appreciating the differences in the course and presentation of Alzheimer's disease in people with Down syndrome and how that differs from the typically developing populations will inform diagnosis and interventions, which at present are predominately modifications to a person's living environment and style of support, but may eventually include more effective treatments that prevent or ameliorate the course of Alzheimer's disease. Whilst focusing on Alzheimer's disease, as the most commonly occurring form of dementia, we will include studies with evidence of the link between frontotemporal dementia in people with Down syndrome.

Down syndrome

Down syndrome is a genetic disorder which in 95 per cent of cases arises from the triplication of Human Chromosome 21 – HSA21 (Lamb *et al.*, 1996), with the remaining 5 per cent of cases being caused by either Robertsonian Translocation or a mosaicism of healthy and aneuploid cells (Bandyopadhyay *et al.*, 2002). There are estimated to be approximately 60,000 people with Down syndrome living in the UK (Down Syndrome Association, 2013), with an incidence of Down syndrome in approximately 1 in every 700–1000 live births internationally (Bittles *et al.*, 2007; Roizen and Patterson, 2003). Over the last 30 years, advances in health and social care have led to exponential improvements in the quality of life of people with Down syndrome (Roizen and Patterson, 2003). In 1983, the life expectancy of a person with Down syndrome in the USA was 25 years of age (Yang *et al.*, 2002), whereas in developed countries today the life expectancy of the Down syndrome population exceeds 50 years, with 20 per cent or more of adults now being aged 55 years or older (Yang *et al.*, 2002; Zigman and Lott, 2007).

However, these improvements in the quality of life and increased life expectancy have had unexpected consequences, as early onset Alzheimer's disease has now become endemic amongst people with Down syndrome. It is clear that individuals with Down syndrome are more prone to age-related cognitive decline and are at high risk of developing dementia that resembles Alzheimer's disease at a much earlier age in comparison to typically developing individuals (Beacher *et al.*, 2010). A global study by Ferri *et al.* (2005) estimated that even in later life, that is over the age of 85, the prevalence of dementia in the general population in western Europe is 24.8 per cent. This is still lower than, or at the very least equal to, the proposed prevalence rates for Alzheimer's disease in the much younger population of people with Down syndrome. Importantly though, the prevalence of Alzheimer's disease in people with Down syndrome does not appear to reach 100 per cent as may be expected if Alzheimer's disease was a fully penetrant genetic disorder.

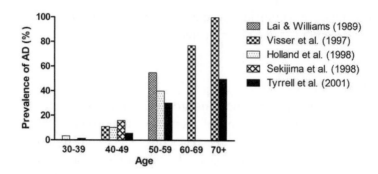

Figure 2.1: Variation in the reported prevalence of Alzheimer's disease in Down syndrome across studies

Studies have reported a similar prevalence of Alzheimer disease in the fourth and fifth decades of life in people with Down syndrome. However, as age increases, so does the variance in the reported prevalence across studies, with estimates ranging from 50–100 per cent by the eighth decade of life.

It can be seen that all studies reported a similar prevalence of Alzheimer's disease in the third decade of life in people with Down syndrome. However, as age increases, so does the variance in the reported prevalence of Alzheimer's disease across all studies, with estimates ranging from 70 to 100 per cent by the seventh of life.

Over the last 30 years, numerous studies have been conducted in an attempt to explain the association between Down syndrome and early development of Alzheimer's disease pathology from both a clinical and neuropathological standpoint. Given the current knowledge base in Alzheimer's disease pathology and complete mapping of the human genome, including HSA21, the strongest and most widely accepted candidate theory for this striking association is the amyloid cascade hypothesis.

Alzheimer's disease in Down syndrome and the amyloid cascade hypothesis

The pathological hallmarks of Alzheimer's disease were first described by Alois Alzheimer in 1907 following the post-mortem examination of a 51-year-old woman, who had experienced severe memory loss and developed strange behaviours (Alzheimer *et al.*, 1995). We now know these pathological changes to be beta-amyloid (Aβ) plaques and neurofibrillary tangles composed of hyperphosphorylated tau, although little is still known about how or why these proteins become irregular and lead to Alzheimer's disease. In spite of this, current evidence indicates that beta-amyloid and/or particular versions of it may be central to the development of Alzheimer's disease, which has led to the development of the amyloid cascade hypothesis (Hardy and Higgins, 1992; Selkoe, 1991).

The amyloid cascade hypothesis suggests that the abnormal metabolism of amyloid precursor protein is the initiating event in Alzheimer's disease pathogenesis, subsequently leading to progressive accumulation of misfolded insoluble fibrous material, composed of Aβ peptides, in the ageing brain (Hardy and Higgins, 1992). Aβ peptides are derived from a large, transmembrane glycoprotein called amyloid precursor protein (APP), the gene for which resides on HSA21 (Caricasole et al., 2003). There are two distinct biochemical pathways involved in APP proteolysis, one of which produces Aβ that is believed to trigger the pathological cascade leading to the development of Alzheimer's disease. A non-amyloidogenic pathway involves sequential enzymatic cleavage of APP by an α-secretase and γ-secretase, which generates the harmless extracellular peptide p3 and amyloid intracellular domain (AICD) as the end products. However, the cleavage of the APP by beta-site amyloid precursor protein-cleaving enzyme-1 (BACE-1), followed by subsequent enzymatic cleavage by γ-secretase, constitutes the pathological or amyloidogenic pathway, producing the aggregation prone Aβ peptide and intracellular AICD (Cole and Vassar, 2007; Querfurth and LaFerla, 2010).

APP can undergo proteolytic processing via two pathways. Cleavage by α-secretase occurs within the Aβ domain and generates a large soluble APP (sAPPα) ectodomain and an 83-residue C-terminal fragment C83. Further cleavage of C83 by γ-secretase generates the non-amyloidogenic extracellular peptide p3 and the amyloid intracellular domain (AICD). Alternatively, cleavage of APP by beta-site amyloid precursor protein-cleaving enzyme 1 (BACE-1) occurs at the beginning of the Aβ domain, liberating a shorter soluble APP (sAPPβ) and longer C-terminal fragment C99. Further proteolytic digestion of C99 by γ-secretase generates the amyloidogenic soluble Aβ peptide and AICD. AICD is a short tail of approximately 50 amino acids that is released into the cytoplasm and targeted to the nucleus for transcription activation. Inner-membrane proteolytic cleavage of sAPPβ by γ-secretases results in C-terminal heterogeneity of Aβ to produce either 40 amino acid (Aβ40) or 42 amino acid (Aβ42) long Aβ peptides (Querfurth and LaFerla, 2010).

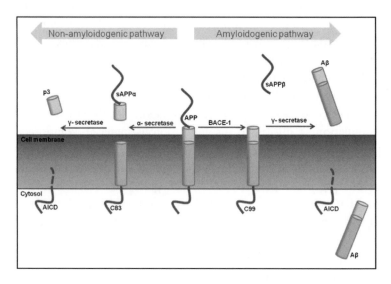

Figure 2.2: Intracellular processing of amyloid precursor protein

The Aβ peptide can be between 38 and 43 amino acids long, with peptide length affecting both the behaviour and the toxicity of the protein (Querfurth and LaFerla, 2010). Aβ42 is the species of beta-amyloid that is particularly prone to self-aggregate into multiple different physical forms which are presumed to be toxic (Yan and Wang, 2007). One form of Aβ42 presents in insoluble fibrillar form and by self-arranging into beta-sheet structure, forms the core of the circular amyloid plaques that are visible with light-microscopy (De Strooper, 2010). Aβ42 can also exist in the form of oligomers (2–6 peptides), which evidence indicates to be more neurotoxic than fibrillar plaques as they cause disruption of synapses and eventually neuronal death. Furthermore, examination of the total brain Aβ load (or at least Aβ40 and Aβ42) using enzyme linked immunoabsorbant assay (ELISA) reveals a positive correlation between the level of Aβ and the severity of Alzheimer's disease, which experiments based on manually counting the number of plaques present in post-mortem brains of people with Alzheimer's disease have failed to demonstrate (Braak and Braak, 1991; Naslund *et al.*, 2000).

However, evidence has emerged to suggest that accumulation of a small yet critical concentration of Aβ fibrils induces the formation of toxic Aβ oligomers, and indirectly damages the nearby neuronal structures. Cohen and colleagues (2013) have demonstrated that once a small amount of plaques have formed, these plaques cause other Aβ monomers to form oligomers via a secondary nucleation process. This is thought to cause an exponential increase in the amount of Aβ42 oligomers, which not only aggregate into toxic insoluble plaques, but also cause synaptic disruption and cell death whilst in their soluble, oligomeric form (Cohen et al., 2013). This is supported by the observation of Aβ plaques being surrounded by a halo of Aβ oligomers, and further evidence, which shows that the amount of damage to dendrites surrounding Aβ plaques depends on the distance between the dendrite and the plaque (Cohen et al., 2013; Koffie et al., 2009).

Despite these facts, it has been noted that the toxicity of Aβ alone cannot explain the vast loss of neurons in the brain affected by Alzheimer's disease (Hardy, 2009). Evidence has demonstrated tau pathology to be the primary cause of neuronal damage in Alzheimer's disease (Wolfe, 2009) as the level of tau in the form of neurofibrillary tangles (NFTs) correlates better with clinical dementia ratings in comparison to Aβ load (Braak and Braak, 1991). Tau is a soluble microtubule associated protein which plays a role in stabilising microtubules, thus supporting axonal transport of vesicles and organelles. Hyperphosphorylation of tau, as happens in Alzheimer's disease, attenuates its affinity for microtubules and promotes its assembly into paired helical filaments, which further aggregate to form the neurotoxic NFTs. However, the reasons as to why tau becomes hyperphosphorylated have yet to be understood. Interestingly, a gene that resides on chromosome 21 (DYRK1A–dual specificity tyrosine-phosphorylation-regulated kinase 1A) has been implicated in the formation of NFTs in the brains of people with Down syndrome (Liu et al., 2008). The DYRK1A gene encodes for a serine/threonine kinase, and has been shown in vitro to contribute to hyperphosphorylation of tau, suggesting its possible contribution to Alzheimer's disease pathology in this group. In spite of this, research in mice shows that tau pathology in Alzheimer's disease is driven by Aβ pathology (Götz et al., 2001), emphasising once again the importance of amyloid in the process of dementia.

Evidence from studies using cortical neurons generated and maintained in culture dish derived from either trisomy 21 embryonic stem cells or from induced pluripotent stem cells from the skin of adults with Down syndrome has clearly demonstrated that there is an excessive production of Aβ (Shi *et al.*, 2012). Using a γ-secretase inhibitor, this production of Aβ42 was suppressed. Furthermore, neurons were also found to contain hyperphosphorylated tau. This model system appears to recapitulate features of Alzheimer's disease and is likely to be useful for drug discovery.

Association between Down syndrome and Alzheimer's disease

Independent of the presence of clinical symptoms of Alzheimer's disease, post-mortem studies in people with Down syndrome, who died when aged 40 years or older, suggest that individuals with Down syndrome invariably develop neuropathological features similar to the hallmarks of Alzheimer's disease (Mann *et al.*, 1984; Wisniewski *et al.*, 1985). These characteristic neuropathological features include cerebral neuritic plaques, primarily composed of the pathogenic Aβ peptide, Aβ in meninges and cerebral blood vessels, and presence of neurofibrillary tangles (Wisniewski *et al.*, 1985; Zigman and Lott, 2007). Strikingly, soluble Aβ42 has been found even in the brains of those with Down syndrome from as early as 21 weeks gestational age (Teller *et al.*, 1996). As mentioned earlier, one possible explanation to account for the striking association between Down syndrome and an early development of Alzheimer-like neuropathology is that the gene for APP is mapped on HSA21, which is inherited in triplicate in the majority of individuals with Down syndrome (Goldgaber *et al.*, 1987). Increasing evidence suggests that the presence of an extra copy of APP leads to overproduction of the Aβ protein in the brain and plasma and thereby contributes to the development of Alzheimer's disease pathology (Zigman and Lott, 2007). As a result, amyloid plaques and neurofibrillary tangles may appear in the brains of people with Down syndrome as early as in the teens, and almost universally by the age of 40 years or older (Mann *et al.*, 1984; Wisniewski *et al.*, 1985). Furthermore, mutations in the APP gene have been linked to early onset familial Alzheimer's disease in the general population, indicating the importance of this gene in the development of Alzheimer's disease. On the other hand, Jonsson and colleagues (2012) have described a coding mutation (A673T) in the APP gene that encodes a suboptimal BACE-1 cleavage site and thereby results in approximately 40 per cent reduction in the formation of amyloidogenic Aβ in vitro. The families described with mutations at this site are not only protected against Alzheimer's disease, but also against cognitive decline, providing further evidence in favour of the amyloid cascade hypothesis and the important role of the APP gene in the development of Alzheimer's disease pathology. The presence of the APP gene in triplicate as a homogeneous cause and a single major factor for causing clinical Alzheimer's makes Down syndrome a unique and powerful model in support of the amyloid cascade hypothesis.

Braak and Braak (1991) were the first to demonstrate that both Aβ deposition and neurofibrillary tangle formation follow a sequential distribution pattern, which for Aβ deposition commences both before tau pathology and before the appearance of clinical symptoms of dementia (pre-clinical phase). In the absence of Aβ plaques, conditions directly linked to tau pathology are known as 'tauopathies' and include frontotemporal dementia (with or without Parkinsonism), sporadic corticobasal degeneration and progressive supranuclear palsy (Lee *et al.*, 2001). Furthermore, mutations in genes associated with the proteolytic processing of APP are causative of Alzheimer's disease, whereas mutation in tau are not as they lead to frontotemporal dementia – 17T as described by Hutton *et al.* (1998).

Thus, despite the gaps in our knowledge about how Aβ causes neurotoxicity, all of the above offers compelling evidence in support of the hypothesis that excessive production of Aβ may be a shared mechanism for the cause of Alzheimer's disease in both the typically developing and Down syndrome populations. Although evidence from neuropathological studies suggests that individuals with Down syndrome experience exactly the same pathological process in earlier life, as normally developing individuals with Alzheimer's disease much later, it is likely that the triggers for the pathological cascade, as well as presentation of clinical symptoms of dementia, are markedly different between the two populations.

In vivo measurement of fibrillar Aβ and biomarkers of Alzheimer's disease

The diagnosis of Alzheimer's disease can currently only be confirmed at post-mortem, when the presence of the classic neuropathology is confirmed. However, it is now possible to detect the presence of fibrillar Aβ plaques *in vivo* with the use of positron emission tomography (PET). This is a technique whereby a patient is injected with a radioactive ligand capable of crossing the blood–brain barrier. This ligand then binds to the fibrillar Aβ in the brain and emits a positron as it decays. This travels a very short distance before colliding with an electron, emitting a gamma ray, which is detected by the positron emission tomography (PET) scanner. When combined with anatomical data from magnetic resonance imaging (MRI), this technique allows accurate localisation and quantification of amyloid plaques in the cortex. Several radioligands with similar properties are now available and are currently being used in a great number of trials.

The first ligand of this kind to become available was a modified version of the histological dye Thioflavin-T – a carbon-11 labelled tracer called Pittsburgh compound-B, or PiB (Klunk *et al.*, 2004). PiB has been used widely in studies of Alzheimer's disease since its inception, including two large international initiatives; the Alzheimer's Disease Neuroimaging Initiative (ADNI) and the Dominantly Inherited Alzheimer Network (DIAN) study (Bateman *et al.*, 2012; Weiner *et al.*, 2010). However, as a carbon-labelled radioactive compound, PiB has a half-life of around 20 minutes, meaning that the time from production to injection is very short. For this reason, the use of PiB requires an on-site cyclotron, which limits the availability of this compound to many PET scanning centres. However, fluorine-based ligands such as florbetapir (Wong *et al.*, 2010) have a much longer half-life and therefore can be produced off-site and shipped to nearby PET centres, allowing a greater number of researchers to study Alzheimer's disease pathology *in vivo*.

Several PET studies involving people with Down syndrome have been published. A small pilot study by Landt *et al.* (2011) sought to first determine the safety, feasibility and tolerability of such techniques in people with Down syndrome. The research team found that PET scanning was safe and acceptable for this population of people and, furthermore, taking part in the research proved to be an enjoyable experience for them. The ethical and methodological challenges of doing such a study were considered in a paper by d'Abrera *et al.* (2011), where examples of the positive feedback given by the participants with Down syndrome in this study can be found.

The study by Landt and colleagues found substantial differences in amyloid binding between younger and older participants with Down syndrome. All those over the age of 45 (n = 5) were found to have amyloid binding in at least five of the six regions of interest investigated. Four of these participants already had a diagnosis of Alzheimer's disease. Younger participants with Down syndrome between 25 and 36 years of age (n = 3) were negative for PiB binding. A study of similar size was conducted by Handen *et al.* (2012); however, only adults with Down syndrome who did not have dementia were included. Nevertheless, two participants of this study were found to have increased PiB retention, when compared with non-Down syndrome cognitively normal controls. These were participants aged 38 and 44. Similar to the findings of Landt *et al.* (2011), the younger subjects (aged between 20 and 35) did not show an increase in PiB retention.

Both of these studies, in addition to research conducted in the general population, have confirmed that Aβ deposition increases with age and can be present even in the absence of cognitive symptoms. This evidence suggests that deposition of Aβ in the brain may be one of the earliest indicators that Alzheimer's disease will manifest clinically (Jack *et al.*, 2012). Early pre-clinical detection has become an important goal if therapies to modify or stop the process of Alzheimer's disease are going to be developed. In 2011, the National Institute on Aging and the Alzheimer's Association commissioned a workgroup to determine research criteria for the diagnosis of early Alzheimer's disease (Sperling *et al.*, 2011). These criteria were based on putative biomarkers of Alzheimer's disease, including high PET amyloid tracer retention, levels of Aβ42 and tau in CSF, atrophy in structural MRI images and cognitive decline, and it was proposed that they could be used to identify three stages of pre-clinical Alzheimer's disease. Jack *et al.* (2012) provided some validation of these criteria, managing to distinguish all three stages of pre-clinical Alzheimer's disease in otherwise typically developing individuals. However, these results require further validation and whether they are applicable to the Down syndrome population is difficult to determine. This is mainly due to the stage three criteria which are largely based on symptoms of cognitive decline, and in those with Down syndrome this does not always follow the pattern typically associated with Alzheimer's disease.

The clinical presentation of Alzheimer's disease in Down syndrome

Alzheimer's disease is the most common type of dementia, accounting for up to 56 per cent of dementia cases at post-mortem examination (Querfurth and LaFerla, 2010). Typically preceded by a syndrome known as mild cognitive impairment, patients with Alzheimer's disease usually present with anterograde amnesia, a condition causing problems with remembering recent events and other newly learned information (Reed et al., 2007). However, Alzheimer's disease is more than just an amnestic syndrome. Other cognitive problems such as executive dysfunction are often seen later in the course of the illness, and indeed both DSM-5 and ICD-10 criteria require at least one other cognitive deficit, including aphasia, apraxia or executive dysfunction, to be present for a diagnosis. Most importantly these deficits, together with the memory impairment, must amount to a significant decline from previous levels of functioning and must have an impact on a person's social or occupational functioning.

Unfortunately, the diagnosis of Alzheimer's disease in people with Down syndrome is rarely straightforward and is made more difficult by the presence of intellectual disability, particularly in cases where the clinician assessing for dementia is not aware of the patient's previous levels of functioning (Strydom et al., 2010). Furthermore, it appears the first symptoms often noticed are not deficits in memory but changes in behaviour and personality (Ball et al., 2006a; Holland and Oliver, 1995; Holland et al., 1998; Holland et al., 2000). A study by Holland and colleagues (1998) investigated the prevalence of dementia in Down syndrome using a modified version of the Cambridge Examination for Mental Disorders of the Elderly (since published under the name CAMDEX-DS). This involves conducting a detailed interview with someone who knows the participant with Down syndrome, such as a carer or parent, in order to determine whether or not the person has declined from a previous level of functioning. The questionnaire seeks to identify a person's abilities at their best level of functioning and any changes that have been noticed by the caregiver in areas of memory and orientation, language, praxis, executive functioning, personality and behaviour, and self-care.

The possibility of any other psychiatric disorders being present in the individual with Down syndrome is also assessed, including depression, paranoid illness and delirium, as well as physical health problems that could confound a diagnosis of Alzheimer's disease, such as hypothyroidism and cerebrovascular problems. Holland and colleagues found that the most frequently reported changes during their initial population-based study were those pertaining to personality and behaviour, such as increased apathy, decreased empathy or concern for other people and perseveration. A follow-up study 18 months later demonstrated that people previously diagnosed with what they term as 'a frontotemporal-like dementia' were likely to progress to a full diagnosis of Alzheimer's disease. The study also indicated that the highest incidences of frontotemporal dementia were in younger groups of people with Down syndrome, whereas the peak incidences of Alzheimer's disease were in the older groups, again indicating that a frontal-like syndrome precedes dementia in this population.

There are several possible reasons for this finding. In the first instance, as suggested by Aylward *et al.* (1997), it may be the case that in individuals with an intellectual disability, baseline functioning is so low that the initial changes of Alzheimer's disease, such as memory loss, are not obvious. Therefore, carers and family members would be more likely to report changes in behaviour and personality as the first changes they have perceived. In addition, the patients themselves may be less able to report symptoms of memory loss compared to patients with Alzheimer's disease from the general population due to their intellectual disability.

However, findings from Ball *et al.* (2006a) suggest that this may not be the case. In this study, patients were assessed for changes in behaviour and personality by means of an interview with a caregiver, as well as on a battery of neuropsychological tests designed to probe both executive function and memory. The benefit of this study is that it sought to correlate changes in personality and behaviour with a neuropsychological measure, in this case executive function, that can be compared with the measures for memory. However, executive function can be difficult to define as it is often seen to encompass a great many things. As Stuss (2007) writes, the term is vague and difficult to apply consistently to a given set of functions as it is a psychological construct with no definite anatomical correlates, and it is applied inconsistently in the scientific literature. However, he does furnish us with a definition of 'executive cognitive functions', as 'high-level cognitive functions, believed to be mediated primarily by the LPFC [lateral prefrontal cortex], that are involved in the control and direction, for example: planning, monitoring, energizing, switching, inhibiting, of lower-level more automatic functions' (Stuss, 2007, p. 293). Ball *et al.* (2006b) found that participants, who showed changes in behaviour and personality sufficient for a diagnosis of frontotemporal dementia, had a significant impairment in executive function, but no significant impairment in memory, indicating that the frontotemporal-like symptoms seen in this population are probably not just an artefact of comorbidity for intellectual disability. Incidentally, this also found that those with a diagnosis of frontotemporal dementia were significantly more likely to have progressed to a diagnosis of Alzheimer's disease than those without. Additionally, individuals identified as displaying changes in personality and behaviour not quite sufficient for a diagnosis of frontotemporal dementia were also more likely to have progressed to a diagnosis of frontotemporal dementia or Alzheimer's disease over the course of five years. Both of these findings provide support for the hypothesis that frontotemporal like symptoms are a pre-clinical manifestation of Alzheimer's disease in individuals with Down syndrome.

Further evidence for this forewarning of frontotemporal-type manifestation of Alzheimer's disease in people with Down syndrome was provided by Adams and Oliver (2010). They demonstrated that deficits in executive function were only present in people with Down syndrome who had declined cognitively over a period of 16 months. In contrast, those not showing any cognitive decline did not experience deficits in executive function. Furthermore, impairments in executive function were associated with behavioural changes but were not associated with a decline in memory, again indicating that changes in behaviour and executive function occur prior to amnestic symptoms in Alzheimer's disease in Down syndrome. It has been demonstrated in the general population that, although a minority may have a greater deficit in executive function than in memory (around 10%), the vast majority of people with Alzheimer's disease present with a low memory profile with executive function being significantly less impaired (Reed *et al.*, 2007).

The frontal lobes and Alzheimer's disease in Down syndrome

With the findings of these multiple studies in mind, we can begin to appreciate that the early changes in behaviour and personality, as well as deficits in executive function, are unlikely to be due to comorbidity for intellectual disability but in fact represent a true difference in the progression of dementia in this population. However, theories that attempt to explain the appearance of frontotemporal-type symptoms so early in the course of Alzheimer's disease in the Down syndrome population remain speculative. It has been widely proposed that the changes in personality, behaviour and executive function seen in people with Down syndrome result from an acquired deficit in frontal lobe functioning, which may be due to the frontal lobes being preferentially affected by the accumulation of amyloid (Ball *et al.*, 2006a; Holland *et al.*, 1998, 2000; Lott and Head, 2001). Why the frontal lobes are preferentially affected by Alzheimer's disease in Down syndrome, but not in the typically developing population, is far from clear.

It is well known that the frontal lobes in people with Down syndrome are underdeveloped compared with typically developing age-matched controls. In a comprehensive review of neurodevelopmental abnormalities and cognitive disabilities in Down syndrome, Contestabile *et al.* (2010) cite multiple studies that have confirmed the tendency towards incomplete development in the frontal lobes of those with Down syndrome. Their review highlights that neuroanatomical deficiencies are present in people with Down syndrome from very early in life and persist throughout, only to be further exacerbated with ageing. To illustrate, evidence from Lu *et al.* (2012) suggests that the reduction in total brain volume in people with Down syndrome may be due to impairments in neuronal proliferation during foetal development. It is possible that the overexpression of the oligodendrocyte transcription factor OLIG2 (for which the gene is located on HSA21) may be a large contributor to this. Lu and colleagues claim that the high concentrations of this transcription factor can impair the differentiation of neural progenitors into neurons by promoting oligodendroglial features in a greater number of these cells at an early gestational age (14–18 weeks), as well as by impairing the expression and function of potassium ion channels. These early deficiencies mean that there is a lack of grey matter in the brain of individuals with Down syndrome relative to the typically developing population, and evidence from several studies confirms that this is the case for the frontal lobes of the brain, amongst other areas, throughout the lifespan of a person with Down syndrome (Beacher *et al.*, 2010; Menghini *et al.*, 2011; Suzuki, 2007; Teipel *et al.*, 2004).

In addition to this inherent difference throughout life, Beacher *et al.* (2010) have demonstrated a greater tendency for age-related change in the brain of a person with Down syndrome. Thirty-nine adults with Down syndrome who did not have dementia underwent an MRI scan in this study and were compared to typically developing controls. It was found that not only did the individuals with Down syndrome have reduced volume of the left and total prefrontal regions bilaterally, but these areas also showed a greater age-related reduction in volume when compared with controls.

Thus, it is clear that the frontal lobes of those with Down syndrome are premorbidly abnormal and it is possible that for this reason the frontal areas are at a greater risk of damage from neuropathology relative to other structures in the brain. This theory was proposed by Holland and colleagues (1998, 2000) to explain why changes in personality and behaviour might be the first presenting clinical symptoms of Alzheimer's disease in people with Down syndrome. It was subsequently cited by Ball *et al.* (2006b) as the possible reason for the deficit in executive function in people with Down syndrome with preserved memory functions. Ball *et al.* (2010) have proffered a theoretical explanantion that goes beyond the reserve capacity hypothesis and draws on ideas put forward by Tekin and Cummings (2002) regarding the functional architecture of the basal ganglia thalamocortical networks. These are separable circuits in the brain connecting the frontal lobes, striatum, globus pallidus and substantia nigra, and are suggested to govern several behaviours and cognitive functions typically designated as 'frontal'. Ball *et al.* (2010) expanded upon the work by Tekin and Cummings by suggesting that, during the course of Alzheimer's disease in people with Down syndrome, these networks become disrupted, with the orbitofrontal circuit, thought to play a role in inhibition, emotional stability and empathy, being disproportionally affected by the illness. However, while this would offer a neat explanation, it is yet to be investigated, although a thorough understanding of this could be of benefit when considering targeted therapeutic interventions.

Conclusion

Although our knowledge of Alzheimer's disease as it affects people with Down syndrome has significantly increased, we are still very far from finding treatments for this condition. From a more preventative perspective, the concern is that once the clinical symptoms have developed to the level that fits the diagnostic criteria for Alzheimer's disease, the neuropathology in the brain has already reached the point of no return. Therefore, more basic research is needed to pinpoint the window of intervention in which something can be done to prevent the development of Alzheimer's disease in people with Down syndrome. The advent of tools for imaging Aβ and NFTs *in vivo* may prove to be of immense value, as they may help determine precisely when pathology begins to accumulate. Once this is determined, perhaps trials to find a treatment that prevents the accumulation of Aβ in the parenchyma will prove fruitful. Even though we still have a long way to go, collaborative efforts between people with Down syndrome, their families, scientists and clinicians continue to take us closer to our goal of defeating dementia in people with Down syndrome.

References

Adams, D. and Oliver, C. (2010) The relationship between acquired impairments of executive function and behaviour change in adults with Down's syndrome. *Journal of Intellectual Disability Research 54*, 5, 393–405.

Alzheimer, A., Stelzmann, RA., Schnitzlein, HN. and Murtagh, FR. (1995) An English translation of Alzheimer's 1907 paper, 'Uber eine eigenartige Erkankung der Hirnrinde.' *Clinical Anatomy 8*, 6, 429–431.

Aylward, EH., Burt, DB., Thorpe, LU., Lai, F. and Dalton, A. (1997) Diagnosis of dementia in individuals with intellectual disability. *Journal of Intellectual Disability Research 41*, 2, 152–164.

Ball, SL., Holland, AJ., Watson, PC. and Huppert, FA. (2010) Theoretical exploration of the neural bases of behavioural disinhibition, apathy and executive dysfunction in preclinical Alzheimer's disease in people with Down's syndrome: Potential involvement of multiple frontal-subcortical neuronal circuits. *Journal of Intellectual Disability Research 54*, 4, 320–336.

Ball, SL., Holland, AJ., Hon, J., Huppert, FA., Treppner, P. and Watson, PC. (2006a) Personality and behaviour changes mark the early stages of Alzheimer's disease in adults with Down's syndrome: Findings from a prospective population-based study. *International Journal of Geriatric Psychiatry 21*, 7, 661–673.

Ball, SL., Holland, AJ., Huppert, FA., Treppner, P. and Dodd, K. (2006b) *The CAMDEX-DS: The Cambridge Examination for Mental Disorders of Older People with Down's Syndrome and Others with Intellectual Disabilities*. Cambridge: Cambridge University Press.

Bandyopadhyay, R., Heller, A., Knox-Dubois, C. *et al.* (2002) Parental origin and timing of De Novo Robertsonian Translocation Formation. *The American Journal of Human Genetics 71*, 6, 1456–1462.

Bateman, RJ., Xiong, C., Benzinger, TLS. *et al.* (2012) Clinical and biomarker changes in dominantly inherited Alzheimer's disease. *New England Journal of Medicine 367*, 9, 795–804.

Beacher, F., Daly, E., Simmons, A. *et al.* (2010) Brain anatomy and ageing in non-demented adults with Down's syndrome: an in vivo MRI study. *Psychological Medicine 40*, 4, 611–619.

Bittles, AH. Bower, C., Hussain, R. and Glasson, EJ. (2007) The four ages of Down's syndrome. *European Journal of Public Health 17*, 2, 221–225.

Braak, H. and Braak, E. (1991) Neuropathological staging of Alzheimer-related changes. *Acta Neuropathologica 82*, 4, 239–259.

Caricasole, A., Copani, A., Causo, A. *et al.* (2003) The Wnt pathway, cell-cycle activation and beta-amyloid: novel therapeutic strategies in Alzheimer's disease? *Trends in Pharmacological Sciences 24*, 5, 233–238.

Cohen, SI., Linse, S., Luheshi, LM. et al. (2013) Proliferation of amyloid-beta42 aggregates occurs through a secondary nucleation mechanism. *Proceedings of the National Academy of Sciences USA 110*, 24, 9758–9763.

Cole, SL. and Vassar, R. (2007) The Alzheimer's disease beta-secretase enzyme, BACE1. *Molecular Neurodegeneration 2*, 2, 22.

Contestabile, A., Benfenati, F. and Gasparini, L. (2010) Communication breaks-Down's: From neurodevelopment defects to cognitive disabilities in Down's syndrome. *Progress in Neurobiology 91*, 1, 1–22.

d'Abrera, JC., Holland, AJ., Landt, J., Stocks-Gee, G. and Zaman, SH. (2011) A neuroimaging proof of principle study of Down's syndrome and dementia: Ethical and methodological challenges in intrusive research. *Journal of Intellectual Disability Research 57*, 2, 105–118.

De Strooper, B. (2010) Proteases and proteolysis in Alzheimer disease: A multifactorial view on the disease process. *Physiological Reviews 90*, 2, 465–494.

Down's Syndrome Association (2013) *Key Facts and Frequently Asked Questions*. Available at www.downs-syndrome.org.uk/about-us/key-facts-and-faqs.html, accessed 4 December 2013.

Ferri, CP., Prince, M., Brayne, C. *et al.* (2005) Global prevalence of dementia: A Delphi consensus study. *The Lancet 366*, 9503, 2112–2117.

Goldgaber, D., Lerman, MI., McBride, WO., Saffiotto, U. and Gajdusek, DC. (1987) Isolation, characterization, and chromosomal localization of human brain cDNA clones coding for the precursor of the amyloid of brain in Alzheimer's disease, Down's syndrome and aging. *Journal of Neural Transmission 24*, 23–28.

Götz, J., Chen, F., Van Dorpe, J. and Nitsch, RM. (2001) Formation of neurofibrillary tangles in p301l tau transgenic mice induced by Aβ42 fibrils. *Science 293*, 1491–1495.

Handen, BL., Cohen, AD., Channamalappa, U. *et al.* (2012) Imaging brain amyloid in nondemented young adults with Down's syndrome using Pittsburgh compound B. *Alzheimer's and Dementia 8*, 6, 496–501.

Hardy, J. (2009) The amyloid hypothesis for Alzheimer's disease: A critical reappraisal. *Journal of Neurochemistry 110*, 4, 1129–1134.

Hardy, J. and Higgins, G. (1992) Alzheimer's disease: The amyloid cascade hypothesis. *Science 256*, 5024, 184–185.

Holland, AJ. and Oliver, C. (1995) Down's syndrome and the links with Alzheimer's disease. *Journal of Neurology, Neurosurgery, and Psychiatry 59*, 2, 111–114.

Holland, AJ., Hon, J., Huppert, FA. and Stevens, F. (2000) Incidence and course of dementia in people with Down's syndrome: Findings from a population-based study. *Journal of Intellectual Disability Research 44*, 2, 138–146.

Holland, AJ., Hon, J., Huppert, FA., Stevens, F. and Watson, P. (1998) Population-based study of the prevalence and presentation of dementia in adults with Down's syndrome. *British Journal of Psychiatry 172*, 6, 493–498.

Hutton, M., Lendon, CL., Rizzu, P. *et al.* (1998) Association of missense and 5'-splice-site mutations in tau with the inherited dementia FTDP-17. *Nature 393*, 6686, 702–705.

Jack, CR., Knopman, DS., Weigand, SD. *et al.* (2012) An operational approach to National Institute on Aging – Alzheimer's Association criteria for preclinical Alzheimer disease. *Annals of Neurology 71*, 6, 765–775.

Jonsson, T., Atwal, JK., Steinberg, S. *et al.* (2012) A mutation in APP protects against Alzheimer's disease and age-related cognitive decline. *Nature 488*, 7409, 96–99.

Klunk, WE., Engler, H., Nordberg, A. *et al.* (2004) Imaging brain amyloid in Alzheimer's disease with Pittsburgh Compound-B. *Annals of Neurology 55*, 3, 306–319.

Koffie, RM., Meyer-Luehmann, M., Hashimoto, T. *et al.* (2009) Oligomeric amyloid β associates with postsynaptic densities and correlates with excitatory synapse loss near senile plaques. *Proceedings of the National Academy of Sciences 106*, 10, 4012–4017.

Lai, F. and Williams, RS. (1989) A prospective study of Alzheimer disease in Down's syndrome. *Archives of Neurology 46*, 8, 849–853.

Lamb, NE., Freeman, SB., Savage-Austin, A. *et al.* (1996) Susceptible chiasmate configurations of chromosome 21 predispose to non-disjunction in both maternal meiosis I and meiosis II. *Nature Genetics 14*, 4, 400–405.

Landt, J., d'Abrera, JC., Holland, AJ. *et al.* (2011) Using positron emission tomography and Carbon 11-labeled Pittsburgh Compound B to image brain fibrillar beta-amyloid in adults with Down's syndrome: Safety, acceptability, and feasibility. *Archives of Neurology 68*, 7, 890–896.

Lee, VM., Goedert, M. and Trojanowski, JQ. (2001) Neurodegenerative tauopathies. *Annual Review of Neuroscience 24*, 1121–1159.

Liu, F., Liang, Z., Wegieil, J. *et al.* (2008) Overexpression of Dyrk1A contributes to neurofibrillary degeneration in Down's syndrome. *The FASEB Journal 22*, 9, 3224–3233.

Lott, IT. and Head, E. (2001) Down's syndrome and Alzheimer's disease: A link between development and aging. *Mental Retardation and Developmental Disability Research Review 7*, 3, 172–178.

Lu, J., Lian, G., Zhou, H. *et al.* (2012) OLIG2 over-expression impairs proliferation of human Down's syndrome neural progenitors. *Human Molecular Genetics 21*, 10, 2330–2340.

Mann, DM., Yates, PO. and Marcyniuk, B. (1984) Alzheimer's presenile dementia, senile dementia of Alzheimer type and Down's syndrome in middle age form an age related continuum of pathological changes. *Neuropathology and Applied Neurobiology 10*, 3, 185–207.

Menghini, D., Costanzo, F. and Vicari, S. (2011) Relationship between brain and cognitive processes in Down's syndrome. *Behavior Genetics 41*, 3, 381–393.

Naslund, J., Haroutinian, V., Mohs, R. *et al.* (2000) Correlation between elevated levels of amyloid beta-peptide in the brain and cognitive decline. *Journal of the American Medical Association 283*, 12, 1571–1577.

Querfurth, HW. and LaFerla, FM. (2010) Alzheimer's Disease. *New England Journal of Medicine 362*, 4, 329–344.

Reed, BR., Mungas, DM., Kramer, JH. *et al.* (2007) Profiles of neuropsychological impairment in autopsy-defined Alzheimer's disease and cerebrovascular disease. *Brain 130*, 3, 731–739.

Roizen, NJ. and Patterson, ND. (2003) Down's syndrome. *Lancet 361*, 9365, 1281–1289.

Selkoe, D. J. (1991) The molecular pathology of Alzheimer's disease. *Neuron 6*, 6, 487–498.

Shi, YC., Kirwan, P., Smith, J., Maclean, G., Orkin, SH. and Livesey, FJ. (2012) A human stem cell model of early Alzheimer's disease pathology in Down's syndrome. *Science Translational Medicine 4*, 124, 29.

Sekijima Y. et al. (1998) Prevalence of dementia of Alzheimer type and apolipoprotein E phenotypes in aged patients with Down's syndrome. *European Journal of Neurology 39*, 4, 234–237.

Sperling, RA., Aisen, PS., Beckett, LA. *et al.* (2011) Toward defining the preclinical stages of Alzheimer's disease: Recommendations from the National Institute on Aging – Alzheimer's Association workgroups on diagnostic guidelines for Alzheimer's disease. *Alzheimer's and Dementia 7*, 3, 280–292.

Strydom, A., Shooshtari, S., Lee, L. *et al.* (2010) Dementia in older adults with intellectual disabilities – epidemiology, presentation, and diagnosis. *Journal of Policy and Practice in Intellectual Disabilities 7*, 2, 96–110.

Stuss, DT. (2007) New approaches to prefrontal lobe testing. In BL. Miller and LCJ. Cummings (eds) *The Human Frontal Lobes: Functions and Disorders*. New York, NY: The Guilford Press.

Suzuki, K. (2007) Neuropathology of developmental abnormalities. *Brain and Development 29*, 3, 129–141.

Teipel, SJ., Alexander, GE., Schapiro, MB., Moller, HJ., Rapoport, SI. and Hampel, H. (2004) Age-related cortical grey matter reductions in non-demented Down's syndrome adults determined by MRI with voxel-based morphometry. *Brain 127*, 4, 811–824.

Tekin, S. and Cummings, JL. (2002) Frontal–subcortical neuronal circuits and clinical neuropsychiatry: An update. *Journal of Psychosomatic Research 53*, 1, 647–654.

Teller, JK., Russo, C., Debusk, LM. *et al.* (1996) Presence of soluble amyloid beta-peptide precedes amyloid plaque formation in Down's syndrome. *Nature Medicine 2*, 1, 93–95.

Visser, FE., Aldenkamp, AP., van Huffelen, AC. and Kuilman, M. (1997) Prospective study of the prevalence of Alzheimer-type dementia in institutionalized individuals with Down's syndrome. *American Journal on Mental Retardation 101*, 4, 412.

Weiner, MW., Aisen, PS., Jack, CR. Jr. *et al.* (2010) The Alzheimer's Disease Neuroimaging Initiative: Progress report and future plans. *Alzheimer's and Dementia 6*, 3, 202–211.

Wisniewski, KE., Wisniewski, HM. and Wen, GY. (1985) Occurrence of neuropathological changes and dementia of Alzheimer's disease in Down's syndrome. *Annals of Neurology 17*, 3, 278–282.

Wolfe, MS. (2009) Tau mutations in neurodegenerative diseases. *Journal of Biological Chemistry 284*, 10, 6021–6025.

Wong, DF., Rosenberg, PB., Zhou, Y. *et al.* (2010) In vivo imaging of amyloid deposition in Alzheimer disease using the radioligand 18F-AV-45 (Flobetapir F 18). *Journal of Nuclear Medicine 51*, 6, 913–920.

Yan, Y. and Wang, C. (2007) Aβ40 protects non-toxic Aβ42 monomer from aggregation. *Journal of Molecular Biology 369*, 4, 909–916.

Yang, Q., Rasmussen, SA. and Friedman, JM. (2002) Mortality associated with Down's syndrome in the USA from 1983 to 1997: A population-based study. *Lancet 359*, 9311, 1019–1025.

Zigman, WB. and Lott, IT. (2007) Alzheimer's disease in Down's syndrome: neurobiology and risk. *Mental Retardation and Developmental Disability Research Review 13*, 3, 237–246.

3

The Outpatient Clinic for Adults with Down Syndrome

A Model to Diagnose Dementia

Antonia M.W. Coppus

Introduction

Down syndrome is the most commonly identified cause of intellectual disability and is caused by a triplication of chromosome 21, except in rare instances of translocation (4–5%) or mosaicism (2–4%). Individuals with Down syndrome show many age-related changes in health and functional status at a significantly younger age than those without Down syndrome. This includes early menopause in women (Coppus *et al.*, 2010; Schupf *et al.*, 1997; Seltzer *et al.*, 2001), early onset of visual and hearing impairment, mobility restrictions (Evenhuis *et al.*, 2001; van Schrojenstein Lantman-de Valk *et al.*, 1994), hypothyroidism (Prasher, 1999), obesity (Prasher, 1995), depression (Coppus *et al.*, 2006), an early decrease in functioning (Carmeli *et al.*, 2004) and an increased risk in developing Alzheimer's disease (Coppus *et al.*, 2006; Holland *et al.*, 2000; Oliver *et al.*, 1998; Schupf and Sergievsky, 2002).

In Down syndrome, Alzheimer's disease is assumed to be caused by the triplication and overexpression of the gene for amyloid precursor protein (APP), located on chromosome 21 and leading to the accumulation of cerebral beta-amyloid. There is an ongoing debate on the percentage of persons who will eventually develop dementia in old age. In response to changing need for diagnosis and support of people with Down syndrome, the first multidisciplinary outpatient clinic for adults with Down syndrome in the Netherlands started in January 2007.

The outpatient clinic

In this clinic, an annual multidisciplinary Down syndrome Health Watch programme is available. The participants, all adults with Down syndrome, receive a complete assessment, including a general physical and psychological examination. Blood samples are obtained for standardised measurements and are preserved for future research. Ethical approval for this study was obtained from the medical ethical committee of the Elkerliek Hospital and the Radboud University Nijmegen, with written consent from all representatives.

The multidisciplinary team consists of a medical doctor who specialises in intellectual disability medicine, the director of the clinic, an ear, nose and throat specialist, a psychologist, an ophthalmologist, an audiologist and a nutritionist. The full facilities of the hospital are available for use as required, such as echocardiography or X-ray. Each individual with Down syndrome sees each health care provider on the same day at the clinic, and a brief verbal summary of the findings is discussed together at the end of the day. A written report, including the findings and recommendations, is sent to parents or carers and the primary physician.

Diagnosis of dementia

To diagnose dementia, the ICD-10 symptom checklist for mental disorders (World Health Organization, 1992) is used alongside the guidelines produced by the Ageing Special Interest group of the International Association for the Scientific Study of Intellectual Disabilities (IASSID) (Aylward et al., 1997; Burt and Aylward, 2000).

Before visiting the clinic, the participants and their carers receive an information pack that includes detailed clinical information and comprehensive medical and psychological questionnaires. The use of baseline dementia screening questionnaires starts at the age of 40. The prescreen dementia checklist is used at the first visit (National Task Group, 2013). To support a diagnosis of dementia, two observer-rated questionnaires are used, the Dementia Questionnaire for Persons with Mental Retardation (Evenhuis, 1992, 1996), and/ or the Dementia Scale for Down Syndrome (Gedye, 1995) and the Social Competence Rating Scale (Kraijer et al., 2004). Those who screen positive also receive an extra clinical work-up, in accordance with the guidelines of the Dutch National Institute of Health

(Centraal BegeleidingsOrgaan, 2005). The clinical evaluation has been focused on obtaining a chronology of symptoms, a description of functional and behavioural changes, the findings in the physical examinations and the mental status examination. The basic laboratory work-up includes a complete blood count, renal and liver function tests, blood levels of folate, vitamin B12, calcium, glucose and thyroid-stimulating hormone. Where possible, supplementary tests are included, such as a CT-scan (computerised tomography), MRI or lumbar puncture. EEG is recommended in the differential diagnosis of atypical clinical presentations of dementia (electroencephalogram to record brain activity).

A final general dementia diagnosis is given based on the pattern of annual observations and findings. Each new diagnosis is discussed in a diagnostic panel consisting of the members of the multidisciplinary team, the person's main carer and their general practitioner.

Results

Since the clinic opened in 2007, an average of 100 participants have visited the outpatient clinic annually, with an average follow-up period of 4.2 years. The average age of the participants was 37 years (18–64 years), of whom 45 (43%) were 40 years and older at the first visit. Most of those attending (38%) lived with family members, or in small group homes with support (55%), 7 per cent lived in settings with 24-hour support. The severity of intellectual disability was classified using the International Classification of Diseases (World Health Organization, 1992), 73.3 per cent had a moderate level (IQ 35–50), 11.4 per cent had a severe level (IQ <35) and 15.2 per cent had a mild level of intellectual disability (IQ 50–70).

Physical health

A general neurological and physical examination is performed as assessment of comorbidity is important in ageing people with Down syndrome. Middle-aged and older adults are known to show age-related changes in health and functional capacity at an earlier age. As a result, particular attention has to be given to physical and psychiatric disorders which can cause or mimic a decline in functioning.

Hearing and visual evaluation should be part of any diagnosis of cognitive function in Down syndrome as visual impairments and eye abnormalities are common (McCarron *et al.*, 2005; van Splunder *et al.*, 2003). Spectacles to correct refraction errors were widely used in the clinic, but 30 per cent of those who attended were not using the correct prescription for their glasses. A diagnosis of cataracts was made in 40 per cent and of keratoconus in 8 per cent. Hearing loss is very common in adults (van Buggenhout *et al.*, 1999; Evenhuis *et al.*, 1992; Evenhuis *et al.*, 2001). The ear, nose and throat specialist/ audiologist diagnosed a hearing loss in 70 per cent of the group; 30 per cent needed a hearing aid immediately, although 6 per cent chose not to accept or use one when supplied.

As in the general population without an intellectual disability, age affects the frequency of thyroid abnormalities in people with Down syndrome; this frequency increases with age and is possibly a sign of precocious ageing (Prasher, 1999; Prasher and Gomez, 2007). Thyroid function was tested with half of the participants having abnormal thyroid-stimulating hormone levels. Most of the abnormalities were subclinical: 25 per cent of the participants, in the age category of 40 and above, were using thyroid hormone replacement therapy. Overt hypothyroidism is associated with a complex range of symptoms that can cause a functional decline with symptoms similar to Alzheimer's disease. Most guidelines recommend two to five yearly screening for thyroid disease in adults with Down syndrome (Prasher *et al.*, 2011).

The rate of seizures increases with age, especially for those who have comorbid dementia. In the clinic, 12 per cent of the patients had a history of epilepsy, 7 per cent developed late-onset epilepsy during follow-up, at a mean age onset of 40.1 years. It was observed that some anti-convulsive medication could cause cognitive and behavioural deterioration, yet conversely other anti-convulsants such as Tegretol and valproic acid often decreased behaviour that proved challenging to others.

Sleep problems were observed in 12 per cent of the patients, especially difficulties associated with ritual and obsessive behaviour. Obstructive sleep apnea was only determined in 4 per cent of the patients, in contrast with other studies in Down syndrome (Trois *et al.*, 2009). The frequency of other conditions, associated with ageing in the general population such as acquired cardiac diseases, diabetes, hypertension and cancer was very low (1–5%).

Pharmacology

Pharmacological reviews were carried out for each individual and included assessment of their medication history, and present use of prescribed drugs. Particular attention was given to sleep medication, psychotropic drugs and pain medication with chronic medication use decreased from 50 per cent in the first year to 30 per cent after four years of follow-up. The advice given was that use of psycho-active medications for behavioural control should be limited to acute situations for time limited periods. Sleep medication, pain medication and other routine medication was restricted in line with an established diagnosis.

Mental health

People with Down syndrome show more mental health and psychological problems starting at the age of 40, younger than those with other types of intellectual disabilities (Haveman et al., 1994). Many older people with Down syndrome were referred to the clinic because of an existing suspicion of dementia, rather than for routine screening.

Behavioural changes such as loss of skills, loss of energy, loss of interest, loss of self-care skills, and withdrawal from social activities occur frequently from the age of 40 (20%). It was interesting that these patients did not initially meet the criteria of dementia, although showed a decline in cognitive and functional skills during follow-up. It has yet to be identified if this decline, or change in functioning, can be diagnosed as mild cognitive impairment, as the result of preclinical onset of Alzheimer's disease, or of normal ageing in people with Down syndrome, although the results were comparable with those found in a previous study (Coppus et al., 2008).

Psychiatric symptoms were identified in 30 per cent of the patients aged 40 years and over, including a possible diagnosis of depression (25%) and dementia (27%). Twenty-nine per cent of the patients had a previous history of depression with 8 per cent having a documented diagnosis of delirium. Both of these overlap between, and are often mistaken for, the symptoms of dementia. Individuals with both dementia and depression were closely followed up to ensure that depression was not misdiagnosed as dementia. Any sudden change in mood or behavioural patterns always warrants further investigation and a thorough physical examination.

Conclusion

The first results of this Health Watch programme show a relatively high rate of sensory impairment with subclinical hypothyroidism and behavioural disturbances, especially in the group aged 40 years and older. These findings are consistent with other reports, but emphasise the need for appropriate health and care support. Health care providers should be informed of health conditions that are more common among adults with Down syndrome as they age, including, but not exclusively, dementia.

The risk of dementia is certainly an important issue for relatives and carers. Screening for dementia, and excluding all other factors that can also cause a decline, is of utmost importance in the population of people with Down syndrome. At this moment, there are well-accepted criteria with which to diagnose dementia in adults with an intellectual disability (Aylward *et al.*, 1997; Burt and Aylward, 2000; Strydom and Hassiotis, 2003; Strydom *et al.*, 2013). Nevertheless, the assessment and diagnosis of dementia remains difficult. In the clinic, individuals were systematically and annually screened for dementia, to check for signs of neurocognitive or neurobehavioural decline, with each person acting as his or her own control over the years. Those diagnosed with dementia met the ICD-10 criteria and experienced a steady progressive course of the condition.

There has been an increasing interest in mild cognitive impairment. This has been suggested as a transitional stage between typical functioning and dementia. There are no exact criteria to diagnose mild cognitive impairment in people with an intellectual disability (Jenkins *et al.*, 2012; Petersen, 2004; Strydom *et al.*, 2010); although a change in behaviour and a decrease in functioning was recognised in some participants, especially in the age category between 35 and 55 years. Whilst this initial group is small, the ongoing follow-up of this programme will inform of the progression of symptoms from mild cognitive impairment into dementia.

It is hoped that as therapeutic interventions become available, treatments for specific prodromal forms of cognitive impairment and dementia in this group of people with Down syndrome will be available. Unfortunately, trials of anti-dementia medication have not reported positive results in the population with Down syndrome (Hanney *et al.*, 2012; Lott *et al.*, 2011; Mohan *et al.*, 2009a, 2009b, 2009c). Medical, behavioural and psychiatric problems are common among adults with Down syndrome and require a full and early assessment to treat remediable causes and to improve wellbeing and quality of life. This specialised Health Watch programme, incorporating different aspects of a person's heath, in a multidisciplinary approach, appears to be a positive model in which to assess functional and cognitive decline.

References

Aylward, EH., Burt, DB., Thorpe, LU., Lai, F. and Dalton, A. (1997) Diagnosis of dementia in individuals with intellectual disability. *Journal of Intellectual Disabilities Research 41*, 2, 152–164.

Burt, DB. and Aylward, EH. (2000) Test battery for the diagnosis of dementia in individuals with intellectual disability, Working Group for the Establishment of Criteria for the Diagnosis of Dementia in Individuals with Intellectual Disability. *Journal of Intellectual Disabilities Research 44*, 2, 175–180.

Carmeli, E., Kessel, S., Bar-Chad, S. and Merrick, J. (2004) A comparison between older persons with Down's syndrome and a control group: Clinical characteristics, functional status and sensorimotor function. *Down's Syndrome Research and Practice 9*, 1, 7–24.

Centraal BegeleidingsOrgaan (CBO), Kwaliteitsinstituut voor de Gezondheidszorg (2005) Diagnostiek en medicamenteuze behandeling van dementie. In Vereniging van Klinische Geriatrie (ed.) *Geriatrie*. Utrecht: Van Zuiden Communications BV.

Coppus, A., Evenhuis, H., Verberne, GJ. *et al.* (2006) Dementia and mortality in persons with Down's syndrome. *Journal of Intellectual Disabilities Research 50*, 10, 768–777.

Coppus, AM., Evenhuis, HM., Verberne, GJ. *et al.* (2010) Early age at menopause is associated with increased risk of dementia and mortality in women with Down's syndrome. *Journal of Alzheimer's Disease 19*, 2, 545–50.

Coppus, AMW., Verberne, GJ., Visser, FE. *et al.* (2008) Survival in elderly persons with Down's syndrome. *Journal of Intellectual Disabilities Research 52*, 12, 649–649.

Evenhuis, HM. (1992) Evaluation of a screening instrument for dementia in ageing mentally retarded persons. *Journal of Intellectual Disabilities Research 36*, 4, 337–347.

Evenhuis, HM. (1996) Further evaluation of the Dementia Questionnaire for Persons with Mental Retardation (DMR). *Journal of Intellectual Disabilities Research 40*, 4, 369–373.

Evenhuis, HM., Theunissen, M., Denkers, I., Verschuure, H. and Kemme, H. (2001) Prevalence of visual and hearing impairment in a Dutch institutionalised population with intellectual disability. *Journal of Intellectual Disabilities Research 45*, 1, 457–464.

Evenhuis, HM., van Zanten, GA., Brocaar, M. P. and Roerdinkholder, WH. (1992) Hearing loss in middle-age persons with Down's syndrome. *American Journal of Mental Retardation 97*, 4, 47–56.

Gedye, A. (1995) *Dementia Scale for Down's Syndrome Manual*. Vancouver, BC: Gedye Research and Consulting.

Hanney, M., Prasher, V., Williams, N. *et al.* (2012) Memantine for dementia in adults older than 40 years with Down's syndrome (MEADOWS): A randomised, double-blind, placebo-controlled trial. *Lancet 379*, 9815, 528–536.

Haveman, MJ., Maaskant, MA., van Schrojenstein Lantman, HM., Urlings, HF. and Kessels, AG. (1994) Mental health problems in elderly people with and without Down's syndrome. *Journal of Intellectual Disabilities Research 38*, 3, 341–355.

Holland, AJ., Hon, J., Huppert, FA. and Stevens, F. (2000) Incidence and course of dementia in people with Down's syndrome: Findings from a population-based study. *Journal of Intellectual Disability Research 44*, 2, 138–146.

Jenkins, EC., Ye, L., Velinov, M., Krinsky-McHale, SJ. *et al.* (2012) Mild cognitive impairment identified in older individuals with Down's syndrome by reduced telomere signal numbers and shorter telomeres measured in microns. *American Journal of Medical Genetics Part B: Neuropsychiatric 159B*, 598–604.

Kraijer, D., Kema, G. and de Bildt, AA. (2004), *SRZ/SRZ-i, Sociale Redzaamheidsschalen. Handleiding.* Amsterdam: Harcourt Test Publishers.

Lott, IT., Doran, E., Nguyen, VQ., Tournay, A., Head, E. and Gillen, DL. (2011) Down's syndrome and dementia: A randomized, controlled trial of antioxidant supplementation. *American Journal of Medical Genetics A 155A*, 1939–1948.

McCarron, M., Gill, M., McCallion, P. and Begley, C. (2005) Health co-morbidities in ageing persons with Down's syndrome and Alzheimer's dementia. *Journal of Intellectual Disabilities Research 49*, 7, 560–566.

Mohan, M., Bennett, C. and Carpenter, PK. (2009a) Galantamine for dementia in people with Down's syndrome. *Cochrane Database of Systematic Reviews 1*, CD007656.

Mohan, M., Bennett, C. and Carpenter, PK. (2009b) Rivastigmine for dementia in people with Down's syndrome. *Cochrane Database of Systematic Reviews 1*, CD007658.

Mohan, M., Carpenter, PK. and Bennett, C. (2009c) Donepezil for dementia in people with Down's syndrome. *Cochrane Database of Systematic Reviews 1*, CD007178.

National Task Group (NTG) (2013) *National Task Group on Intellectual Disabilities and Dementia Practices Prescreen Dementia List.* Available at www.aadmd.org/ntg/screening, accessed on 5 December 2013.

Oliver, C., Crayton, L., Holland, A., Hall, S. and Bradbury, J. (1998) A four year prospective study of age-related cognitive change in adults with Down's syndrome. *Psychological Medicine 28*, 6, 1365–1377.

Petersen, RC. (2004) Mild cognitive impairment as a diagnostic entity. *Journal of Internal Medicine 256*, 3, 183–194.

Prasher, VP. (1995) Overweight and obesity amongst Down's syndrome adults. *Journal of Intellectual Disabilities Research 39*, 5, 437–441.

Prasher, VP. (1999) Down's syndrome and thyroid disorders: A review. *Down's Syndrome Research and Practice 6*, 1, 25–42.

Prasher, VP. and Gomez, G. (2007) Natural history of thyroid function in adults with Down's syndrome 10-year follow-up study. *Journal of Intellectual Disabilities Research 51*, 4, 312–317.

Prasher, VP., Ninan, S. and Haque, S. (2011) Fifteen-year follow-up of thyroid status in adults with Down's syndrome. *Journal of Intellectual Disabilities Research 55*, 4, 392–396.

Schupf, N. and Sergievsky, GH. (2002) Genetic and host factors for dementia in Down's syndrome. *British Journal of Psychiatry 180*, 405–410.

Schupf, N., Zigman, W., Kapell, D., Lee, J. H., Kline, J. and Levin, B. (1997) Early menopause in women with Down's syndrome. *Journal of Intellectual Disabilities Research 41*, 3, 264–267.

Seltzer, GB., Schupf, N. and Wu, HS. (2001) A prospective study of menopause in women with Down's syndrome. *Journal of Intellectual Disabilities Research 45*, 1, 1–7.

Strydom, A. and Hassiotis, A. (2003) Diagnostic instruments for dementia in older people with intellectual disability in clinical practice. *Aging and Mental Health 7*, 6, 431–437.

Strydom, A., Chan, T., Fenton, C., Jamieson-Craig, R., Livingston, G. and Hassiotis, A. (2013) Validity of criteria for dementia in older people with intellectual disability. *American Journal of Geriatric Psychiatry 21*, 3, 279–288.

Strydom, A., Shooshtari, S., Lee, L. *et al.* (2010) Dementia in older adults with intellectual disabilities-epidemiology, presentation, and diagnosis. *Journal of Policy and Practice in Intellectual Disabilities 7*, 2 96–110.

Trois, MS., Capone, GT., Lutz, JA. *et al.* (2009) Obstructive sleep apnoea in adults with Down's syndrome. *Journal of Clinical Sleep Medicine 5*, 4, 317–323.

van Buggenhout, GJ., Trommelen, JC., Schoenmaker, A. *et al.* (1999) Down's syndrome in a population of elderly mentally retarded patients: Genetic-diagnostic survey and implications for medical care. *American Journal of Medical Genetics 85*, 4, 376–384.

van Schrojenstein Lantman-de Valk, HM., Haveman, MJ., Maaskant, MA., Kessels, AG., Urlings, HF. and Sturmans, F. (1994) The need for assessment of sensory functioning in ageing people with mental handicap. *Journal of Intellectual Disabilities Research 38*, 3, 289–298.

van Splunder, J., Stilma, JS., Bernsen, RM., Arentz, TG. and Evenhuis, HM. (2003) Refractive errors and visual impairment in 900 adults with intellectual disabilities in the Netherlands. *Acta Ophthalmologica Scandinavica 81*, 2, 123–129.

World Health Organization (1992) *ICD-10: International Statistical Classification of Diseases and related Health Problems, 10th Revision.* Geneva: WHO.

4

Medication Treatment of Dementia in People with Intellectual Disabilities

Ken Courtenay, Nicole Eady

Introduction

Dementia is a long-term condition that poses challenges to health and social care services in providing good quality care (Department of Health, 2009). Treatments offered to people with dementia include socially oriented approaches, and psychological and pharmacological interventions. The principle purpose of medication is to slow cognitive decline and to maintain the person's level of functioning. Medication is also used to manage the behavioural difficulties and psychiatric disorders associated with dementia using anti-depressant or anti-psychotic drugs.

The evidence base for drug therapy in the management of the cognitive and behavioural difficulties associated with dementia in the general population has grown over the decades. The aim of anti-dementia medication is to maintain the person's level of functioning for as long as possible in the absence of medical cure for dementia. In maintaining a person's level of functioning for as long as possible, the secondary gain to health and social care services from using medication is to help the person maintain their independence for as long as possible.

The use of anti-dementia medication among adults with an intellectual disability is recommended by the National Institute for Clinical Excellence (NICE, 2011). However, the evidence to support their prescription is small. The reasons for this include the difficulty in making a diagnosis of dementia early in the condition, the presence of existing cognitive impairment, comorbid illness, for example epilepsy, or lack of awareness and experience among health care professionals of the potential benefits of medication on behavioural difficulties and psychiatric disorders associated with dementia. The chemical theories of dementia will be presented along with the actions of anti-dementia drugs in the brain, the potential for drugs to enhance cognitive function, the role of non-dementia medication in care, and the issues for people with an intellectual disability and dementia using medication.

The chemistry of dementia

The human nervous system is made up of two parts: the central nervous system and the peripheral nervous system. The central nervous system is the brain and spinal cord. The peripheral nervous system consists of the nerves that supply all areas of the body to help the person feel touch, pain, temperature, vibration and joint position. Sensory information from the peripheral nervous system feeds back to the brain through the spinal cord informing the brain on how the body is working and about its environment. The changes occurring in dementia affect the central nervous system.

Nerve cells

The building block for both the central nervous system and peripheral nervous system is the nerve cell or neuron. Neurons are similar to other cells in the body containing cytoplasm and a nucleus that is surrounded by a membrane. They are different from cells in other parts of the human body in that they have spiky projections on them, dendrites. They increase the surface area of the cell enabling it to communicate with its neighbouring cells. In this way information is passed from one cell to another to form thoughts, feelings and memories (cognitive functions) that can lead to behavioural changes. Therefore, damage to the nerve cells can lead to disordered brain functioning.

Neurotransmitters

Neurons communicate with each other using neurotransmitters. A neurotransmitter is a chemical that is released by one cell, then absorbed by another through a receptor on the wall of the neighbouring cell. There are different types of neurotransmitter of which glutamate is the most common. The connection point between neurons is the synapse where the transmitting and receiving cells are very close together. This enables rapid transfer of information from one cell to another.

The transmission of information between cells occurs as follows. The electrical charges on the two sides of the nerve membrane differ where one is more negatively charged than the other. When the charges on the two sides equalise, channels in the membrane open to allow positively charged calcium ions to enter the cell, returning the membrane to a neutral charge. The increase in calcium ions causes packets, or vesicles, of neurotransmitters (pre-made stores of neurotransmitters) to fuse with the membrane of the cell releasing their contents of neurotransmitter into the synaptic cleft (the small gap between the cells). The neurotransmitter diffuses into the synapse away from the pre-synaptic neuron connecting with a receptor on a neighbouring cell, or the post-synaptic neuron. The responding action of the receiving cell depends on the type of neurotransmitter and receptor it is connected to.

The principle neurotransmitter affected in dementia is acetylcholine (ACh). It is important in creating memories, maintaining attention, acquiring language and applying reasoning. A reduction in ACh results in memory loss, loss of language and reduced attention span. The nucleus basalis of Meynert is the centre for the production of ACh (Casanova *et al.*, 1985). Acetylcholine is broken down in the synapse by the enzyme acetylcholinesterase (AChe) which prevents the accumulation of ACh in the synaptic cleft, allowing for the effective and efficient transmission of impulses from one neuron to others (Casanova *et al.*, 1985).

Palmer and Gershon (1990) suggested the theoretical roles of acetylcholine and glutamate in dementia. The loss of ACh-producing neurons and the excessive action of glutamate in destroying cells provide the neurochemical basis of dementia (Danysz and Parsons, 2003). In dementia, plaques made of amyloid protein and fibrillary tangles accumulate in the neurons over many years leading to impairment in function or cell death and thus a reduction in neurotransmitters.

The decline in the amount of ACh is gradual over time as a person ages, reaching significance when memory disorder is evident. The activity of AChe in breaking down ACh in the synapse is maintained but the reduced amount of ACh results in impaired function between the neurons. These changes occur earlier in the lives of people with Down syndrome (Lott and Head, 2005). Therefore, the rationale of drug treatment is to either increase the amount of ACh produced by the neuron, or to enhance the action of what ACh is available by inhibiting its breakdown by AChe and maintaining communication between neurons.

Anti-dementia medication

The purpose of anti-dementia medication is to slow the progress of dementia by acting on the neurotransmitters in the brain involved in memory, attention and language. The drugs can be classified into two groups:

- Cholinesterase inhibitors (AChe) – donepezil (Aricept); rivastigmine; galantamine
- N-methyl-D-aspartate antagonist (NMDA) – memantine.

The cholinesterase inhibitors stop the breakdown of the enzyme in the synaptic cleft allowing more ACh to be available. Donepezil and galantamine only inhibit the enzyme acetylcholinesterase. Rivastigmine inhibits two enzymes, acetlycholinesterase (AChe) and butyrylcholinesterase (BChe). Memantine blocks off the NMDA receptor, thus antagonising the action of glutamate (Danysz and Parsons, 2003).

Donepezil

Donepezil is useful in slowing the progress of dementia and is safe to use in people with dementia in the general population (Rogers and Friedhoff 1996; Rogers *et al.*, 1998). It is recommended by NICE guidance (2011) as first-line drug treatment in the management of Alzheimer-type dementia. It can be used in treating vascular dementia that is caused by impaired blood supply to the brain. It is given once a day up to 30mg in dose (British National Formulary (BNF), 2013).

Rivastigmine

Rivastigmine is given in either tablet form or as a daily patch for people who cannot tolerate tablets. The tablets are taken twice a day. The dose is variable allowing the most effective dose to be achieved that the person can tolerate. The maximum dose is 12mg per day (BNF, 2013).

Galantamine

Galantamine is indicated in people with mild to moderate dementia. It is given twice a day in tablet form and the maximum daily dose is 24mg (BNF, 2013).

Memantine

Glutamate amino acid is the chemical involved in the glutamergic system of neurotransmission that excites nerve cells (Danysz *et al.*, 1995). Glutamate destroys the cells because of excessive action as it is not counterbalanced by protective chemicals (Rothman and Olney, 1987). Memantine blocks the N-methyl DA receptor (NMDA) and thus reduces the destructive action of glutamate on the nerve cell. It is taken in tablet form and used once a day at a maximum dose of 20mg (BNF, 2013).

The evidence for anti-dementia medication in people with intellectual disabilities

The general literature in dementia supports the effectiveness of anti-dementia medication in people with dementia by improving cognitive functioning, which is evident after three months of use (Rogers and Friedhoff, 1996).

In comparison to the general adult population, there is a small evidence base for the pharmacological treatment of dementia in people with intellectual disabilities. The gold standard of medical evidence is the randomised controlled trial comparing a large number of people both with and without treatment to establish its effectiveness and to identify the frequency of adverse effects. To find statistically significant differences between two groups, large numbers of participants are required as part of a randomised controlled trial. Finding acceptable numbers of people with an intellectual disability and dementia who could participate in drug trials can be challenging because the incidence – the number of new cases per year – of intellectual disability and dementia is relatively low, despite the higher prevalence when compared with the general population (Strydom *et al.*, 2007). Therefore, any trial would have to be conducted through a number of trial centres in order to recruit sufficient participants.

The evidence on the effectiveness of anti-dementia drugs in people with intellectual disabilities is through case reports that have been followed up with randomised controlled trials. The evidence has become stronger over time as more people use anti-dementia medication. Much of the evidence for using anti-dementia drugs in people with intellectual disabilities refers to adults with Down syndrome. This is not surprising because of the prevalence of dementia in people over 40 years of age in this population, and the difficulties of diagnosing dementia in people who do not have Down syndrome. Therefore, most case series and randomised controlled trials refer to people with Down syndrome.

Donepezil

Lott *et al.* (2002) suggested that donepezil is effective in people with Down syndrome, a finding that was supported by Prasher *et al.* (2002) in a 24-week randomised controlled trial. The findings did not reach statistical significance and therefore could not confirm the effectiveness of donepezil in dementia in people with intellectual disabilities. A follow-up study over a longer period of time demonstrated the effectiveness of donepezil in people with intellectual disabilities (Prasher *et al.*, 2003). The study was limited by its small numbers but is a valuable contribution to our knowledge of anti-dementia medication use in people with intellectual disabilities. Kondoh *et al.* (2011) undertook a randomised controlled trial of donepezil in 21 women with Down syndrome and dementia. The findings, also with small numbers, showed that the level of function had improved in the treated group after 24 weeks of the trial.

Rivastigmine and galantamine

Prasher *et al.* (2005) reviewed the case notes of people with Down syndrome with dementia who used rivastigmine and compared them with people with Down syndrome treated with a placebo. Rivastigmine led to a slower decline in global functioning and adaptive behaviour over 24 weeks, but it was not statistically significant. Haessler (2006) reported the positive effects of rivastigmine in a case series of three people with Down syndrome and dementia. On the basis of the evidence, a Cochrane Review could not recommend rivastigmine for dementia in Down syndrome (Mohan *et al.*, 2009a). Specific evaluation of the effect of galantamine in people with intellectual disabilities has not been reported. Mohan *et al.* (2009b) in their review did not elicit strong evidence to support its use in people with intellectual disabilities.

Memantine

Hanney *et al.* (2012) completed a randomised controlled trial of people with Down syndrome over 40 years of age using memantine. The aim was to ascertain the effect of memantine on cognitive function. It was not necessary for participants to have a firm diagnosis of dementia since the prevalence of dementia in people with Down syndrome over 40 years is approximately 40 per cent (Prasher, 1995). A total of 176 people were included in the trial but the findings did not reach statistical significance and therefore did not support the effectiveness of memantine in people with Down syndrome.

There are many case reports and some randomised controlled trials in people with Down syndrome that do not reach significance, providing conflicting evidence. Many of these have had positive outcomes suggesting the use of anti-dementia medication in this group is effective and safe. However, there is not sufficient published evidence for the statistical results of the trials to be combined in a meta-analysis to support one conclusion at present. The overall impression is that anti-dementia medication is effective in people with Down syndrome, but effect size cannot be demonstrated because of the small numbers involved in trials.

The authors have not found published studies on the treatment outcomes for people with an intellectual disability (other than Down syndrome) and dementia. Prescribing guidance advises that medication can be offered to people with an intellectual disability with dementia as part of a treatment plan (NICE/SCIE 2006) and initiated by specialists in dementia care rather than a general medical practitioner.

Acquiring the evidence

In order to expand the evidence base, the challenge is to diagnose dementia early in people with intellectual disabilities. People with an intellectual disability and dementia are more likely to have other medical problems, for example seizures and sensory impairments, which can complicate the presentation of dementia. They may also have mental health and behavioural difficulties, for example, related to autistic spectrum disorders or depression. Both physical and psychiatric problems can exclude people from taking part in anti-dementia drug trials.

It can be difficult to know what to measure in a trial, or which trial group the participant should move into. When separating individuals into treatment groups or diagnostic groups, such uncertainty can reduce the power of the results to show a significant difference in applying an intervention. There is also a requirement to measure the differences in cognitive and social functioning in the participants in the trial. Whilst a number of tools and scores to measure dementia in intellectual disabilities are available, many of them have not been fully validated or are not adequately sensitive to detect small changes. It can be difficult to compare the results between trials when different instruments are used in trials. There can be a misconception that because of a person's intellectual disability, their memory difficulties do not require treatment or would not respond to it. Such views could indirectly affect efforts to broaden the evidence base in this area.

Adverse effects of anti-dementia medication

In common with all medication, anti-dementia drugs have side effects. There is much debate in the literature on the side effects experienced by people with an intellectual disability who use donepezil. Hemingway-El Tomey and Lerner (1999) reported cases of urinary incontinence and aggression in a case series that led to stopping the drug. Cipriani et al. (2003) had to cease using donepezil because of side effects in its small study of four adults with dementia. Prasher et al. (2002) also reported that people with intellectual disabilities experience side effects commonly when using donepezil. Kishnani et al. (2001) did not observe this in their experience of using the drug and in a larger study, Lott et al. (2002) reported side effects that were temporary.

The Maudsley prescribing guidelines (Taylor *et al.*, 2011) report that tolerability is more closely related to the rate of titration, the increase in dose over time, than the dose prescribed. Donepezil and galantamine are metabolised by the liver and their effectiveness could be affected by any other medication that increases or decreases the action of enzymes within the liver. In people with an intellectual disability, it is recommended that medication is started at a low dose and increased slowly, if indicated. Most side effects are secondary to an excess in cholinergic stimulation. Common side effects of all anti-dementia medications include nausea, vomiting, reduced appetite and diarrhoea, whilst some notice a change in their sleeping pattern. Acetylcholinesterase inhibitors should be used cautiously in people with breathing problems because they can precipitate spasm in the airways in some people. The drugs can slow the heart rate causing dizziness and falls and so heart function should be assessed when medication is first started.

Cognitive enhancing drugs

In considering the role of drug therapy in dementia it is important to refer to drugs that aim to improve a person's cognitive function and to explore their potential to enhance a person's memory and level of functioning. Cognitive enhancers are a varied group of compounds that appear to improve the memory skills of people with dementia and, more importantly, in people who do not have dementia but are at high risk of developing the condition. Certain compounds have been noted to improve memory in people with intellectual disabilities. Some are recognised medications, for example, donepezil, while others are naturally occurring compounds such as Vitamin E.

Donepezil

Johnson *et al.* (2003) conducted a randomised controlled trial of donepezil in 19 adults with Down syndrome, but without dementia. There was no effect on cognitive function but a positive impact on language with either improvement or no apparent decline in the person's language skills. Kishnani *et al.* (2004) also observed an improvement in language skills.

Acetyl-L-carnitine

Pueschel (2005) conducted a double-blind control trial of acetyl-L-carnitine among 40 young male adults with Down syndrome to test its effect on memory and other cognitive skills. None in the matched groups had dementia. In both groups there were significant changes in their results, but the overall finding from the study was that acetyl-L-carnitine did not improve mental function in male adults with Down syndrome.

Anti-oxidants

The metabolism in the nerve cell leads to the release of free radicals that can cause damage to the cell because of the accumulation of amyloid peptide in the cell. Anti-oxidant compounds such as Vitamin E are thought to help to absorb the toxic-free radicals and protect the cell from damage and to slow the progress of dementia (Behl, 1997). Aisen *et al.* (2005) reported on a multi-centre trial of the effect of Vitamin E on memory in adults with Down syndrome but did not find a significant effect on cognitive function. Similarly, Lott *et al.* (2011) completed a two-year randomised controlled trial of 53 adults with Down syndrome to assess the impact of Vitamin E in cognition. The conclusion was that anti-oxidants are safe to use at the trial doses, but do not provide benefit in cognitive function to the person. Other anti-oxidant compounds, for example, aspirin, could be explored for their effects on preserving or enhancing cognitive function.

Non-dementia medication

In addition to anti-dementia medications, people with dementia often use a variety of drugs to manage behavioural difficulties, mental health and physical health problems. As a consequence, the potential for drug interactions to occur is high. Such drugs do not delay the progression of dementia but are used to treat symptoms that commonly occur and cause distress in those with dementia. When prescribing such medications the prescriber must balance the benefit of additional medication versus the side effects that such a medication may cause. Often the proposed benefit would be to reduce distress, or to help the person remain in their home in familiar surroundings.

Anti-depressants can be useful in treating depression that can occur in people with dementia. They are beneficial in treating dementia-associated apathy and some behavioural disturbance. Geldmacher *et al.* (1997) support the use of selective serotonin re-uptake inhibitors (SSRI) anti-depressants to treat functional decline, aggression, social withdrawal and compulsive behaviours in a case series of six adults with Down syndrome. SSRIs are generally well tolerated but the common side effects include gastrointestinal disturbance and a change in sleep pattern.

Stevens *et al.* (2012) described the occurrence of a serious neurological disorder, neuroleptic malignant syndrome, in a person with Down syndrome and dementia when rivastigmine was used with olanzapine, an anti-psychotic. The person recovered, but it highlights the need for prescribers to be aware of the drug interactions associated with drug combinations and their potential for lethal effects.

Anti-psychotic drugs are sometimes used, for example risperidone and olanzapine, to manage behavioural difficulties that people with dementia present. Their use is not advocated because of the increased risk of stroke affecting the brain (Ballard *et al.*, 2008). Where people are using it when dementia is diagnosed, it is advisable to reduce the dose with a view to withdrawing the drug.

Preparing to start anti-dementia medication

In people with intellectual disabilities, clinicians should commence the drug at a low dose and increase it according to the clinical response. Measuring cognitive function and behaviour prior to starting medication is good practice that helps to assess the effect of the drug on the person's memory and behaviour. A physical examination should be completed by a doctor before starting the drugs, paying attention to the cardiovascular system by measuring blood pressure and heart rate. The acetylcholinesterase inhibitors can slow the heart rate and therefore a pre-treatment assessment of the heart rate and rhythm using an electrocardiogram (ECG) is advisable.

Other physical investigations to complete prior to starting medication include kidney and liver function to ensure that they are working within normal limits. Blood tests are important because donepezil and galantamine are broken down by the liver and the kidney removes the drugs from the body. Regular monitoring of the person's physical health, including heart rate, should continue whilst they are using anti-dementia medication.

Measuring outcomes of treatment

Clinical interventions should be clear on the desired outcome of treatment. To assess the effectiveness of drug treatment on the person's level of functioning and quality of life, clinical response needs to be measured using objective tools. Objective measurements are often combined with the overall clinical impression of the person's response by the clinician. The tools need to measure what they intend to measure (validity) and to be repeatable (reliability) in their application. Choosing a measurement tool is up to the clinician and depends on what they intend to measure, whether it is quality of life or cognitive function. Examples of tools used in practice include: Neuropsychiatric Inventory (NPI) (Cummings *et al.*, 1994) and Dementia in Learning Disability (DLD) (Evenhuis *et al.*, 2007). However, not all measurement tools are applicable or have been validated in people with an intellectual disability and results need to be interpreted with caution. The tools used in the general population could be used to measure outcomes in adults with mild intellectual disability, for example the Mini-Mental State Examination (Folstein *et al.*, 1975).

Capacity to consent

A principle of good medical care is partnership in decision-making between the clinician and the person receiving treatment. The capacity of the person to take a decision on proposed treatment is an essential component in this relationship. Mental capacity might be compromised in people with intellectual disabilities because of their lifelong level of cognitive functioning or because of dementia in older age or during periods of ill health. Clinicians are obliged to undertake an assessment of the person's mental capacity to give their consent to drug treatment. To achieve this, guidelines on assessing mental capacity can be followed. Legislation in the UK provides a framework under which decisions in care can be taken (Adults with Incapacity (Scotland) Act 2000; Mental Capacity Act 2005). Where a person does not have the mental capacity to take a decision on anti-dementia treatment and where efforts have been made to enhance their level of understanding, provision is made to decide in the person's best interests. The process should involve carers, family and professionals in reaching a decision that weighs up the advantages and disadvantages of treatment. It should take into account the person's expressed wishes before they lost mental capacity, if any had been stated. In spite of the benefits to using anti-dementia medication, the person has the right not to accept treatment. In the absence of mental capacity legislation, clinicians should follow such principles and be guided by their professional codes of practice.

The future of anti-dementia medication

Research

Much of the evidence base for using anti-dementia medication in people with intellectual disabilities is based on trials and experience in practice in the general population. The current evidence is limited randomised controlled trial data and case reports. Clinical guidance does not have a strong base on which to create guidance for clinicians working with people with intellectual disabilities. Acquiring good evidence on the effectiveness of medication in people with intellectual disabilities and dementia is difficult because of the complexities associated with intellectual disabilities, for example coexistent epilepsy or cerebral palsy.

The barriers to research on medication in people with intellectual disabilities include capacity to consent to take part in drug trials, accurate and timely diagnosis of dementia, and the impact of other disorders on the response to anti-dementia medication. The difficulties of identifying people with intellectual disabilities who have dementia impacts upon achieving adequate numbers of participants in trials. For this reason, larger populations of people with intellectual disabilities need to be recruited. The population most at risk are adults with Down syndrome, who should be considered separately from adults without Down syndrome to exclude it as a confounding variable. Research in the future needs to establish the effectiveness of clinical interventions applied to people with intellectual disabilities that would provide a good evidence base, and thus enhance clinical practice, whilst guarding people from harm when exposed to medication that would not be effective as part of their care. Acquiring funding to conduct research with people who have intellectual disabilities can be difficult due to the small numbers affected when compared with the general population without an intellectual disability.

Disease modification

Cummings (2006) refers to 'disease modification' where a drug slows down the process of cell death in dementia, and neuroprotective agents could act by enhancing cell health. Bullock and Dengiz (2005) suggest that acetylcholinesterase inhibitors can modify the course of dementia. It is accepted, however, that AChe drugs lose their benefit over time (Doody *et al.*, 2001; Winblad and Jelic, 2006). Therefore, alternative strategies to the cholinergic model could be considered that include drugs acting directly on the accumulation of amyloid peptide in the nerve cells (Aisen *et al.*, 2005).

Carers

The role of caring for a person with intellectual disabilities who has dementia often falls on carers (Courtenay *et al.*, 2010). Therefore, efforts to raise awareness of dementia in people with intellectual disabilities among carers and family members could facilitate people seeking help earlier in the condition to avail of evidence-based medical interventions. The presence of a pre-existing cognitive disorder can mask the subtle signs of memory difficulties until the diagnosis is more apparent when behavioural difficulties are present (McKenzie *et al.*, 2002). For this reason, enhanced knowledge of dementia among carers could enable access to timely, appropriate care.

Conclusion

Anti-dementia medications are a useful intervention in the management of people with intellectual disabilities who have dementia. They offer the potential to improve memory function, skills used in daily living, and to improve a person's quality of life. They are potent drugs that require skilled assessment and prescribing for people who have complex health conditions. The drugs need to be monitored by clinicians during treatment because of the higher risk in people with intellectual disabilities of developing side effects.

The evidence base to support the use of anti-dementia medication in people with intellectual disabilities and dementia is not robust or broad compared with that available to the general population. There have been a limited number of randomised controlled trials completed in people with intellectual disabilities and dementia and some case reports that provide the evidence for their efficacy. The complexity of physical and mental health difficulties of people with intellectual disabilities add other dimensions to the management of dementia on which the generic evidence cannot always provide guidance. Despite this, and the differences outlined, clinicians and carers often need to infer from the generic evidence base in dementia when applying current knowledge in the care of people with intellectual disabilities and dementia.

The challenge to the research community and those supporting people with an intellectual disability and dementia is to develop research strategies that will answer questions about the use of anti-dementia medication in this population, especially in people with Down syndrome. With limited budgets in health care research most money is directed towards research that may benefit the large cohorts of a population. To achieve such numbers, collaboration between research groups will be essential in order to establish a good evidence base. In conjunction with research efforts is the necessity to educate families and carers on the early signs of dementia. This can offer the person the potential benefit of using medication to help slow progression that could enhance their quality of life and allow them to age in their existing surroundings, if this is desired. It is hoped that advances in knowledge of dementia in people with intellectual disabilities will offer new treatments to arrest the condition.

References

Adults with Incapacity (Scotland) Act (2000). Available at www.legislation.gov.uk/asp/2000/4/contents, accessed 5 December 2013.

Aisen, PS., Dalton, AJ., Sano, M., Lott, IT., Andrews, HF. and Tsai, W. (2005) Design and implementation of a multicenter trial of Vitamin E in aging individuals with Down's syndrome. *Journal of Policy and Practice in Intellectual Disabilities 2*, 2, 86–93.

Ballard, CG., Waite, J. and Birks, J. (2008) Atypical antipsychotics for aggression and psychosis in Alzheimer's disease. *Cochrane Database of Systematic Review, Issue 1. CD003476.* doi: 10.1002/14651858.CD003476.pub2.

Behl, C. (1997) Amyloid B-protein toxicity and oxidative stress in Alzheimer's disease. *Cell Tissue Research 290*, 3, 471–480.

British National Formulary (BNF) (2013) *BNF 65 The Authority on the Selection and Use of Medicines.* London: BMJ Publishing Group Ltd and Pharmaceutical Press.

Bullock, R. and Dengiz, A. (2005) Cognitive performance in patients with Alzheimer's disease receiving cholinesterase inhibitors for up to 5 years. *International Journal Clinical Practice 59*, 7, 817–822.

Casanova, MF., Walker, LC., Whitehouse, PJ. and Price, DL. (1985) Abnormalities of the nucleus basalis in Down's syndrome. *Annals of Neurology 18, 3,* 310–313.

Cipriani, G., Bianchetti, A. and Trabucchi, M. (2003) Donepezil use in the treatment of dementia associated with Down's syndrome. *Archives of Neurology 60,* 2, 292.

Courtenay, K., Jokinen, NS. and Strydom, A. (2010) Caregiving and adults with intellectual disabilities affected by dementia. *Journal of Policy and Practice in Intellectual Disabilities 7,* 1, 26–33.

Cummings, JL. (2006) Challenges to demonstrating disease-modifying effects of Alzheimer's disease clinical trials. *Alzheimer's and Dementia 2,* 4, 263–271.

Cummings, JL., Mega, M., Gray, K., Rosenberg-Thompson, S., Carusi, DA. and Gornbein, J. (1994) The Neuropsychiatric Inventory: Comprehensive assessment of psychopathology in dementia. *Neurology 44,* 12, 2308–2314.

Danysz, W. and Parsons, CG. (2003) The NMDA receptor antagonist memantine as a symptomatological and neuroprotective treatment for Alzheimer's disease: Preclinical evidence. *International Journal of Geriatric Psychiatry 18,* 1, S23–S32.

Danysz, W., Parsons, CG., Bresink, I. and Quack, G. (1995) Glutamate in CNS disorders – a revived target for drug development. *Drug News Perspective 8,* 261–277.

Department of Health (2009) *Living Well With Dementia: A National Dementia Strategy.* Available at www.gov.uk/government/publications/living-well-with-dementia-a-national-dementia-strategy, accessed on 5 December 2013.

Doody, RS., Dunn, JK., Clark, CM. *et al.* (2001) Chronic donepezil treatment is associated with slowed cognitive decline in Alzheimer's disease. *Dementia Geriatric Cognitive Disorders 12,* 4, 295–300.

Evenhuis, HM., Kengen, MMF. and Eurlings, HAL. (2007) *Dementia Questionnaire for People with Learning Disabilities (DLD) UK adaptation.* San Antonio, TX: Harcourt Assessment.

Folstein, MF., Folstein, SE. and McHugh, PR. (1975) 'Mini-Mental State': A practical method for grading the cognitive state of patients for the clinician. *Journal Psychiatric Research 12,* 3, 189–198.

Geldmacher, DS., Lerner, AJ., Voci, JM., Noelker, EA., Somple, LC. and Whitehouse, PJ. (1997) Treatment of functional decline in adults with Down's syndrome using selective serotonin-reuptake inhibitor drugs. *Journal of Geriatric Psychiatry and Neurology 10,* 3, 99–104.

Haessler, F. (2006) Rivastigmine in the therapy of dementia in patients with mental retardation. *Psychopharmakotherapie 13,* 5, 205–209.

Hanney, M., Prasher, VP., Williams, N. *et al.* (2012) Memantine for dementia in adults older than 40 years with Down's syndrome (MEADOWS): A randomised, double-blind, placebo-controlled trial. *The Lancet 379,* 9815, 528–536.

Hemingway-El Tomey, JM. and Lerner, AJ. (1999) Adverse effects of donepezil in treating Alzheimer's disease associated with Down's syndrome. *American Journal of Psychiatry 156,* 156, 1470–1470.

Johnson, N., Fahey, C., Chicone, B., Chong, G. and Gitelman, D. (2003) Effects of donepezil on cognitive functioning in Down's syndrome. *American Journal on Mental Retardation 108,* 6, 367–372.

Kishnani, PS., Spiridigliozzi, GA., Heller, JH., Sullivan, JA., Murali Doraiswamy, P. and Ranga Rama Krishnan, K. (2001) Donepezil for Down's syndrome. *American Journal of Psychiatry 158,* 1, 143.

Kishnani, PS., Sullivan, JA., Spiridigliozzi, GA., Heller, JH. and Crissman, BG. (2004) Donepezil use in Down's syndrome. *Archives of Neurology 61,* 4, 606.

Kondoh, T., Amamoto, N., Doi, T. *et al.* (2011) Dramatic improvement in Down's syndrome-associated cognitive impairment with donepezil. *The Annals of Pharmacotherapy 39,* 3, 563–566.

Lott, IT. and Head, E. (2005) Alzheimer disease and Down's syndrome: factors in pathogenesis. *Neurobiology of Aging 26,* 3, 383–389.

Lott, IT., Osann, K., Doran, E. and Nelson, L. (2002) Down's syndrome and Alzheimer's disease: Response to Donepezil. *Archives of Neurology 59*, 7, 133–1136.

Lott, IT., Doran, E., Nguyen, VQ., Tournay, A., Head, E. and Gillen, DL. (2011) Down's syndrome and dementia: A randomized controlled trial of antioxidant supplementation. *American Journal of Medical Genetics, Part A, 155*, 1939–1948.

McKenzie K., Baxter S., Paxton D. and Murray G. (2002) Picking up the signs. *Learning Disability Practice 5*, 3, 16–19.

Mental Capacity Act (2005) Available at www.legislation.gov.uk/ukpga/2005/9/contents, accessed on 5 December 2013.

Mohan, M., Bennett, C. and Carpenter, PK. (2009a) Rivastigmine for dementia in people with Down's syndrome. *Cochrane Database of Systematic Reviews 1, CD007658.* doi: 10.1002/14651858.CD007658.

Mohan, M., Bennett, C. and Carpenter, PK. (2009b) Galantamine for dementia in people with Down's syndrome. *Cochrane Database of Systematic Reviews 1, CD007656.* doi: 10.1002/14651858.CD007656.

National Institute for Health and Care Excellence (NICE)/Social Care Institute for Excellence (SCIE) (2006) *Dementia: Supporting people with dementia and their carers in health and social care.* London: The Stationery Office.

NICE (2011) *Alzheimer's Disease – Donepezil, Galantamine, Rivastigmine and Memantine (TA217).* Available at http://guidance.nice.org.uk/TA217, accessed on 19 March 2014.

Palmer, AM. and Gershon, S. (1990) Is the neuronal basis of Alzheimer's disease cholinergic or glutamatergic? *Federation of American Studies for Experimental Biology Journal 4*, 10, 2745–2752.

Prasher, VP. (1995) Age-specific prevalence, thyroid dysfunction and depressive symptomatology in adults with Down's syndrome and dementia. *International Journal of Geriatric Psychiatry 10*, 1, 25–31.

Prasher, VP., Adams, C. and Holder, R. (2003) Long-term safety and efficacy of donepezil in the treatment of dementia in Alzheimer's disease in adults with Down's syndrome: Open label study. *International Journal of Geriatric Psychiatry 18*, 6, 549–551.

Prasher, VP., Fung, N. and Adams, C. (2005) Rivastigmine in the treatment of dementia in Alzheimer's disease in adults with Down's syndrome. *International Journal of Geriatric Psychiatry 20*, 5, 496–497.

Prasher, VP., Huxley, A. and Haque, MS. (2002) A 24-week, double-blind, placebo controlled trial of donepezil in patients with Down's syndrome and Alzheimer's disease: Pilot study. *International Journal of Geriatric Psychiatry 17*, 3, 270–278.

Pueschel, SM. (2005) The effect of acetyl-L-carnitine administration on persons with Down's syndrome. *Research in Developmental Disabilities 27*, 6, 599–604.

Rogers, SL. and Friedhoff, LT. (1996) The efficacy and safety of donepezil in patients with Alzheimer's disease: Results of a US multicentre, randomized, double-blind, placebo-controlled trial. *Dementia 7*, 6, 293–303.

Rogers, SL., Farlow, MR., Doody, RS., Mohs, R. and Friedhoff, LT. (1998) A 24-week, double-blind, placebo-controlled trial of donepezil in patients with Alzheimer's disease. *Neurology 50*, 1, 136–145.

Rothman, SM. and Olney, JW. (1987) Excitotoxicity and the NMDA receptor. *Trends in Neurosciences 10*, 7, 299–302.

Stevens, DL., Lee, MR. and Padua, Y. (2012) Olanzapine-associated neuroleptic malignant syndrome in a patient receiving concomitant rivastigmine therapy. *Pharmacotherapy 28*, 3, 403–405.

Strydom, A., Livingston, G., King, M. and Hassiotis, A. (2007) Prevalence of dementia in intellectual ability using different diagnostic criteria. *British Journal of Psychiatry 191*, 2, 150–157.

Taylor, D., Paton, C. and Kapur, S. (eds) (2011) *The Maudsley Prescribing Guidelines.* 11th edition. London: Wiley Blackwell.

Winblad, B. and Jelic, V. (2006) Treating the full spectrum of dementia with memantine. *International Journal of Geriatric Psychiatry 18*, 1, S41–S46.

5

Non-Pharmacological Interventions

Nancy S. Jokinen

Introduction

Many practice guidelines in dementia care recommend the use of various non-pharmacological interventions to alleviate behavioural and psychological symptoms of Alzheimer's disease and other dementias, alongside or prior to the introduction of pharmacological treatments. Drug therapies should be used with caution given their reported limited efficacy and potential for adverse drug reactions. Non-pharmacological strategies may also serve to maintain or enhance quality of life, alleviate some of the stress experienced by caregivers, and forestall relocation of the person affected by dementia. The scientific evidence supporting non-pharmacological alternatives is ambiguous, although this is often as a result of criteria used for judging efficacy. Non-pharmacological interventions are examined, first from the general dementia-related literature and research with older people, followed by specific interventions with people who have an intellectual disability.

Worldwide, Alzheimer's disease and other dementias are a major concern for families, practitioners, service providers and policy-makers (World Health Organization, 2012). In the field of intellectual disabilities, similar concerns are now being echoed (National Task Group on Intellectual Disabilities and Dementia Practice, 2012). Adults ageing with intellectual disabilities live in a variety of settings: with family, alone, or within different residential settings in both intellectual disability and older care. The ability of their formal and informal supports to accommodate age-related changes and dementia care varies. The early onset of symptoms related to dementia may or may not be recognized, and if so are disconcerting to family members as well as support staff. Yet, it is evident that some families and intellectual disability service providers have long been encouraged to proactively plan for the potential that dementia will affect some adults with intellectual disabilities, although many continue to struggle in providing appropriate supports (Janicki *et al.*, 1996; Wilkinson and Janicki, 2002).

Alzheimer's disease and other dementias have a tremendous impact on the individual, family and friends as well as on direct and indirect support staff. Dementia changes a person's abilities and, over time, additional assistance becomes necessary, for example with personal care and support for palliative and end of life care. The challenge is to be responsive to the individual's needs and support them to live well throughout the course of dementia (Cayton, 2004). Enacting concepts and ideas ideally associated with dementia care, however, may be challenging for both organizations and individual carers. Worldwide, many intellectual disabilities organizations are faced with other priorities, for example deinstitutionalization, or youth transitions to adult services. Family carers, in the midst of providing care, may become discouraged as they are confronted with conflicts or lack of information and training. While the heart of dementia care occurs at the personal level in the interactions between the person affected by dementia and the persons responsible for support, the quality of that care is influenced by organizational and inter-organizational factors (Courtenay *et al.*, 2010).

Most intellectual disability services tend to focus on and promote enhancement of skills for independent living, self-determination and employment opportunities. Dementia care requires a shift in that focus to one in which the priorities attend to maintaining abilities and quality of life for as long as is possible. This is in the face of progressive loss of functional and cognitive abilities and growing dependence. Although the behavioural and psychological symptoms associated with dementia are individually experienced and vary with the progression and stage, some of these symptoms create daily challenges to family and other carers. Many service providers will need to fundamentally change to accommodate dementia as it affects persons with intellectual disabilities (Jokinen *et al.*, 2013). Without forethought, problems that arise might prompt a reactive rather than a planned relocation (Jokinen *et al.*, 2012) of the individual with dementia to an alternative living arrangement, or a withdrawal from day program supports.

In order to cope with increased caregiving demands, carers sometimes request pharmacological treatments to ameliorate the symptoms of dementia and the resultant stress in providing care. Yet, medications and polypharmacy are major issues for older-aged adults (Blozik *et al.*, 2013) as well as for adults ageing with intellectual disabilities (British Psychological Society, 2009; Jokinen *et al.*, 2013) and a regime of additional pharmaceuticals to treat behavioural and psychological symptoms of dementia likely exacerbates these concerns. Guidelines do exist for treatment of various symptoms associated with dementia such as agitation or aggression using pharmacological agents (British Psychological Society, 2009; Gauthier *et al.*, 2012; National Institute for Health and Clinical Excellence (NICE), 2012). Commonly, there are cautions given with the use of such treatments and the drugs may have limited, short-term efficacy and potential for adverse effects (Ballard *et al.*, 2008). For all individuals, a pharmacological intervention necessitates prudent ongoing evaluation of the drug's benefits as well as risks (NICE, 2012).

Categories and types of non-pharmacological interventions in the general ageing population

Non-pharmacological interventions consist of an array of approaches that generally aim to promote quality of life, proactively or reactively address symptomatic issues that arise over the course of dementia, and/or provide support to family and other carers. The terms psychosocial and non-pharmacological are occasionally used synonymously in literature, and interventions are categorized in a variety of ways in the absence of a standardized classification system (Maslow, 2012). For instance, the National Institute for Health and Clinical Excellence (NICE, 2012) categorizes non-pharmacological interventions according to use: for cognitive symptoms, non-cognitive symptoms and behaviour, comorbid emotional conditions and carer support. On the other hand, de Merdeiros and Basting (2013) grouped non-pharmacological interventions as either psychosocial or cultural and arts based in relation to an outcome category: either cognition or quality of life. Furthermore, non-pharmacological approaches may also be identified and reported in terms of specific problems that arise in providing care, for example interventions at mealtimes (Liu *et al.*, 2013) or sleep problems (Brown *et al.*, 2013).

This variation in classification and identification makes it difficult to discern the approach choices to use under different circumstances. As Maslow (2012) reported, a uniform classification would be helpful and should be a priority.

There are a variety of non-pharmacological interventions associated with 'best practice' in dementia care that, at minimum, have evidence of beneficial short-term impact, such as music and recreational activities (Vink *et al.*, 2012). The use of these interventions is dependent on the resources available to the individual, family and/or organization. For instance, the use of music might easily be incorporated to create a calm ambience in the individual's home living environment, yet access to a music therapist may be beyond the financial resources of the individual, family or service provider. Additionally, music therapists may not practise in or have limited availability within a particular community. Table 5.1 identifies non-pharmacological interventions commonly found in the literature.

Table 5.1: Examples of non-pharmacological interventions

Intervention	Examples	Rationale
Counselling and group supports	Individual, family and significant others	Address psychosocial/ emotional needs of individual affected and carers
Culture or arts based and other therapies	Dance/movement, music/music therapy, art, pet, massage	Enhance quality of life, maintain interests/ abilities, address behaviours
Environmental design and home modifications	Safe walking paths, use of colour, lighting, and furniture style and placement	Promote independence, safety, security, or reduce perceived behavioural issues
Education and skills training for carers	Dementia information, communication strategies, other specific interventions	Modify carer interactions, reduce behavioural reactions/ stress
Health related	Physical exercise, dining strategies	Maintain health and improve diet, nutrition and hydration of person

Multi-sensory approaches	Snoezelen, Montessori	Stimulate yet calm the individual
Programmatic adaptations	Changes to content and implementation	Encourage active participation
Technology-based strategies	Assistive devices, monitoring	Maintain independence, safety

Design and modification of the physical space in which the person with dementia interacts has been shown to be an appropriate starting point for non-pharmacological interventions in the ageing population generally. Architectural design and other features of the environment play an important role in supporting individuals affected by dementia in terms of daily functioning, orientation and way finding (Marquardt, 2011). Modification of the environment is amongst the least intrusive and restrictive options for intervening. Some modifications are relatively inexpensive to introduce such as the use of colour as a camouflage or cue. Another essential and early non-pharmacological intervention involves the education and training of carers. Carers who understand the nature of dementia and how interactions can be altered to better meet the needs of the person with dementia, are better prepared to continue in their caregiving role. Brodaty and Arasaratnam (2012) found that family carers employed non-pharmacological interventions that were effective in lessening behavioural and psychological symptoms associated with dementia, provided they were given sufficient and individually tailored in-home support with follow-up. Yet, there are a number of barriers in providing training for family carers including systemic issues, current knowledge of various interventions that work, and cultural issues (Gallagher-Thompson *et al.*, 2012). There is also an increasing interest in the use of multi-sensory approaches in dementia care. These types of interventions, where individualized, are non-directive, pleasurable or entertaining, with few if any demands placed on the person to perform in a specific given way. Evidence suggests such approaches have positive short-term impact on mood and behavioural challenges associated with dementia, although the long-term benefits and efficacy have yet to be determined (Sánchez et al., 2013).

Another category of non-pharmacological interventions that is becoming prominent in dementia care is the use of technologies that may assist people to remain in their own homes and more easily manage day-to-day living (Mokhtari et al., 2012). Technological interventions that are individually tailored may help support as well as reduce behavioural and psychological symptoms. These interventions include the use of video prompting (Perilli et al., 2013) and the creation of personal DVDs (Hatakeyama et al., 2010). There are a number of ethical and practical concerns about the use of technologies in dementia care (Schermer, 2007), and their use for surveillance purposes raises additional issues. Niemeijer and colleagues (2010) critiqued the international literature pertaining to surveillance in dementia care and thematically categorized issues such as conflict of interests, human rights, privacy and consent. The authors suggested the themes identified in their review could form the basis of policies that give clear direction for the use of surveillance technologies in support of vulnerable populations. The views of people with dementia must also be considered with many promoting the use of global positioning systems (GPS) from a 'safe walking' perspective, because of the reassurance that they know it gives their spouse or carer.

Many practice guidelines for dementia care pertaining to the general population espouse the use of non-pharmacological interventions as a first recourse in supporting persons affected by dementia and their carers (Hogan et al., 2008; NICE, 2012). Although there is variation across guidelines, non-pharmacological interventions targeting the carer and physical activity for persons with dementia are most commonly recommended (Vasse et al., 2012). Non-pharmacological interventions also complement and are incorporated into a person-centred approach (Alzheimer Society of Canada, 2011). Depending on circumstance, such approaches can be used solo, in combination with one another or arranged in conjunction with a pharmacological treatment. Non-pharmacological interventions may also be pre-planned with the individual and become an integral part of daily life and routine. Yet, at other times, carers introduce such interventions to try to resolve issues that arise with changes in ability or mood experienced by the person affected by dementia which create challenges to caregiving. A selected intervention may therefore be introduced on a trial basis and monitored to determine its usefulness in alleviating the situation. Predominately across guidelines, it is evident that non-pharmacological interventions should be individualized with continuation based on response to that intervention.

Evidence supporting use of non-pharmacological interventions

Evidence supporting the use of non-pharmacological interventions in dementia care generally appears ambiguous. Commonly, many reviews and reports examining the efficacy of non-pharmacological interventions utilize inclusion and exclusion criteria that give credence to randomized controlled trials, considered a gold standard in rigorous research. Yet, many studies examining the implementation and impact of a non-pharmacological intervention employ alternative study designs and are of a qualitative nature with a smaller number of participants. While these studies may adhere to rigorous standards, they are not randomized controlled trials and are excluded from most reviews of efficacy. Adjusting such evaluative criteria may be necessary to gain a fuller understanding and better assess evidence pertaining to the effectiveness of various non-pharmacological interventions (de Medeiros and Basting, 2013; Maslow, 2012).

There are also other concerns regarding the evidence supporting non-pharmacological interventions that need to be taken into consideration. Many study samples with older people, for instance, involve persons with dementia living in residential care settings, their spousal caregivers, or staff. Fewer studies focus on people with dementia living in the community, where the majority of persons affected live (Gallagher-Thompson et al., 2012). Additionally, although there are many principles, goals and interventions reported in the literature regarding environmental design, few studies actually examine their efficacy within the private homes of persons with dementia (van Hoof et al., 2010). This means that the translation of evidence-based practices from research to community settings is not as straightforward as it might appear; it requires committed partnerships, sustained funding and evaluation over time (Teri et al., 2012). Maslow (2012) points to the particular lack of evidence in regards to marginalized populations, such as people with an intellectual disability or minority ethnic groups. However, evidence for a particular intervention found to be 'inconclusive' does not necessarily mean that it is not effective. The collective evidence gathered on various non-pharmacological interventions can be used to guide development of policy and practice in dementia care.

Non-pharmacological interventions and people with intellectual disabilities

Guidelines for the provision of community support to people with intellectual disabilities affected by dementia incorporate notions of non-pharmacological interventions (British Psychological Society, 2009; Jokinen *et al.*, 2013). However, research and reports on specific non-pharmacological interventions used to support persons with an intellectual disability experiencing dementia or their carers is sparse (Courtenay *et al.*, 2010). The evidence supporting use has generally been extrapolated from studies conducted within the general population affected by dementia. These circumstances are very different from the context within which many adults with an intellectual disability live. Some service providers have made modifications within the confines of the resources available to them in order to accommodate the needs of adults experiencing dementia (Janicki *et al.*, 2005; Kerr, 2007), often using this evidence base from dementia care generally. Yet other service providers are just beginning to acknowledge the challenges ahead and consider future needs. Several reports in the literature do indicate positive benefits related to the use of non-pharmacological interventions in the field of intellectual disability. Belleth (1995) reported benefits of using music therapy for people with Down syndrome and dementia, whilst Rosewarne (2001) discussed various non-pharmacological strategies successfully used in developing support groups. Lynggaard and Alexander (2004) also found benefits to small group sessions held with co-residents of persons with intellectual disabilities and dementia using strategies such as visual aids and role-play. Furthermore, Kalsy *et al.* (2007) found that staff education and training on behavioural changes in dementia had a positive influence on staff's understanding of the condition. De Vreese *et al.* (2012) reported a number of non-pharmacological interventions that were incorporated in the planning and development of a specialist unit for persons with intellectual disabilities experiencing decline. These interventions targeted staff education and skills training, environmental design and programmatic adjustments to engage people in daily activities and routines. Initial findings from this longitudinal study suggest positive outcomes in taking such an approach.

One factor that may sway the use of non-pharmacological interventions is whether an intellectual disability service provider has engaged in strategic planning to become 'dementia capable'. Dementia capable refers to a notion of being knowledgeable and skilled in providing supports to individuals affected by dementia and their families, as well as knowledgeable of other available services that may assist (Janicki and Dalton, 2000; Jokinen et al., 2013). Strategic planning of this nature should also be considered as a non-pharmacological intervention. It has direct bearing on the quality and type of supports provided by a service agency to the individual affected by dementia and to family or staff carers. The potential for the design of the physical environment and communication strategies will both be considered further as little, if any, additional demand is placed on the person with an intellectual disability and dementia to change or perform in a specific way. Rather, the onus is on the organization and/or carers to alter the physical environment or change their interpersonal communication strategies.

Physical environment design and modifications

Various aspects of the built environment can influence physical and psychological health, as well as ability to perform activities of daily living. Resources are available that provide suggestions on home design and modification to support people with dementia generally (van Hoof and Kort, 2009). This includes floor plans to promote access, interior design elements such as plant selection, furniture, managing cable cords, lighting and use of assistive technologies. Within the field of intellectual disability, there are also resources regarding environmental modifications that can be made in dementia care. Watchman (2007) offers a number of succinct suggestions visually depicted that may be easily incorporated within the home setting. This includes colour contrasts of food, plate and placemat in dining to enhance visibility and promote independence and food intake. Kerr (2007) offers suggestions on creating the right environment, one that is calm, familiar, predictable, makes sense, and is stimulating. Jokinen et al. (2013) suggests taking a stage-based approach, for example de-cluttering is a low cost modification used in early stage dementia to create a calm environment.

Clearly, a range of environmental designs and modifications can be employed to assist in providing dementia care for people with intellectual disabilities. These non-pharmacological interventions can potentially promote independence and the maintenance of skills, provide for safety and security, stimulate yet calm individuals with dementia, and ease carer stress. Adults ageing with intellectual disabilities affected by dementia reside and interact in a range of community settings, some of which are more easily modified than others. Two overall strategies would support and create change using environmental design and modification interventions. First, on a macro level, there are growing numbers of people affected by Alzheimer's disease and other dementias (World Health Organization, 2012; National Task Group on Intellectual Disabilities and Dementia Practice, 2012) with a resultant need for housing and other buildings to be adequately designed for people with dementia. Intellectual disability organizations and service providers should join forces with older persons groups to advocate for such designs. Working with local housing authorities as well as architects and developers will begin to meet this forthcoming demand for affordable appropriately designed housing.

Second, on a micro level, carers not only need information about environmental modifications but must also recognize the necessity and benefits of changing the environment. Often carers become accustomed to, and complacent about, the environment within which they work and support someone with dementia. Aspects of the environment such as the pile of papers in the corner, placement of furniture or ornaments, lighting, noise or wall colour go unrecognized yet potentially influence mood, behaviour or the abilities of the person with an intellectual disability and dementia. Under these circumstances, photographs taken of the everyday environment may remind carers to objectively reflect on the reality of their surroundings and consider modifications that can enhance care and function. With forethought, environmental design and modifications can negate the need to transition the person to a different living environment, thus supporting ageing in place.

Communication strategies

As dementia progresses, individuals commonly lose their abilities to converse and verbally communicate needs. Whilst these losses are individually experienced, receptive and expressive communication skills tend to initially fluctuate and eventually diminish. These losses create frustrations for the person with intellectual disabilities, as well as for family and staff carers, which can affect relationships and ultimately the provision of care. Communication strategies used to manage these changes are also a form of non-pharmacological intervention, and should be routinely incorporated as part of information and training sessions for carers and staff.

There are a number of dementia-specific resources available offering suggestions for communication (Alzheimer's Society, 2013). Resources within the field of intellectual disability are also available and suggest strategies for effective communication (Jokinen *et al.*, 2013; McCallion, 1999; Murphy and Boa, 2012; Watchman *et al.*, 2010). Common strategies across both fields of dementia care and intellectual disability are evident. These include the use of body language, such as facial expressions and gestures, keeping an amenable tone of voice, use of short sentences, taking advantage of long-term memories held by the individual, and taking time to allow for response. Memory aids may also stimulate communication. For instance, the creation of memory boxes, life story work or individual life stories prior to late stage dementia may help communicate with the individual, provided that this does not stir negative memories, particularly if the person experienced institutional care when younger. This provides opportunity for reminiscence and, later, for familiar and valued topics, people or events to be discussed (Webster and Fels, 2013). Whilst staff working with people with an intellectual disability may be familiar with alternative communication styles, they need to remain vigilant for changes in communication abilities that occur with the progression of dementia and open to adjusting communication over time, as required.

One of the dilemmas faced by many carers in communicating with a person who has dementia is managing altered reality: beliefs that are held despite appearing delusional. For instance, the person may believe a parent is coming to pick them up for a visit, although the parent has been dead for years. In waiting, the person becomes distressed and agitated. Dementia care advocates accepting the person's perceived reality, perhaps managing the situation with a distracting activity. This is perceived to be kinder and preferred to a reality orientation approach reminding the person of the parent's death, which may relive the grief and loss previously felt. Hertogh and colleagues (2004) discuss moral tensions that arise in dementia care and, in particular, whether this strays into deception. Dodd (2010) also discusses situations where long-term memories are spoken of as if they are in the present, although she acknowledges individuality and that there is no one solution for every situation. Commonly, carers want to avoid confrontations that increase a person's confusion or agitation level, yet remain truthful. Carers need to discuss these types of situations and, with support, decide how best to manage them given the individual and particular context.

Conclusion

Non-pharmacological interventions used in the support of people with dementia have been considered, drawing on the literature pertaining to the ageing population generally. Despite a myriad of interventions, few are seen in a specific evidence base relating to people with intellectual disabilities and dementia. There is a lack of studies reporting efficacy of such interventions with this population, and dementia care practices within intellectual disability service providers draw heavily on general population research and best practices. This is commendable in terms of adopting a proactive approach. However, the very nature of intellectual disability service provision, the care setting, and differences in background and familial supports experienced by adults with an intellectual disability may well contribute to unique responses in relation to non-pharmacological interventions that have yet to be realized. Non-pharmacological interventions do provide viable options in the provision of dementia care, yet carers need education and training for effective implementation. A service provider's actions or inactions to provide this education and training affects the abilities of carers to provide quality care, which in turn directly influences the daily life of the person affected by dementia.

References

Alzheimer's Society (2013) *Factsheet: Communicating.* Available at www.alzheimers.org.uk/site/scripts/download_info.php?fileID=1789, accessed on 5 December 2013.

Alzheimer Society of Canada (2011) Guidelines for care: Person-centred care for people living with dementia in care homes. Available at www.alzheimer.ca/~/media/Files/national/Culture-change/culture_change_framework_e.ashx, accessed 5 December 2013.

Ballard, C., Day, S., Sharp, S., Wing, G. and Sorensen, S. (2008) Neuropsychiatric symptoms in dementia: Importance and treatment considerations. *International Review of Psychiatry* 20, 4, 396–404.

Belleth, J. (1995) Music therapy for adults with Down's syndrome and dementia of the Alzheimer-type: A study of active and passive task sequencing. *Canadian Journal of Music Therapy 3,* 1, 35–51.

Blozik, E., Rapold, R., Overbeck, J. and Reich, O. (2013) Polypharmacy and potentially inappropriate medication in the adult, community-dwelling population in Switzerland. *Drugs and Aging 30,* 7, 561–568.

British Psychological Society (2009) *Dementia and People with Learning Disabilities: Guidance on the Assessment, Diagnosis, Treatment and Support of People with Learning Disabilities who Develop Dementia.* Available at www.rcpsych.ac.uk/files/pdfversion/cr155.pdf, accessed on 5 December 2013.

Brodaty, H. and Arasaratnam, C. (2012) Meta-analysis of nonpharmacological interventions for neuropsychiatric symptoms of dementia. *American Journal of Psychiatry 169,* 9, 946–953.

Brown, CA., Berry, R., Tan, MC., Khoshia, A., Turlapati, L. and Swedlove, F. (2013) A critique of the evidence base for non-pharmacological sleep interventions for persons with dementia. *Dementia 12,* 2, 210–237.

Cayton, H. (2004) Telling stories: Choices and challenges on the journey of dementia. *Dementia The International Journal of Social Research and Practice 3,* 2, 9–17.

Courtenay, K., Jokinen, NS. and Strydom, A. (2010) Caregiving and adults with intellectual disabilities affected by dementia. *Journal of Policy and Practice in Intellectual Disabilities 7,* 1, 26–33.

de Medeiros, K. and Basting, A. (2013) 'Shall I compare thee to a dose of donepezil?': Cultural arts interventions in dementia care research. *The Gerontologist.* doi: 10.1093/geront/gnt055.

De Vreese, LP., Mantesso, U., De Bastiani, E., Weger, E., Marangoni, AC. and Gomiero, T. (2012) Impact of dementia-derived nonpharmacological intervention procedures on cognition and behavior in older adults with intellectual disabilities: A 3-year follow-up study. *Journal of Policy and Practice in Intellectual Disabilities 9,* 2, 92–102.

Dodd, K. (2010) Psychological and other non-pharmacological interventions in services for people with learning disabilities and dementia. *Advances in Mental Health and Learning Disabilities 4,* 1, 28–36.

Gallagher-Thompson, D., Tzuang, YM., Au, A. *et al.* (2012) International perspectives on nonpharmacological best practices for dementia family caregivers: A review. *Clinical Gerontologist 35,* 4, 316–355.

Gauthier, S., Patterson, C., Chertkow, H. *et al.* (2012) Recommendations of the 4th Canadian consensus conference on the diagnosis and treatment of dementia (CCCDTD4). *Canadian Geriatrics Journal 15,* 4, 120–126.

Hatakeyama, R., Fukushima, K., Fukuoka, Y. *et al.* (2010). Personal home made digital video disk for patients with behavioral psychological symptoms of dementia. *Geriatrics and Gerontology International 10,* 1, 272–274.

Hertogh, C., The, B., Miesen, B. and Eefsting, J. (2004) Truth telling and truthfulness in the care for patients with advanced dementia: An ethnographic study in Dutch nursing homes. *Social Science and Medicine 59,* 8, 1685–1693.

Hogan, DB., Bailey, P., Black, S. *et al.* (2008) Diagnosis and treatment of dementia: 5. nonpharmacologic and pharmacologic therapy for mild to moderate dementia. *Canadian Medical Association Journal 179*, 10, 1019–1026.

Janicki, MP. and Dalton, A. (2000) Prevalence of dementia and impact on intellectual disability services. *Mental Retardation 38*, 8, 276–288.

Janicki, MP., Heller, T., Seltzer, GB. and Hogg, J. (1996) Practice guidelines for the clinical assessment and care management of Alzheimer's disease and other dementias among adults with intellectual disability. *Journal of Intellectual Disability Research 40*, 4, 3, 374–382.

Janicki, MP., Dalton, A., McCallion, P., Baxley, D. and Zendell, A. (2005) Group home care for adults with intellectual disabilities and Alzheimer's disease. *Dementia 4*, 4, 361–385.

Jokinen, NS., Janicki, MP., Hogan, M. and Force, LT. (2012) The middle years and beyond: Transitions and families of adults with Down's syndrome. *Journal of Developmental Disabilities 18*, 2, 59–69.

Jokinen, N., Janicki, MP., Keller, SM., McCallion, P., Force, LT. and National Task Group on Intellectual Disabilities and Dementia Care Practices (2013) Guidelines for structuring community care and supports for people with intellectual disabilities affected by dementia. *Journal of Policy and Practice in Intellectual Disabilities 10*, 1, 1–24.

Kalsy, S., Heath, R., Adams, D. and Oliver, C. (2007) Effects of training on controllability attributions of behavioural excesses and deficits shown by adults with Down's syndrome and dementia. *Journal of Applied Research in Intellectual Disabilities 20*, 1, 64–68.

Kerr, D. (2007) *Understanding Learning Disability and Dementia.* London: Jessica Kingsley Publishers.

Liu, W., Cheon, J. and Thomas, SA. (2013) Interventions on mealtime difficulties in older adults with dementia: A systematic review. *International Journal of Nursing Studies.* doi: 10.1016/j.ijnurstu.2012.12.021.

Lynggaard, H. and Alexander, N. (2004) Why are my friends changing? Explaining dementia to people with learning disabilities. *British Journal of Learning Disabilities 32*, 1, 30–39.

Marquardt, G. (2011) Wayfinding for people with dementia: A review of the role of architectural design. *HERD 4*, 2, 75–90.

Maslow, K. (2012) *Translating Innovation to Impact: Evidence-based Interventions to Support People with Alzheimer's Disease and their Caregivers at Home and in their Communities. A White Paper.* Alliance for Aging Research and Administration on Aging. Available at www.aoa.gov/AoA_Programs/HPW/Alz_Grants/docs/TranslatingInnovationtoImpactAlzheimersDisease.pdf

McCallion, P. (1999) Maintaining communication. In MP. Janicki and AJ. Dalton (eds) *Dementia, Aging, and Intellectual Disabilities: A Handbook.* Philadelphia, PA: Brunner/Mazel.

Mokhtari, M., Aloulou, H., Tiberghien, T., Biswas, J., Racoceanu, D. and Yap, P. (2012) New trends to support independence in persons with mild dementia – A mini-review. *Gerontology 58*, 6, 554–563.

Murphy, J. and Boa, S. (2012) Using the WHO-ICF with talking mats to enable adults with long-term communication difficulties to participate in goal setting. *Augmentative and Alternative Communication 28*, 1, 52–60.

National Institute for Health and Clinical Excellence (NICE) (2012) *CG 42 Dementia: NICE guideline.* Available at http://guidance.nice.org.uk/CG42/NICEGuidance/pdf/English, accessed on 5 December 2013.

National Task Group on Intellectual Disabilities and Dementia Practice (2012) *'My Thinker's Not working': A National Strategy for Enabling Adults with Intellectual Disabilities Affected by Dementia to Remain in their Community and Receive Quality Supports.* Available at http://aadmd.org/sites/default/files/NTG_Thinker_Report.pdf, accessed on 5 December 2013.

Niemeijer, AR., Frederiks, BJM., Riphagen, II., Legemaate, J., Eefsting, JA. and Hertogh, CMPM. (2010) Ethical and practical concerns of surveillance technologies in residential care for people with dementia or intellectual disabilities: An overview of the literature. *International Psychogeriatrics 22*, 7, 1129–1142.

Perilli, V., Lancioni, GE., Hoogeveen, F. *et al.* (2013) Video prompting versus other instruction strategies for persons with Alzheimer's disease. *American Journal of Alzheimer's Disease and Other Dementias.* doi: 10.1177/1533317513488913.

Rosewarne, M. (2001) Learning disabilities and dementia: A pilot therapy group. *Journal of Dementia Care 9*, 4, 18–20.

Sánchez, A., Millán-Calenti, JC., Lorenzo-López, L. and Maseda, A. (2013) Multisensory stimulation for people with dementia: A review of the literature. *American Journal of Alzheimer's Disease and Other Dementias 28*, 1, 7–14.

Schermer, M. (2007) Nothing but the truth? On truth and deception in dementia care. *Bioethics 21*, 13–22.

Teri, L., McKenzie, G., Logsdon, RG. *et al.* (2012) Translation of two evidence-based programs for training families to improve care of persons with dementia. *The Gerontologist 52*, 4, 452–459.

van Hoof, J. and Kort, H. (2009) Supportive living environments: A first concept of a dwelling designed for older adults with dementia. *Dementia 8*, 2, 293–316.

van Hoof, J., Kort, HS., van Waarde, H. and Blom, MM. (2010) Environmental interventions and the design of homes for older adults with dementia: an overview. *American Journal of Alzheimer's Disease and Other Dementias 25*, 3, 202–232.

Vasse, E., Vernooij-Dassen, M., Cantegreil, I. *et al.* (2012) Guidelines for psychosocial interventions in dementia care: A European survey and comparison. *International Journal of Geriatric Psychiatry 27*, 1, 40–48.

Vink, AC., Zuidersma, M., Boersma, F., De Jonge, P., Zuidema, SU. and Slaets, JPJ. (2012) The effect of music therapy compared with general recreational activities in reducing agitation in people with dementia: A randomised controlled trial. *International Journal of Geriatric Psychiatry 28*, 1031–1038.

Watchman, K. (2007) *Living with Dementia: Adapting the Home of a Person who has Down's Syndrome and Dementia.* Edinburgh: Down's Syndrome Scotland.

Watchman, K., Kerr, D. and Wilkinson, H. (2010) *Supporting Derek: A Practice Development Guide to Support Staff Working with People who Have a Learning Difficulty and Dementia.* Brighton: Pavilion/Joseph Rowntree Foundation.

Webster, G. and Fels, D. (2013) Portraits of people with dementia: Three case studies of creating portraits. *American Journal of Alzheimer's Disease and Other Dementias 28*, 4, 371–376.

Wilkinson, H. and Janicki, MP. (2002) The Edinburgh Principles with accompanying guidelines and recommendations. *Journal of Intellectual Disability Research 46*, 3, 279–84.

World Health Organization (2012) *Dementia: A Public Health Priority.* Geneva: WHO.

6

Living Life with Dementia
Enhancing Psychological Wellbeing

Sunny Kalsy-Lillico

Introduction

Having some sense of what it must be like to live with a life-limiting condition such as dementia is crucial to being able to understand what people with intellectual disabilities with a diagnosis of dementia face in their daily lives. However, it is not only about understanding from a clinical, professional or carer point of view that is important. It is also appreciating the individual's feelings that are engendered through the course of dementia whilst recognising that, alongside commonality or similarity in experience, these will also be unique for each person. This perspective can be encapsulated by attending to psychosocial models of dementia.

The core premise in considering the experience of living well with dementia for an individual with intellectual disabilities is the maintenance of the person, the individual and the centre of their experience. The focus of enhancing psychological wellbeing relates to the social, interpersonal and emotional aspects of living life with dementia. Memory loss is only one experience that contributes to the difficulties faced by people with dementia. Many behavioural, physical, social and emotional activities can be impaired which are just as, or even more, debilitating and there is a growing body of understanding that can provide a powerful insight into what it feels like to live with dementia. If meaningful engagement is to occur, and a true person-centred approach is to be adopted, it is essential that opportunities are grasped that involve, value and respect the experiences of the individuals concerned.

Drawing on the limited research available about the subjective experiences of people with intellectual disabilities and dementia, what follows is a discussion on how the enhancing of psychological wellbeing of individuals can be considered and supported by those people and services around them. Discussion will also consider how psychosocial models of dementia can impact upon practice as well as contributing to frameworks for understanding how the experiences of people with intellectual disabilities and dementia are understood.

Psychosocial models of dementia

Psychosocial models of dementia share a fundamental principle and this is that people with dementia have a range of impairments and are further disabled by the way in which they are treated by, or excluded from, society. With regards to the field of intellectual disabilities, Vanier (1989) has written extensively of the 'wounds' that society can inflict on an individual with intellectual disabilities, through its association of disability and ill health, weakness, difference or inferiority. With the field of dementia, the key proponents of the psychosocial position are Kitwood, who has organised his framework within the notion of 'personhood' and relational processes (Kitwood, 1997) and Buijssen who has highlighted the 'two laws of dementia' (Buijssen, 2005).

It may be helpful to consider Buijssen's work in particular, given its focus on the cognitive impact of dementia upon an individual's psychosocial wellbeing. The first law is the 'law of disturbed encoding', which refers to the individual being unable to transfer successfully information from their short-term memory and store it in their long-term memory. This means that the individual is unable to remember things that have recently happened. Additionally, the person is unable to form any new memories for events that are experienced or information that is told; there is no emotional tagging (or encoding) of events necessary to create a memory. In terms of how this law is then experienced by an individual with intellectual disabilities and dementia, the following observations have been made both in the literature and in clinical practice, the intensity of which is moderated by the stage of dementia. The individual may:

- appear disorientated in an unfamiliar environment
- seem disorientated in time

- ask the same questions repeatedly
- quickly lose track of conversation
- seem less able to learn anything new
- easily lose or misplace things
- be unable to recall people that they have recently met
- forget key dates such as appointments
- experience considerable anxiety and stress.

Buijssen's second law of note is the 'law of roll-back memory'. Fundamentally, long-term memory is the store for all of life's memories. As dementia progresses, the individual will be increasingly unable to form new memories. At first, long-term memories will remain intact and as dementia progresses, these will also begin to dissipate. Deterioration begins with the most recent memories and progresses until typically those of childhood or early adulthood remain. A useful visual way of explaining this law is that of a row of dominoes, with the first domino representing the most recent memory and the last representing the earliest memory. As the first domino is knocked down, it causes the others to fall too, representing the rolling back of memory. Again, it is useful to consider how this law can be experienced by an individual with intellectual disabilities and dementia. The individual may be observed by others to:

- lose the steps or sub-steps of daily living skills
- experience memory loss for events, beginning with the most recent
- make social faux pas or show inappropriate behaviours
- have paucity in their vocabulary or inability to find words
- struggle to recognise family/relatives or see (misconstrue) people from their past
- lose the steps or sub-steps in their personal or self-care skills
- appear to have changes in aspects of their personality traits or preferences so, for example, someone who was calm and relaxed may now become more quickly irritated with others
- believe that they are younger in years than they are and that time has actually 'rolled back'.

It must be noted that psychosocial models do not deny the impact of the physical nature of dementia, the brain–behaviour link. Authors such as Keady *et al.* (2012) have highlighted that a more salient representation of the physical domain of dementia is imperative. The premise is that the recognition of physical wellbeing, physical health and examination, physical care, physical treatment and physical environment presents a holistic and culturally sensitive approach to understanding the experience of living with dementia.

With regards though to the work of Kitwood and Buijssen, the shared perspectives of these psychosocial models are that dementia is not the fault of the individual who has the condition. Both models encourage a strong focus on the remaining skills that the individual has, as opposed to what skills or experiences that have been lost. The models also emphasise that a truly holistic appreciation of the individual must take place so that those around the individual with dementia fully understand their life history and their likes or dislikes. The similarities continue in relation to the recognition that respectful relationships alongside enabling or supportive environments are vital, with appropriate communication and a preponderance of stress-free and failure-free activities in order to maintain and sustain the wellbeing of the person with dementia.

Psychological interventions to enhance wellbeing

With specific reference to the practice responses to presenting need, descriptions are available which highlight assessments and intervention models that have the primary goal of enhancing quality of life for the person with intellectual disabilities with dementia (Adams *et al.*, 2008; Auty and Scior, 2008; British Psychological Society, 2009; Dodd, 2003). Also highlighted are appropriate supports to compensate for losses or changes in ability and circumstances, whilst maintaining personal dignity and respect, as well as the continuity of service delivery with interdisciplinary and cross-agency working that emphasises a long-term service commitment to older adults with intellectual disabilities and their ageing family carers (Adams *et al.*, 2008; Kalsy *et al.*, 2005; Kalsy-Lillico *et al.*, 2012; Oliver *et al.*, 2008).

Psychological interventions described in the general dementia literature can be adapted for use with people with intellectual disabilities, as a similar three-stage model is used to describe the clinical progress of the condition in both populations (Dalton and

Janicki, 1999; Kalsy-Lillico *et al.*, 2012). Interventions must consider multiple systemic influences on behaviour in order to support the individual and carers to understand, cope with and manage behaviour concerns and emotional distress. This consideration of behavioural and systemic contexts alongside a biomedical appreciation (of any associated medical conditions and/or the stages of dementia) enables greater intervention choice. This more person-centred approach is consistent with social models of dementia that emphasise personhood, adjustment and coping, considering contextual influences such as environment and caregiver relationships as influences on behaviour (Kerr, 1997; Kitwood, 1997). It firmly places the responsibility for change on those around the person with dementia. Practically this means that the onus is on others to communicate appropriately with the person with dementia, for the environment to enhance the individual's capability rather than compound their disabilities and recognition that an individual is a valued person who has remaining skills that need to be supported.

Table 6.1 presents a framework for organising psychological interventions and practices into four broad groups.

To reiterate, the core aims of psychological interventions with older adults with intellectual disabilities and dementia are to enable the retention and maintenance of skills, optimise a sense of personhood and emotional wellbeing and compensate for changes in an individual's functional abilities.

These psychological interventions are postulated upon a number of systemic influences, some specific to the person concerned and their circumstances and others more broadly related to general conceptual understanding about dementia. Kalsy *et al.* (2005) provide a stage-defined model of psychological interventions (see Table 6.2).

Table 6.1: A framework for psychological interventions

Behaviour-oriented	A full functional analysis of the behaviour in question will enable a systemic understanding of the behaviour as a form of communication. The best practice principles that should be considered when supporting ageing adults with intellectual disabilities and dementia include simplifying multistep activities/skills, matching the level of demand on the individual with that of their current capacities, employing a range of prompts to facilitate communication and to modify the environment insofar as possible to compensate for deficits and capitalise on the individual's strengths. For carers, recommended practice also encourages the adoption of a proactive approach to identify potential stressors (or triggers) that can lead to distressed behaviours and moderate change as necessary.
Emotion-oriented	The underlying principles for such interventions are to reduce distress, validate a sense of self, enhance emotional wellbeing and support coping strategies. Psychodynamic approaches appear helpful for understanding intrapsychic concerns, cognitive/behavioural techniques assist individuals in the early stage to build coping strategies and reduce distress, reminiscence and life review approaches provide individuals in the mild to moderate stage of dementia with interpersonal connections.
Cognition-oriented	The aim of these techniques is to compensate for cognitive deficits by utilising behavioural approaches to focus on specific cognitive and behavioural impairments and help to optimise remaining abilities. These techniques include skills training.
Stimulation-oriented	These treatments include recreational activities (such as crafts, games, pets) and art therapies (music, dance, art) to provide stimulation and enrichment that will engage the individual's available cognitive and emotional resources. Approaches such as life work that include life stories, valuables and memorable pictures/photographs/objects are powerful ways of relating to the individual with dementia in a person-centred way. Reminiscence work is also important as a process of recalling experiences and events memorable for the individual by using different mediums such as verbal, visual, musical, tactile and smell. Anecdotally, in using reminiscence with groups of ageing adults with intellectual disabilities, Kalsy-Lillico has found that its associative process, that is one memory leads to another so that one person's shared recollection usually sparks off associated recollections or 'memories' in others, has had positive effects on engagement and communication as reminiscence makes connections between a person's past, present and future.

Source: Kalsy-Lillico *et al.*, 2012

Table 6.2: Dementia stage-defined psychological practices

Early stage	Middle stage	Late stage
• Maintaining skills and independence by increasing supervision and prompting • Minimising changes in the environment and daily routine • Structuring and simplifying routines to help orientation • Using multimodal memory aids, for example picture calendars to support understanding • Keeping communication simple and clear, using additional prompts when necessary • Using a prompting system of 'tell' (verbal), 'show' (model), 'guide' (physical) • At times of expressed confusion, offer sensitive reminders of where the person is, what they are doing, as appropriate • Reducing demands by breaking tasks down, easing choice, clutter and noise • Behavioural strategies and validation to manage affective and anxiety symptoms • Encouraging engagement with activity by the individual setting their own pace, for example observing or participating • Psychotherapeutic techniques promoting dignity, self-esteem, emotional wellbeing • Monitoring and documenting change closely	• Preserving abilities, using life story work, reminiscence, favoured activities, low-level behavioural interventions • Monitoring behavioural changes (typically excesses), for example verbal agitation, wandering, stereotyped actions or disturbed sleep • Supporting behaviours that challenge, such as anxiety and agitation, with reassurance, patience, redirection, avoiding confrontation • Offering alternative means of communication incorporating visual images, pictures and objects, touch, sounds and smells • Offering appropriately stimulating and failure-free activities that promote cognition, physical health, social roles, emotional wellbeing and self-care • Offering activities that balance sensory stimulation with sensory calming/relaxing • Maintaining environments that are safe, calm, predictable, familiar, suitably stimulating and make sense for the individual • Working with caregivers and peers with intellectual disabilities on understanding the individual's condition • Monitoring and documenting change closely	• Contributing to multidisciplinary, family and other care providers planning of end of life care • Supporting and working with families, other care providers and peers with intellectual disabilities around issues of loss and bereavement • Working with families, other care providers and peers with intellectual disabilities around reminiscence and remembering • Contributing to multidisciplinary, family and other care providers' ethical decision-making around further physical health interventions such as percutaneous endoscopic gastronomy (PEG) feeds

Source: Kalsy *et al.*, 2005

The premise of psychosocial interventions is that neurological conditions such as dementia will affect each individual differently. The individual biography, life history and personality of the person with intellectual disabilities and dementia will serve as moderating factors. Furthermore, the presence of coexisting physical and mental health problems such as anxiety and depression and the extent and type of dementia will also shape the experience in an individual with intellectual disabilities. In addition to this, a consideration should be made of the social relationships of the individual concerned, the physical environment of their care system (such as home, day centre, employment or college) in conjunction with the community and cultural understandings of, and tolerance for, confusion and frailty.

The COPE model

It may be useful to consider at this point a conceptual representation that has been developed by the author and which is based on a review of clinical practice and psychological formulations related to clinical presentations. This representation has enabled the facilitation of staff and carer understanding of the rationale underpinning psychological interventions. The key tenets of this representation combine to form the acronym COPE:

- **Compensate:** for the skills, abilities, opportunities, relationships and experiences that are being lost and/or changing.

- **Optimise:** the strengths, resources, skills, abilities, opportunities, relationships and experiences that are to be maintained and sustained.

- **Person-centred:** so all approaches whilst broadly encapsulating the tenets are individualised according to the needs, wants, desires and qualities of the person concerned.

- **Enable:** the care situation around the individual to enhance and enable their emotional wellbeing, engagement and skills in order to avoid the likelihood of the individual with intellectual disabilities and dementia being further disabled by their environment and the people within it.

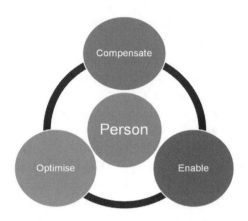

Figure 6.1: COPE: a conceptual representation of the philosophy behind psychological interventions

In practical terms, the following principles of care are reiterated:

- Understand and know the person.
- Understand dementia and its consequences.
- Use proactive approaches that predict 'stressors'.
- Ensure that the person with dementia has stress-free, failure-free and individualised care that is consistent and without time pressures.
- Maintain all the elements of usual daily living to retain skills for as long as possible.
- Consider life story work and reminiscence approaches in order to enhance understanding.
- Most environments where people with intellectual disabilities live are not dementia enabled.
- Balance calmness with stimulation so as to minimise unhelpful stress.

Remember me as a person, not a case

The research on subjective experiences of the individual with intellectual disabilities and dementia is still sparse in comparison to mainstream dementia literature (Lloyd *et al.*, 2007; Watchman, 2012). The insight of service users and other people with intellectual disabilities should be considered, as issues of interdependency between older adults with intellectual disabilities and dementia, their co-residents and family caregivers do impact on the understanding of changes taking place (Lloyd *et al.*, 2007; Lynggaard and Alexander, 2004). Similarly, life after diagnosis should be given a higher priority. The main thrust of published literature has been on recognising signs, assessment and diagnosis of dementia in people with intellectual disabilities. There is limited information available on what happens after diagnosis, including issues such as the process of diagnostic counselling, continuing care, the needs of ageing caregivers, accessing day, residential and respite services, residential supports and future life planning to determine needs and wishes (Kalsy *et al.*, 2005; Thompson and Wright, 2001; Watchman, 2003). However, the wider detrimental effects include the probable moving of a person with dementia to alternative (but potentially inappropriate) accommodation (Thompson and Wright, 2001; Wilkinson *et al.*, 2004).

A further area of development in dementia care generally is the use of touchscreen technology, also as yet unexplored among people with intellectual disabilities and dementia but worthy of further attention. Upton *et al.* (2011) highlighted its use in care settings for individuals with dementia, which included:

- **Supporting reminiscence:** the potential to evoke early memories, which were associated with positive emotions.

- **Aiding recall:** an external memory aid to assist procedural memory, for example in choosing what to eat.

- **Exercising memory:** supported increasingly complex cognitive exercises.

- **Increasing interpersonal interactions:** encouraged residents to engage with others around them.

- **Enhancing communication:** used as a tool for communication; for example, Skype provided a means for keeping in touch with family who were living too far away to visit regularly.

Working with carers and families

A range of practical principles of care practices that aim to facilitate more enabling care experiences and supportive interventions for the carers of ageing adults with intellectual disabilities and dementia are available (British Psychological Society, 2009; Dodd *et al.*, 2006; Kerr *et al.*, 2006). The common five key principles that are highlighted are positive philosophies of care, life story perspective, carer characteristics, enabling environments and proactive service planning:

- **Positive philosophies of care:** key factors include being person-centred, a flexible and adaptable care system, individualised care, regular and consistent staff, provision of stress- and failure-free individualised activities, creative use of compensatory strategies to support changes in communication, memory, future planning considerations (Kalsy-Lillico *et al.*, 2012).

- **Life story perspective:** by understanding a person's past and knowing their likes and dislikes, carers can endeavour to support people. This background knowledge can also help in the form of reassurances offered to the person with dementia should they become distressed. The main focus is to preserve as much quality of their previous lifestyle as is possible. This not only retains the person's dignity but in the early stages of dementia also helps to maintain orientation and sense of reality (Kalsy-Lillico *et al.*, 2012). It is also relevant in alleviating potential conflict between family and staff, something seen at times in residential dementia care and which is a major stressor that disturbs effective relationships (Kellett *et al.*, 2010). For family carers, reviving memories of their relatives in an holistic manner enables them to see beyond the condition and problem-saturated context, whilst for staff creating possibilities of viewing the resident as part of a family context, it enhances their engagement with the individual with dementia. For the individual with dementia, they benefit from the staff having greater insight in how to engage with them.

Table 6.3 highlights particular dementia stage-specific activities. Although not an exhaustive list, this may support the person with dementia to maintain their skills, facilitate interactions with others and sustain engagement with their environment. The activities should be interchanged, depending on the needs, abilities and interests of the person, and should always be meaningful, whether an individual or group activity.

Table 6.3: Suggested dementia stage-specific activities

Early stage	Early–middle stage	Middle stage	End stage
• Board games: card games such as snap are good, as are large-sized dominoes • Ball games: throwing soft balls to each other, standing or sitting • Discussions: about people, places and things • Relaxation: progressive relaxation, massage or aromatherapy activities • Arts and crafts: painting, colouring in, making bean bags, posters • End-product activities – anything where there is an immediate end result such as flower arranging, drawing, cooking, baking • Use visual planner and cues to structure activities/day	• Music – play something that resonates, is liked by the person and has a good bass and beat • Dance – chair dancing is good, swaying and rocking in time to music • Art and 'pottery' – working with dough, clay, plasticine or sand • Movement – guided walks, progressive relaxation • Drama • Reminiscence – using familiar items, mementoes touch, taste, smells, sounds, pictures or photos that remind people of times gone by • Story-telling – talking about old friends, stories about special times, memories or what's on TV • Spiritual or religious activity	• Movement and exercise – can be done standing or sitting • Multi-sensory environments – use lights, sounds, smells, touch, Snoezlen • Massage – hand and feet spa treatments • One-step cooking tasks – such as mixing items, peeling food • One-step gardening tasks – such as watering plants, digging pots • One-step daily living tasks – such as plumping up cushions • Walking – along routes that are circular with focus points • Stacking and folding – clothes, papers, magazines • Soft toys – touch can help anxious feelings • Balls, bubbles, balloons – remind people of fun	• Smiling and laughing – don't underestimate this as an activity • Singing – humming along to popular tunes, radio jingles or TV adverts • Stroking – positive touch of people and objects that have different textures • Gentle rocking – can relax and establish physical contact • Holding – as above • Cuddling – as above

Source: Kalsy-Lillico *et al.*, 2012

- **Carer characteristics:** the key characteristics include the carer's ability to understand and properly know the person they are caring for, to understand issues in ageing and dementia and crucially to proactively work to support the individual to cope with the challenges that dementia causes, for example by predicting potential stressors that may challenge the individual and lead to distressing behaviours (Kalsy *et al.*, 2007; Kalsy-Lillico *et al.*, 2012; Lloyd *et al.*, 2008).

- **Enabling environments:** the main constituents of these environments are that they are calm, predictable, familiar, suitably stimulating and safe. The impact of an environment upon a person's wellbeing, particularly for those people who may have dementia, has also been acknowledged. There is increasing evidence that 'dementia unfriendly' environments further disable people whereas 'dementia friendly' environments help people with intellectual disabilities to maintain levels of independence as well as remain in their own homes if this is a preferred, and viable, option (Hutchings *et al.*, 2000; Kalsy-Lillico *et al.*, 2012; Marshall 2001; Wilkinson *et al.*, 2004).

- **Proactive service planning:** the key factor is a consideration of the person's current needs alongside their future changing needs. Considerations such as taking a wider quality of life perspective and discussions of palliative and end of life issues must be carefully thought about. Furthermore, services need to plan ahead for their sustainability and capacity to meet future demand over the coming years (British Psychological Society, 2009; Department of Health, 2009).

Systematic reviews of the literature have also indicated that there is a clear need for greater support after diagnosis, including advice, social and psychological support, access to community care and respite (Bunn *et al.*, 2012; de Boer *et al.*, 2007; Robinson *et al.*, 2011). The information needs of individuals with intellectual disabilities and dementia and their carers varies over time, and information provision needs to be ongoing, with flexibility in timing and format (Kalsy-Lillico *et al.*, 2012).

In addition to this, there is a particular consideration needed in relation to the support required from professionals and services. The adoption of strategies to manage the condition, minimise losses, reduce social isolation, and maintain a 'normal' lifestyle was common (MacQuarrie, 2005). This included practical strategies such as using reminders or prompts, social strategies such as relying on family support, and emotional strategies such as using humour or finding meaningful activity and peer support (Bunn *et al.*, 2012; Wolverson *et al.*, 2010). Support needs to be ongoing, flexible and sensitive to the needs of different groups, such as those with early onset dementia or minority ethnic groups (Bowes and Wilkinson, 2003); it has to take into account the needs for continuity of care and to manage care needs and safety whilst being aware of the person's sense of identity and dignity.

Indeed, it is clear from the literature that the needs of people with dementia and their carers are complex and varied, and those making decisions about the timing and delivery of services need appropriate advice or expertise and training.

Taking the time to talk, taking the time to listen

There are various techniques that can be used to meaningfully communicate and connect with a person with intellectual disabilities and dementia, with creativity and sensitivity to the individual needs and preferences of the person concerned.

Recognise the communication challenge

Dementia is a progressive condition which inevitably changes and worsens over time and this, in addition to the individual having pre-existing lifelong intellectual disabilities, adds a further challenge to those providing support. A reasonable prediction to make is that people with dementia will gradually have a more difficult time understanding others, as well as communicating in general.

Have the right conversation at the right time and in the right place

Try to find a place and time to talk when there are not a lot of distractions. This creates an optimal space for the individual with intellectual disabilities and dementia to focus their abilities, and harness their energy on the conversation.

Speak out but not too loud

It is important to speak clearly while looking at the person, using a calm voice. Be mindful of any eye conditions or sight deterioration that may affect where you need to stand in order for the person to see you. Don't be afraid to add, as one of my colleagues called it, 'bling' to your voice so it is enhanced with warmth, humour, care and indeed affection. Remember at all times that the conversation is adult-to-adult.

Say my name

Names are important when speaking to or greeting an individual with intellectual disabilities and dementia: 'Hi, Joyce. It's me, Sunny,' is preferable to 'Hi. It's me.' Remember the COPE model: compensating for a deteriorating ability to process information means minimising the amount of information the person has to make sense of. So avoiding pronouns like 'he', 'she', and 'they' during conversation helps the individual to connect with what is being said in a more respectful and less stress-provoking way.

Take your time and keep it focused

For some, multi-tasking and multi-communicating about a range of issues at one time is a way of life but for others it leads to overburdening of their cognitive and emotional state. A person with intellectual disabilities and dementia may not be able to engage in the mental gymnastics and flexibility of thought that is involved in maintaining a conversation with multiple threads. Give the individual extra time to process what is being said to them. Don't let your desire for a response lead to additional pressure on the person to respond.

Speak, show, do

Do not underestimate the power of non-verbal cues and prompts in conversation. The maintaining of eye contact and a smile may help put a person at ease and facilitate mutual understanding.

Appropriate touch to help gain a person's attention in order to begin a conversation is also invaluable, as it helps to engage the person and initiate the conversation.

Listen actively

If you don't understand something that is spoken, politely let the person know. But remember, if you don't understand the words but can understand the feelings or sentiment being expressed, then acknowledge this. So, for example, in the case of an individual resident in a care unit who consistently says that they want to go home, the challenge is to listen to what is underpinning the words. It may be that the individual is expressing a wish to feel comfortable and safe as they were in the past, when they were at home. Instead of responding 'This is your home now,' a more sensitive, relational response could be 'We like having you here.'

Question sensitively

Asking targeted questions that can be answered with a few words instead of open-ended questions is helpful. A question calling for a short answer gives the individual a chance to feel successful. A question calling for a long answer may cause the individual to feel embarrassed and frustrated over their inability to formulate and keep in mind a lengthy answer. So instead of asking 'What did you have for lunch?', the individual with intellectual disabilities and dementia could be asked 'Did you enjoy lunch?', to which they can offer a yes or no response.

Divert don't debate

Interactions will stall if one person is consistently trying to correct each inaccurate statement made. We are used to trusting what our brains tell us, and will do so even if the information it gives us is not correct. When the brain is further damaged by dementia, in addition to a pre-existing intellectual disability, the person is even more likely to be relying on inaccurate information. So instead of arguing or debating, change the subject.

Understand there will be good days and bad days

While the general trend of dementia is a downward decline, people with dementia will have ups and downs just like anyone else. Remember that the individual may compensate by making greater use of remaining abilities, for example earlier memories. The individual may not be oriented to the present day. Avoid blanket 'reality orientation' as this will compound the feeling of stress or distress.

Consider the focus of all interactions

The focus is not on learning new skills, achieving goals or facing change, but rather it is about maintaining health and wellbeing, quality of life and the person's happiness, comfort and security. Finally, communication does not always involve words alone – appropriate touch is incredibly powerful.

Conclusion

In order to support individuals with dementia and their carers, greater consideration needs to be given for effective involvement to take place. In order to really engage people with dementia, a commitment to greater involvement needs to be explicit and planned. The reciprocal nature of sharing experiences and being listened to with a view to decision-making together provides real involvement and empowerment for the person.

The premise of psychosocial interventions is that neurological conditions such as dementia will affect each individual differently. The individual biography, life history and personality of the person with intellectual disabilities and dementia will serve as moderating factors. Furthermore, the presence of coexisting physical and mental health problems, such as anxiety or depression, and the extent and location of the condition will also shape the experience of dementia in an individual with intellectual disabilities. Thus, in addition, consideration should be given to the social relationships of the individual, the physical environment of their care system in conjunction with the community and cultural understandings of, and tolerance for, confusion and frailty.

The core aims of psychological interventions with older adults with intellectual disabilities and dementia have been demonstrated as enabling the retention of skills, optimising a sense of personhood and emotional wellbeing and compensating for changes in an individual's functional abilities. However, the key point is to assess each situation individually. Always allow the person with dementia to set the pace and 'go with the flow', make it a safe environment both physically and psychologically and don't be afraid to be creative and imaginative!

References

Adams, D., Oliver, C., Kalsy, S. *et al.* (2008) Behavioural characteristics associated with dementia assessment referrals in adults with Down's syndrome. *Journal of Intellectual Disability Research 52*, 4, 358–368.

Auty, E. and Scior, K. (2008) Psychologists' clinical practices in assessing dementia in individuals with Down's syndrome. *Journal of Policy and Practice in Intellectual Disabilities 5*, 4, 259–268.

Bowes, A. and Wilkinson, H. (2003) 'We didn't know it would get that bad': South Asian experience of dementia and the service response. *Health and Social Care in the Community 11*, 5, 387–396.

British Psychological Society (2009) *Dementia and People with Learning Disabilities: Guidance on the Assessment, Diagnosis, Treatment and Support of People with Learning Disabilities who Develop Dementia.* Available at www.rcpsych.ac.uk/files/pdfversion/cr155.pdf, accessed on 5 December 2013.

Buijssen, H. (2005) *The Simplicity of Dementia.* London: Jessica Kingsley Publishers.

Bunn, F., Goodman, C., Sworn, K. *et al.* (2012) Psychosocial factors that shape patient and carer experiences of dementia diagnosis and treatment: A systematic review of qualitative studies. *PLoS Med 9*, 10, e1001331. doi:10.1371/journal.pmed.1001331.

Dalton, AJ. and Janicki, MP. (1999) Ageing and dementia. In MP. Janicki and AJ. Dalton (eds) *Dementia, Aging and Intellectual Disabilities: A Handbook.* Philadelphia, PA: Bruner/Mazel.

de Boer, ME., Hertogh, C., Droes, RM. *et al.* (2007) Suffering from dementia – the patient's perspective: A review of the literature. *International Psychogeriatrics 19*, 6, 1021–1039.

Department of Health (2009) *Living Well With Dementia: A National Dementia Strategy.* London: The Stationery Office.

Dodd, K. (2003) Supporting people with Down's syndrome and dementia. *Tizard Intellectual Disability Review 8*, 4, 14–18.

Dodd, K., Kerr, D. and Fern, S. (2006) *Down's Syndrome and Dementia Workbook for Carers.* Teddington: Down's Syndrome Association.

Hutchings, BL., Olsen, RV. and Ehrenkrantz, ED. (2000) Modifying home environments. In MP. Janicki and EF. Ansello (eds) *Community Supports for Aging Adults with Lifelong Disabilities.* Baltimore, MD: Paul H Brookes.

Kalsy, S., Heath, R., Adams, D., and Oliver, C. (2007) Effects of training on controllability attributions of behavioural excesses and deficits shown by adults with Down's syndrome and dementia. *Journal of Applied Research in Intellectual Disabilities 20*, 1, 64–68.

Kalsy, S., McQuillan, S., Adams, D. *et al.* (2005) A proactive psychological screening strategy for dementia in adults with Down's syndrome: Preliminary description of service use and evaluation. *Journal of Policy and Practice in Intellectual Disabilities 2*, 2, 116–125.

Kalsy-Lillico, S. Adams, D. and Oliver, C. (2012) Older adults with intellectual disabilities: Issues in ageing and dementia. In E. Emerson, C. Harton, K. Dickson, R. Gone, A. Caine and Jo Bromley (eds) *Clinical Psychology and People with Intellectual Disabilities.* 2nd edition. Chichester: John Wiley and Sons.

Keady, J., Jones, L., Ward, R. *et al.* (2012) Introducing the bio-psycho-social-physical model of dementia through a collective case study design. *Journal of Clinical Nursing.* doi: 10.1111/j.1365-2702.2012.04292.x.

Kellett, U., Moyle, W., McAllister, M., King, C. and Gallagher, F. (2010) Life stories and biography: A means of connecting family and staff to people with dementia. *Journal of Clinical Nursing 19*, 11–12, 1707–1715.

Kerr, D. (1997) *Down's Syndrome and Dementia: A Practitioner's Guide.* London: Venture Press.

Kerr, D., Cunningham, C. and Wilkinson, H. (2006) *Responding to the Pain Experiences of Older People with a Learning Difficulty and Dementia.* York: Joseph Rowntree Foundation.

Kitwood, T. (1997) *Dementia Reconsidered: The Person Comes First.* Buckingham: Open University Press.

Lloyd, V., Kalsy, S. and Gatherer, A. (2007) The subjective experience of individuals with Down's syndrome living with dementia. *Dementia: The International Journal of Social Research and Practice 6*, 6, 63–88.

Lloyd, V., Kalsy, S. and Gatherer, A. (2008) The impact of dementia upon residential carers for individuals with Down's syndrome. *Journal of International Policy, Practice in Intellectual Disabilities 5*, 1, 33–38.

Lynggaard, H. and Alexander, N. (2004) Why are my friends changing? Explaining dementia to people with learning disabilities. *British Journal of Learning Disabilities 32*, 1, 30–39.

MacQuarrie, CR. (2005) Experiences in early stage Alzheimer's disease: understanding the paradox of acceptance and denial. *Aging and Mental Health 9*, 5, 430–441.

Marshall, M. (2001) Care settings and the care environment. In C. Cantley (ed.) *A Handbook of Dementia Care.* Buckingham: Open University Press.

Oliver, C., Adams, S. and Kalsy, S. (2008) Ageing, dementia and people with intellectual disability. In B. Woods and L. Clare (eds) *Handbook of the Clinical Psychology of Ageing.* Chichester: John Wiley and Sons.

Robinson, L., Gemski, A., Abley, C. *et al.* (2011) The transition to dementia – individual and family experiences of receiving a diagnosis: A review. *International Psychogeriatrics 23*, 1026–1043. doi: 10.1017/S1041610210002437.

Thompson, D. and Wright, S. (2001) *Misplaced and Forgotten? People with Learning Disabilities in Residential Services for Older People.* London: Mental Health Foundation.

Upton, D., Upton, P., Jones, T., Juthia, K. and Brooker, D. (2011) *Evaluation of the Impact of Touch Screen Technology on People with Dementia and their Carers within Care Home Settings.* Worcester: University of Worcester Press.

Vanier, J. (1989) *Community and Growth.* New York, NY: Paulist Press.

Watchman, K. (2003) Critical issues for service planners and providers of care for people with Down's syndrome and dementia. *British Journal of Learning Disabilities 31*, 2, 81–84.

Watchman, K. (2012) Reducing marginalisation in people with learning disabilities and dementia. *Journal of Dementia Care 20*, 5, 35–39.

Wilkinson, H., Kerr, D., Cunningham, C. and Rae, C. (2004) *Home for Good? Preparing to Support People with Learning Difficulties in Residential Settings when They Develop Dementia.* Brighton: Pavilion Publishing/Joseph Rowntree Foundation.

Wolverson EL., Clarke, C. and Moniz-Cook, E. (2010) Remaining hopeful in early-stage dementia: a qualitative study. *Aging and Mental Health 14*, 4, 450–460.

PART 2

Experiences of Dementia in People with Intellectual Disabilities

How Do We Know?

7

The Perspective of People with Intellectual Disabilities

Noelle Blackman, David Thompson
Written in consultation with GOLD group members Betty
Steingold, John Phillips, Sylvia Hibbit, Michael and Sylvia
Brookstein, Pat Charlesworth and Roger Brooksby

Introduction

This chapter describes the experiences of dementia among a group of older people with intellectual disabilities who have been meeting together since 1998. It is written by the facilitators of the group and includes quotes from group members. The chapter was read back to the group for their approval. At the request of the group, names have not been changed.

Background to the Growing Older with Learning Disabilities (GOLD) group

The group was originally formed in order to become a reference group for a four-year research and practice development programme focussing on issues of ageing for people with intellectual disabilities at the Foundation for People with Learning Disabilities. People aged over 50 were recruited from across London. There were nine original members. Most group members did not know each other before coming together for this piece of work, except for a couple who were engaged at the start of the group and have subsequently married.

As well as inputting into the steering group for the programme, the group took part in their own research and found a wide variety of ways to disseminate their findings. By the time the four years of funding had been completed, the group had made a video (GOLD,

2000) and devised two plays, which they performed at national conferences. The themes which we have focussed on include: what sort of settings older people with an intellectual disability live in, keeping healthy while ageing, the importance of friends and family relationships, and how to stay in touch. Dementia has been an unavoidable theme because of how it has affected group members.

Sylvia from the GOLD group sums up what the group is for:

> We meet friends, we talk about getting older and about dementia. We remember people like Corinne, Edna and Tim. We do drama.

Roger says:

> In this group before we start we always tell our own news first; I like hearing other people's news. We talk about Tim, Corinne and Edna. We miss them.

By the end of the original four years of funding, the group had become experts in being able to talk about the lived experience of older people with intellectual disabilities. They had also become good friends and did not want the group to come to an end. We, as facilitators, have therefore found ways to continue to meet at least one afternoon a month since then. The GOLD group is now recognised in the UK as a unique reference group on ageing and intellectual disability. They have often been commissioned by national charities and researchers to carry out specific pieces of work and to speak at conferences. They have also made a short film and contributed to training packs on dementia and intellectual disability.

During the last 15 years there have been some changes to the group membership, all of these connected to significant issues linked to ageing. One group member had a very disabling stroke and has advanced dementia. Two members have died, one suddenly and unexpectedly, the other after a diagnosis of dementia. The stories of the two group members with dementia will be elaborated on during the rest of this chapter. There are now seven group members; this includes a new member who is a sibling of, and lives with, John, one of the original members. She has mild intellectual disabilities and joined following the death of her husband. She had become more dependent on her brother and was anxious about spending time without him. John coming alone was not an option for them.

First encounters with dementia

Case study: Corinne

Towards the end of the first three years of working together, it became noticeable that one member of the group, Corinne, seemed to be sleepier at meetings; we noticed a change in her enjoyment and interest in food at break times. Corinne did not use much verbal communication, but she was extremely sociable and found a variety of ways to clearly make her views known. She was also an extremely creative person: she painted, made pottery and had a great sense of humour; this was best seen in the drama sessions when plays were being devised to take to conferences.

It became clearer as time went on that Corinne was finding it harder and harder to engage in the work. There was one painful and memorable occasion when, after travelling to a conference, Corinne could not take part at all and was clearly in great distress. None of the group really knew what to make of the changes that were being observed. The situation continued with a slow decline, until gradually she needed more and more support, particularly when eating. The mealtimes began to become a big issue and her support worker started to take a much more active role in supporting her in the meetings.

John gets upset when he remembers the anxiety that there was at these times. He says:

> The staff used to force her to eat, I didn't like that. The staff tried to feed her with a spoon and things, I know I didn't like that. It turned out she had dementia, none of us knew.

Gradually, Corinne began to attend the group less and less regularly, however as she had been someone who had loved socialising and had always had big parties on her birthdays, her excellent support staff continued to organise the parties and we all attended them. It was at these gatherings that we could see that Corinne was declining and losing more and more of her skills.

When John was asked how she had changed, he said:

> She'd sleep and things like that.

He also said:

> She was still the same, I still loved the way she was.

When one day one of her support team rang up to let us know that Corinne was in the final stages of dementia, it was a real shock to us as we had not realised how ill she was or, up until that point, that she had dementia. All of the group members made arrangements to visit her regularly during these last few months. Following her death, the whole group attended her funeral and some months later a memorial picnic was held for her in her favourite London park.

John remembers:

We went to sprinkle her ashes on the red roses in the park.

At this memorial picnic, her staff had brought along many pieces of her pottery and other art work and they encouraged each group member to choose a piece of Corinne's work to keep as a reminder of their friendship with her. John chose a pottery box that Corinne had made and he also has a photo of her on his wall at home. He says:

If anyone touches them indoors I go spare, I don't want anyone touching them.

We visit the park sometimes as a group to have a picnic by Corinne's rose bed because, as John reminds us, it gets harder to do this on your own:

I can't get to the park very much now, I'm getting on.

But most importantly he says:

I miss her in the GOLD group now. I was in love with her before she died, that's why I miss her.

Case study: Edna

A year or so later we started to notice some small changes in another member of the group. Edna had always been a quiet group member, but it was clear that she really liked and valued the meetings. She was able to make her choices clearly known and her unique personality shone out. This could particularly be seen in how she chose to dress. Edna had her own individual style of dressing, she liked bright colours and fine patterned fabrics. She preferred dresses and skirts to trousers and would rarely go out without a hat.

When we had first met Edna she was living independently in her own supported flat, she attended a day centre and a college and had a full social life. Then she had a serious fall and a decision was taken that she should no longer live on her own. She was moved into a sheltered housing scheme for older people. Because of the move, she had to stop going to the day centre and to college. The older people's service did not have a culture of facilitating its residents to go out, and staffing levels were not high enough to make it possible for Edna to do this. The other residents were mostly older and frailer than Edna and led sedentary lives. This did not suit Edna and she complained bitterly about the boredom.

The first changes were quite subtle. She became more easily cross and frustrated, which was out of character. It was also clear that some everyday experiences were proving more difficult for her. For example, she had always needed a small amount of support in her personal care, but now it seemed as though she had completely forgotten or lost the skills to do much of this independently. This time we were more proactive and tried to find out what was wrong and very quickly she had a diagnosis of dementia.

Over the next four years her health deteriorated as did her social functioning. She stayed in the sheltered housing scheme until the deterioration was considered too much for the staff. At this point Edna was moved into an assessment unit where she stayed for several months before transferring to a National Health Service specialist dementia unit. She had become at times very resistant to staff's attempts to support her with eating, drinking and personal care. Sadly, in this specialist service some of her basic needs were not being met. For example, despite being given information about Edna's preferences, including her dislike of trousers, she was often found dressed in casual jogging bottoms. Like many people with dementia, Edna had disrupted sleep patterns. Her bedroom curtains were about six inches too short so did not block out the light. Despite our pleas it took many months for correctly fitted curtains to be installed. This seemed such a small but essential thing to get right, and yet it was difficult to get an understanding that it would be important to keep the room dark at night as this would help Edna to differentiate between night and day, and would help her to sleep at night. More seriously, Edna was, on three occasions, found to have heavy bruising when she was visited, with little information available as to how this had happened. Edna stayed in this unit for just under a year until she had a severe stroke which took away her ability to stand or walk. After a couple of months in hospital, she moved to a nursing home, her fifth move since the original signs of dementia.

When Edna first moved from her flat into the older people's service she had a room which was full of art work that she had created over the years. She also had many trinkets and photographs from her sisters who, despite living some distance away, kept in regular contact with her. She also had a wardrobe full of treasured clothing. During each of the moves, Edna lost many of her possessions. By the time she arrived at the nursing home she had virtually nothing left, literally the contents of two black bags.

The loss of her personal possessions and the opportunity to choose her own clothes led to the depersonalisation of Edna. As her dementia worsened, so did the capacity for her carers to see the individual that she was. Each move exacerbated this loss of a sense of identity and self. We often define ourselves through the things we surround ourselves with and the clothes we wear and there was something extremely depersonalising in the loss of Edna's possessions. As she sunk further and further into dementia, the service saw her less and less as the individual that she once was, and were unable to pass on any remnants of her former self to the next service each time she moved.

During this time, Edna became increasingly isolated. Her sisters were themselves frail and unable to visit. Her friends and the staff she knew from college and day centres no longer kept in touch (had they had wanted to, it would have been very difficult to track her down after her multiple moves). However, we have supported the group to stay in touch and we have advocated strongly on Edna's behalf. This included helping to track down some of her missing possessions, putting photographs around her room and her paintings up on the wall and talking to staff about her past life, and about the things that Edna had been involved with previously with the group and about the work they had undertaken together.

Shockingly, the nursing home seemed to expect Edna to spend the rest of her life in bed as she was not able to use the seating available in the home. It was only the GOLD group who thought she deserved a different future. Through persistence, Edna was eventually assessed by an occupational therapist for a properly supportive wheelchair, although it took a further six months to arrive. We arranged for a new coat, hat and shoes to be bought for Edna so that she could be taken for outings to a local coffee shop or visits to old friends, in particular her good friend Betty from the GOLD group who lives nearby.

Betty says:

> We went out with Edna in the park, all the way down to the canal. Edna was trying to talk a bit, not a lot, I couldn't understand, we had a lovely afternoon out. We had a cup of tea in a café.

We also organised for Edna to have a one-to-one support worker twice a week using her unspent welfare benefit entitlement, which was collecting in her account. The consistency of having the same worker who has come to know and understand Edna's likes and needs over the past five years has enabled her to have a much richer and more interesting life. Edna regularly goes out and about in her local community where she has become well known.

Group members find visiting Edna difficult unless we, as facilitators, are there. The difficulty of seeing someone so changed by dementia is shared by many people without intellectual disabilities. To support this, we have arranged to celebrate her birthday together each year bringing party food to the nursing home. At other times, we have shared picnics local to where she lives or made arrangements for her to join a celebration the group is having at Christmas.

All of these simple needs contribute to a meaningful existence, and possibly even to life itself. It is all too easy for an older person with intellectual disabilities, who no longer has family members watching out for them, to become lost in older people's services, their unique identity becomes invisible and they become treated more like an object in receipt of care. Connection with Edna through the GOLD group demonstrates how important it is to work towards keeping a sense of the identity of the person around them at all times, as the temptation for services and staff, involved with someone who has become so frail that they can no longer tell carers anything about themselves, is to depersonalise them.

When a parent gets dementia

Michael had been coming to the group for a long time before it began to dawn on us that his father might have dementia. Michael often talked about his father with great frustration. He would tell of how difficult his visits to see his father were, or how angry his father had made him; but it took a long time for us to put together some of the things that he said and understand what was really going on.

Michael explains in his own words:

Me and my dad we got on as well as a father and son can, then he changed, mainly he didn't want to talk and he was always moody. I thought it was best not to talk too much to him. We were wondering what was up, we just didn't know, we kept thinking it could have been anything, unfortunately we didn't think about dementia. In fact neither my wife Sylvia nor I knew about dementia.

Gradually, we became aware from Michael that his father was wandering off and getting lost and that he wasn't managing to live independently anymore. Michael soon reported that his father had moved into a care home. Michael recalls this time and says:

> I was very reluctant to go and see him because I didn't know what reaction I would get.

His father's mood was unpredictable and it wasn't like going to the family home to visit; now Michael also had to negotiate the staff at the older people's home.

One day Michael seemed particularly distressed about his father. It turned out that he had 'lost' him and no longer knew where he was living. He did not tell us this straight away, perhaps he felt ashamed that such a thing should have happened. But eventually he started to tell us that he had been finding it harder and harder to visit the care home as his father no longer recognised him. Then one day, after a period of time of not visiting, he had gone to the home and found that his father was no longer there. He had not been able to get the staff from the home to give him details as to where his father had been moved to.

Michael recalls:

> The first nursing home, they didn't seem to want to tell me anything...I want to know how my dad is and they wouldn't tell me. I found it very difficult holding on to my temper.

With our support we managed to insist that the care home give Michael forwarding details and we supported him to visit his father in the new nursing home. By this time the GOLD group had begun to focus its work on dementia as it had become such an important part of the group's experience. This made it easier to talk to Michael about what was happening to his father. Until this point he had not understood and he had found this very upsetting. With Michael's permission, we helped him to explain to the manager of the nursing home that he had intellectual disabilities and that he might need their support to understand his father's condition as it deteriorated.

This nursing home was really wonderful at engaging with Michael and Sylvia when they visited. They made them feel really welcome and ameliorated the painfulness of the visits. In Michael's words:

> There was a very big difference between the first place and the second. The doctors talked with us about his condition, that it was advanced dementia and was never going to get better and they were trying their best to look after him and I felt very comforted about that.

He continues:

> We were advised the best thing we could do was just visit him as regularly as we could and support him.

He compares his experience of the two settings that his father was in saying:

> In the first place they wouldn't talk to me, in the second place they couldn't do enough for us and I was really grateful for that.

When eventually his father became too physically frail and was moved to hospital, they called Michael to let him know that his father was seriously ill and advised him to visit. Michael was accompanied to the hospital. His father had a 'do not resuscitate' sign up above his bed, he was asleep and looked very thin and frail. The doctor was asked to come and explain to Michael what the sign meant. This was helpful as it also meant that the ward staff became aware that Michael might need particular support during the time that his father was dying. They were extremely sensitive and open.

Michael says:

> At first I didn't want to go but, as I say, it was an experience and I felt to myself going back there, it was a good thing because I think if he had passed away and I didn't see him I think it would have been worse for me.

Michael has said that he thinks that this helped him to begin to come to terms with his father's death.

Lessons learnt

It has been really important that the GOLD group has been together for so many years. This has allowed everyone to get to know one another really well through creating time to talk together and reflect on lived experiences, as well as sometimes take practical action. Through having focussed time together, the individual group members have been able to make sense of some of the complexities of growing older with intellectual disabilities, to share their hopes and fears; they have taught us as facilitators so much. This important opportunity to enable people to think about and understand some of these difficult issues connected to ageing have helped people to cope in their own lives. This can be seen when Michael talks about how much easier it was to cope with his father's dementia once it was discussed in the group.

However, this does not mean that we don't all worry about getting older and frailer, as John says:

I forget things, that's how I lost my bus pass, I worry about getting dementia.

Dementia is hard to think about, and the group have learnt that in some ways the more you know about it, the less you want to dwell on it. Roger says:

It's sad when the person gets dementia, it's not very nice.

It is relatively unusual for people with intellectual disabilities to be supported to think and talk about uncomfortable life issues, and yet from experiences with this group it has really helped people to have as much knowledge as possible. They know there are things that can help to make sure that people still have a good quality of life and also things that can make the situation worse.

Pat says:

Having memory books is good, it is a good idea to put a picture of a toilet on the door so people can find it.

However, what they know most of all is that having dementia always means that the person will decline and eventually die.

Sylvia says:

I don't want to think about it at the moment. I keep busy doing something. The music and singing is keeping my mind occupied. Michael's dad had dementia, we visited him, he enjoyed the apple pie we took him. Michael's dad stopped talking, it was terrible. I don't think he remembered us anymore, I don't think, I'm not sure.

The importance of talking to people with intellectual disabilities about making plans for the future must be recognised. We have recognised just how important it is to talk to people with an intellectual disability about making plans for the future. We have discussed wills and advance care plans for health in case of loss of capacity and have supported all of the group members to make these plans. In the case of John and his sister Sylv, we worry about what would happen if either of them developed dementia or another condition which challenges their ability to cope. They are each so dependent on each other for everything. Up to the point of Sylv's husband's death they had lived without any input from local services because he had been able to support them both in so many ways. We decided that we should try to get them a bit more support and also make sure that the local social services team were aware of them now rather than wait for a crisis. With John and Sylv's permission, we asked social services to carry out community care assessments and carer's assessment on each of them. This highlighted exactly what each was doing for the other and showed just how mutually dependent they were.

The social worker who carried out the assessment was shocked to see how delicately balanced their situation was, and could see how easily it would fall apart if one of them was taken ill. She assessed them as being eligible for some support, most importantly of all access three days a week each to an older people's day centre. There John is learning to cook. They also have the chance to make individual friends as they each attend on one day a week without the other one. The day centre has widened each of their worlds and networks. It is also helping John to learn new skills which will be vital to him, for example, if he ever needed to cook.

As facilitators, we have learnt how much more vulnerable and isolated people with intellectual disabilities can become as they get older; their own family members will also be ageing and may even have died. This long attachment to all the members of the GOLD group has meant that, as facilitators, we have advocated for them regularly over the years. This has often included addressing deficits in services. How many other people growing older with intellectual disabilities will have experienced the same sorts of changes but without support? We worry about who will be looking out for them.

One of the significant things that the GOLD group has shown is that people with intellectual disabilities are perfectly capable and willing to think and talk about uncomfortable subjects that affect them, and don't want to be 'protected' from difficult truths. Michael has a key message and perhaps this is an important note to end this chapter on. He says:

> I feel it's vital for relatives to be told everything, well everything's a strong word to use, but as much as they can be told that will help them, even if they know that their relative's not going to survive or get better, because otherwise they are not going to know and it's going to make things worse for them. The sooner we are told the better I think.

References

GOLD (2000) *Dementia and People with Learning Disabilities.* London: GOLD (Growing Older with Learning Disabilities) Group/Respond.

8

Towards Understanding Individual Experiences of People Ageing with an Intellectual Disability and Dementia

Karen Watchman

Introduction

We know more of the incidence and prevalence of dementia in people with an intellectual disability and of early signs of physical change. We also have an awareness of the perceptions of carers and of the debate over appropriate accommodation and models of care. We do not have the same understanding of the perception, or the lived experience, of people with an intellectual disability and dementia. This is largely due to the difficulty of including people in research and the changes required in communication as participants become increasingly non-verbal. Gaps in the existing evidence base include:

- understanding the experience of people with an intellectual disability and dementia from their own perspective

- guidance to support people through the progression of dementia, particularly if they are not aware of their diagnosis

- guidance to continue meaningful communication as verbal and cognitive ability change

- examples from research and practice to reduce the inevitability of further marginalisation

- how to blend areas of knowledge from intellectual disability services with aged or dementia care services.

The observations of three people with an intellectual disability in three different accommodation settings will be presented: a shared intellectual disability group home, a generic care home for older people and an individual tenancy with outreach support from intellectual disability support staff. Each person was visited monthly, resulting in a total of 101 hours of visits over a three-year period. This was part of a larger research study that also tracked changes in accommodation post-diagnosis (Watchman, 2008), and investigated awareness of carers (Watchman, 2007). The longitudinal stage involving people with an intellectual disability required flexibility in research methods in order to develop individualised approaches to data collection that incorporated increasingly non-verbal communication. Brief extracts from the three case studies will be presented to show how far people with an intellectual disability and dementia can be enabled not only to participate in research, but have much to share in terms of challenging and changing practice.

Flexibility in research methods

Ethical approval was granted on the condition that each individual was able to give consent to take part at the start of the research and all names have been anonymised. This led to the inclusion criteria of a diagnosis having being made within the previous two years to increase this likelihood, although it is acknowledged that dementia may have been present for longer due to difficulties with confirming the diagnosis among people with an intellectual disability. A further consideration was the need to remain aware that participants were experiencing decline in verbal communication as part of a progressive cognitive condition. Just one of these factors is usually enough for a person to be excluded from research; not uncommon when part of a marginalised group who are not considered to be in a position to share information or contribute to knowledge.

Adopting a flexible approach allowed for non-verbal methods to be introduced such as pictures, photographs and kinaesthetics (tactile and body language as a form of communication). Visits to the home of each participant lasted between 15 minutes and one hour 55 minutes. The content of each was led by each participant based on topics that they wished to discuss, if anything. This adapted narrative method meant that each participant was able to engage with me, sit quietly or look at pictures as appropriate. There was no standardised set of questions; instead a general conversational style was used. With permission, each visit was digitally recorded to ensure accuracy and for ease of analysis. This method also enabled periods of silence to be recorded, plus some spoken observations of the researcher. This became increasingly relevant in terms of identifying responses that were given appropriately, albeit a considerable amount of time later. The individualised communication methods were unique to each person, and were based on Brewster's approach that people respond better in the 'real world in which they live' (2004, p. 35). Factors that supported this approach to communication and inclusion in the research were:

- recognising the importance of adapting communication for individuals, instead of adopting a standard approach to the research

- awareness of the importance of using non-verbal communication

- recognising the importance of the physical environment and meeting each person in their home environment

- not relying on, or seeking, information that was chronological

- recognising that the 'how' aspect of communication was more important than what was said or why.

The following case studies, with only brief detail included here, begin to develop a picture of the lived experience of each individual. Despite differences in methods of communication, location of care and relationships with others, there were similarities in how participants constructed themselves as social beings needing interaction, emotional connection and meaningful activity. It became apparent that meaningful communication was possible even in the end stages of dementia and long after verbal capacity had ceased. Changing or unexpected situations were seen as opportunities rather than challenges to the research, for example the decrease in verbal communication of participants was accepted and included as part of the process.

Case studies

Anna

Anna lived in a group home for people with an intellectual disability with six other residents. Although not living geographically close to her family, after her move from a long-stay institution on its closure, they remained in contact and new cards and photographs were often on display. Her room, decorated bright pink at her request before she moved in, contained many personal items. Anna moved into this group home from another run by the same organisation. Her previous room had been upstairs and her reduced mobility meant that this became untenable. Shortly after she moved, she began using a wheelchair as her mobility deteriorated rapidly.

Based on Anna's enthusiasm for recognising the researcher from the pictorial information sheet provided prior to the research commencing, attempts were made to explore this as a potential means of communication. This was increasingly important as although Anna initially communicated verbally, her speech was very limited and declined quickly. Pictures as a potential means of communication were introduced early in the research, first using emoticons. All were yellow with different facial expressions. Possibly due to failing eyesight, or maybe a lack of ability to interpret facial expressions, Anna recognised them only by their colour and was not able to identify the expression. This mattered to her as she took great pride in 'getting it right'.

The second group of pictures were in the form of real life and still photographs. Anna, familiar with looking at family pictures, immediately tried to recognise those in the images. Rather than cause distress that she was not able to 'get it', this style of picture was discarded. The third set of pictures were free downloadable images available online. Anna immediately identified household items, parts of the body such as feet and teeth and people including a baby.

Anna: Smiles [picture of teeth]

Researcher: Yes a big smile

Anna: [points to picture of baby] Baby, baby, baby, baby boy, I got it, I got it

There were increasing periods of silence in the interactions lasting from between three and 25 seconds. Anna came to associate my visits with looking at the pictures, even asking for some that she couldn't find such as babies and flowers, which were then added to the growing collection. Gradually, Anna became increasingly non-verbal, although reassurance was taken from her responses that she understood what was said.

Researcher: Have you had your hair cut?

Anna: [smiles and touches her hair]

Other residents appeared unaware of how ill Anna was or that her condition would deteriorate to the extent that it did in a relatively short time.

Fellow resident: She's just tired

Anna's deterioration continued and she became increasingly tired during the visits. Whilst I only ever stayed if Anna agreed to this, she continued to hold out her hand and hold tightly to mine during each visit, even if she drifted off to sleep. Anna continued to associate the visits with looking at pictures.

Anna: Pictures

Researcher: Yes I have pictures, maybe you are too tired?

Anna: Baby [drifts back to sleep]

Towards the end of her life, staff engaged in one-sided conversations with Anna, speaking pleasantly, but often rhetorically, not waiting for a response. On a visit to Anna near Christmas time her room was lit with low lighting, a fibre-optic Christmas tree was displayed and her room felt warm and relaxing with a DVD quietly playing Christmas carols, something that she had always enjoyed. Anna was having difficulty in breathing at this point. Her body movements were jerky and she had no control over this, yet still held her hand out to me on arrival. However, it was 23 minutes before she spoke.

[*Field notes:* Based on Anna's body language and positive manner I felt encouraged to stay although was unsure of whether to or not]

Researcher: Will I go now?

[*Field notes:* Anna pulls face, pushes her hand towards me reaching out her fingers]

Researcher: I can stay, are you sure?

Anna: [smiles]

Five days later Anna died. Her funeral was very well attended by residents from her former group home who identified themselves as her friends, although said they had not seen her since she moved. Personal belongings at the front of the church reinforced that the Anna I had got to know at the end of her life, with little verbal interaction, was the same person those present had always known: a lady with an infectious giggle who loved babies and children. It also became apparent at the funeral how shocked staff were at her death, with many appearing unaware that dementia was a condition that would have this ultimate conclusion.

Brian

Brian lived alone and was a tenant with a service provider for people with an intellectual disability. Although aware that he had Down syndrome, he did not know that he had dementia.

The primary method of communication with Brian was verbal, based on his willingness to engage in conversation. Despite this, his clarity of speech was poor and this continued to gradually deteriorate over the research period, whilst his stammer increased. Body language was an indicator of how he was feeling, often showing increased frustration at not being able to find the right words over time. He was visibly more alert and with shorter periods of silence in his conversation when he was talking about a subject that was of interest to him; usually movies or football. Over time, as with Anna, it became important to allow periods of silence as part of the natural dialogue. Brian remained proud of living independently and maintaining his own tenancy. His personal preferences were evident in the flat as, although the decor and furniture were standard issue of the housing association, there were posters and photographs on the walls and doors. Many hundreds of videos and DVDs were visible, some in their original packaging having never been opened.

Staff provided support on four days a week from a nearby office base with the emphasis on minimal intervention and supporting independence. I had concerns about how Brian was functioning in the flat, for example, the heating remaining on high during a warm day with Brian admitting that he didn't remember how to turn it off, suggesting that more appropriate support may have been provided as dementia progressed. Tools were in evidence such as a pictorial staff calendar to inform Brian of which staff would be visiting him. Had this been implemented correctly, it may have supported the principles of ageing in place, addressing his changing needs in his own environment (Janicki et al., 2003). However, it was not reinforced or monitored for effectiveness. It was often poorly printed and difficult to see, or at times the staff rota changed but the calendar was not updated.

> Brian: Sometimes face and different name or the name but different face
>
> Researcher: So you don't know who will walk in the door?
>
> Brian: No

A similar situation was observed with Brian's mobile phone. Although he liked the idea of having this, he did not remember to charge it so was unable to use it. Likewise, his landline telephone often flashed to show that he had an answerphone message but he often asked me how to listen to the messages as he couldn't remember. Brian often took pride in showing photographs of family members and previous holidays. Sometimes the name of the person in the photograph was written on the back, although not the location or venue. This led to frustration for Brian when trying to identify places he, or family members, had visited. Photographs of large groups of people were passed over quickly if they were not labelled, despite his family's best intentions to keep him updated of their activities.

The issue of mealtimes and budget planning gave a further example of the culture of the intellectual disability organisation being about developing, rather than maintaining, skills. Over time, it became apparent that Brian had the same frozen, microwaveable ready-meal in his freezer, one for each day of the week. As evidence of his cooking was seen during early visits, with dishes, pans and cooker in use, this led to the conclusion that there was little support for his shopping, dietary or nutritional needs. It suggested that Brian's relationship with staff had not changed to the extent required. They may have been respecting his choice to buy the same frozen meal every day, yet this was not responsive to his changing capacity and declining ability to shop for himself, cook and plan his meals.

Brian's flat was usually cluttered as a result of his ever-increasing DVD collection, newspapers that he bought daily and sometimes evidence of cooking, as noted by the used crockery and pans. The exception to this was when mice were found in his flat and staff subsequently cleaned it thoroughly. Brian was not aware that the mice should not be encouraged and he was not concerned about their presence. On the contrary, he seemed to enjoy their presence as offering much needed companionship and had been aware that they were there for some considerable time before staff acted to remove them.

Researcher: Did you get a fright when you saw them?

Brian: No

Researcher: Do they come through the night or day?

Brian: Err, night I think

Researcher: Did you see them?

Brian: Yeh, when they are in my bedroom

Researcher: Don't you mind?

Brian: No, I watched them in my room

Brian had been made aware by staff, and kept repeating, that the mice were 'not the kind you can keep', implying that he would have been happy to do so. A further indication of his loneliness became apparent when, on one visit, a large teddy bear was seated in one of the lounge chairs.

Researcher: What made you buy a teddy?

Brian: Company

The bear remained a permanent fixture and was seated on the chair on every visit thereafter. Brian made it clear that he was aware that the bear was not real and could not respond but he enjoyed the feeling of having someone he could talk to.

Brian: Sometimes I talk to myself so I talk to him instead

Researcher: And he won't argue will he?

Brian: [laughs] No

[six seconds]

Brian: I don't argue with him

[seven seconds]

Brian: Doesn't tell me what to do

This may have appeared as evidence of psychotic behaviour or even delusionary. It may have been attributed to having dementia or having an intellectual disability, rather than seeing it for what it was – loneliness.

Clara

Clara had grown up living with her older sister, both in childhood and as an adult. After Clara's hospital admission, her sister's health deteriorated to the extent that Clara was unable to return home. After seven weeks in hospital she was referred out (Janicki *et al.*, 2003) to a generic care home for older people in a different part of the city. Clara was one of 19 residents in her first floor unit; the only person with an intellectual disability.

Clara was non-verbal in her conversation when my visits began, although was still able to sing and hum a tune. She was very tactile and took an interest in my handbag which, on the first visit, she picked up and emptied. Each item was investigated, touched, stroked and examined carefully and gently before it was placed carefully back in the bag. At this point she physically turned and acknowledged me before smiling and handing it back. The handbag became the focus of our time together with Clara proudly holding it over her arm and looking inside. Whilst I took bags in for Clara for her personal use, they were not in evidence on the following visits and staff were unsure what had happened to them.

Clara increasingly made loud noises that appeared to alarm staff who were rarely seen to engage with her. It became apparent during transcription that the noises were attempts at conversation. They were always accompanied by relevant facial expression and were in a tone that conveyed her emotions. Clara's body language changed and she physically relaxed after sitting quietly holding my hand. Clara's understanding was affirmed through her actions and responses, albeit non-verbally.

Researcher: How are your teeth?

[*Field notes:* Clara opens her mouth and leans towards me sticking her chin out]

Clara's room was sparse with little indication of personal belongings. She was always seated in the day room, a lounge area where residents sat in the same chairs and the television was always on. When entering her room her radio was often playing; loud dance music suggesting that others had been listening to it and had not turned it off. The corridor led from the day room to the nurse's station with residents' rooms on either side. Each looked identical with no identifying or distinguishing features to highlight who lived in each room.

It became apparent at an early stage during the research period that staff made assumptions about Clara's ability to eat. This was evidenced when food was taken away, despite her having made no attempt to eat it and even though she was observed making pincer moves with her fingers in the direction of the food. When this happened again, I intervened and offered Clara a small piece of fruit on a fork which she took holding on to my other hand throughout, followed by sips of tea. This continued for 25 minutes until staff removed the fruit and mug, even though Clara was still eating. This left us both sitting in silence as the clatter of the tea trolley disappeared along the corridor and staff moved on to the next task.

On one occasion, Clara's sister was present at the same time as I was and wanted to talk to Clara about family members and neighbours, showing her Christmas cards that had been received. Clara and other residents were seated in the day room whilst scones were being placed in front of residents.

Sister: Do you want it? [to Clara, pointing at scone]

Sister: A bit, take a bit

Researcher: Maybe she needs a bit of help

Sister: What do you mean? She'll do it if she wants it, she won't take it if she doesn't want it, try for yourself

[*Field notes:* I break a small piece of scone and take it to Clara's mouth, which she opens and moves towards the food]

Sister: Well I never, you can do it for her, I never knew to do that

The snack period continued with Clara's sister still talking to her about family. Clara, however, only focused on the food. After she had eaten enough she reached for my handbag and held it tightly, laughing. She leant forward making noises and laughing, as if engaging me in a conversation, but without the words.

Sister: Oh what's she saying?

Researcher: I'm not sure

Sister: Well you seem to be getting on well with her, well I never get that much from her [appears a bit resentful]. Why doesn't she do it for me, after all I'm only her sister?

This reinforced the importance of meeting basic needs such as eating and drinking and of meaningful activity, which for Clara was the handbag. Clara communicated verbally before she had dementia, although she had limited verbal capacity at the start of the study. Our communication methods were developed during the first few weeks based on her interaction with me and the handbag, after touching and stroking the contents. Clara was not interested in the contents of the bag; it was the tactile experience of touching them that she enjoyed. My concern in this care home was for the potential reversion to the same institutional observations recorded by Oswin (1973) with the television always on, a lack of communication with those who had more complex needs, and staff not always speaking in the same language as those they were supporting.

Implications

Thematic and cross-case analysis of the three case studies suggests that formal and family carers of those in an intellectual disability setting view, and respond to, the person as primarily having an intellectual disability rather than focusing on the changes associated with dementia. In the generic care setting for older people, carers did not respond accordingly to Clara's intellectual disability by adapting their approach or the level of support provided. Indeed, at one point I was asked if Clara had been able to talk when she was a child; she had been able to talk when she moved into the care home but very few staff spoke to her.

This concurs with studies of other marginalised groups (Barrientos and Hume, 2008; Devereux *et al.*, 2011) that poor standards of care stem from a combination of prejudice, low expectation and lack of knowledge, plus the notion that people should adapt to services rather than the other way around. As the diagnosis of dementia was not shared with any of the three individuals, life was experienced as normal for the person who had known only the stigma associated with having an intellectual disability, not with dementia. It became a life far less ordinary for carers who had information of the diagnosis of dementia, but no guidance of what to do with this knowledge. Four key issues are explored further:

- the impact of the lack of a shared diagnosis
- the importance of relationship-centred care

- evidence of sense of self
- the importance of adapted communication.

Impact of the lack of a shared diagnosis

A person who is not aware of their diagnosis of dementia cannot position themselves in the way that someone with this knowledge might do. Early in this study it became apparent that the three individuals were not aware of their diagnosis of dementia or of why they were experiencing changes. Increased frustration was observed when Brian was unable to find the correct word or cope with daily activities, although he did not associate this with his changing health. Staff appeared to hold the belief that he would be able to maintain his previous living skills for longer than was the reality, an overestimation perhaps based on his retained verbal capacity. However, the resulting observations were of increased isolation. Clara experienced silence literally as she stopped speaking and being spoken to. Anna was living in a group home among peers who had no knowledge of her condition, and without contact from previous friends who were unaware of where she had moved to.

A challenge in dementia care generally is to provide appropriate post-diagnostic support, and promote awareness that everyone is entitled to know their diagnosis (Scottish Government, 2013). A cultural process that addresses wider inequality is needed in order to acknowledge the human rights of people with an intellectual disability to receive their diagnosis, as part of accessing appropriate support. Top-down rhetoric is needed for specific policy development and communication through all levels, but also a bottom-up approach based on actively involving and including people with an intellectual disability. Kitwood (1997) found that when a person with dementia did not have their individual basic needs met, the result was depersonalisation, a negative process creating withdrawal and social isolation. Whilst this has most commonly been written about in relation to dementia in older people without an intellectual disability, my findings suggest that this process of depersonalisation was evident among Anna, Brian and Clara. This is consistent with a social constructionist approach when labelling is applied at an individual level to explain behaviour viewed as difficult. Contributory factors were the failure to recognise individuality or retained identity, and lack of understanding of what constitutes the norm for each person. For example, Clara was reprimanded for taking a visitor's handbag from the lounge area which caused her distress. Yet, for Clara handbags were both a meaningful activity and a means of social interaction.

How the diagnosis is shared should be based on the capacity of the individual to understand. This may mean that the word 'dementia' is not used, but instead an explanation of a change being experienced as part of an ongoing process, rather than a one-off event using consistent terms, pictures or a form of communication preferred by the individual. There is limited guidance on how to explain dementia to people with intellectual disabilities and this shortage of information increases the potential for individual stereotyping. It also means that until information is shared, we are unable to position people with an intellectual disability and dementia as an authority on their own condition. As a consequence of this, co-production, meaningfully positioning people with intellectual disabilities in the commissioning, design and delivery of ageing and dementia services, remains out of reach and will require a cultural change for many organisations.

Relationship-centred care

Coming from literature on chronic illness, rather than intellectual disabilities or dementia, is the notion that personhood is best understood in the context of relationships, with an appropriate balance needed between dependence, independence and interdependence (MacDonald, 2005). Nolan *et al.* (2006) developed this relationship-centred approach into a senses framework. This maintains that the triad of person, their family, and those who provide paid care should all experience relationships within an appropriate environment that enable a sense of:

- security
- belonging
- continuity
- purpose
- achievement
- significance.

For people with an intellectual disability and dementia it may also be relevant to add a fourth element – friends. Peers, friends or a partner may have had a longer, or more regular relationship with the person than some family members or carers. For example, at Anna's funeral I met some friends from her previous accommodation who had known her for 20 years prior to her first move, as they had all lived in the same long-stay hospital before its closure. They were not aware of why she had moved, or that she had been ill, only that they didn't see her anymore. To maintain the friendships would have required the proactive involvement of staff or carers.

Sense of self

An increasing lack of verbal communication did not result in the loss of self, or sense of identity for Anna, Brian and Clara, reflecting research findings in the general population (Kelly, 2010). Sabat and Harre (1992) distinguished between the 'person' with dementia, as viewed by those around them, and the 'self': the individual with unique circumstances and experiences. Sabat (2002) recorded three types of self:

Self 1: an awareness of 'I or me', which can be retained even in those with profound or advanced impairment.

Self 2: this involves a degree of insight into positive or negative attributes, for example 'I can do that', or 'I am not good at that'. This would be compromised if an additional disability caused the carer to focus on the disability rather than the person (Sabat, 2002).

Self 3: how people present themselves socially in different contexts, usually constructed through interaction with others.

Anna, Brian and Clara all expressed Self 1, 2 and 3 to varying degrees, although this did not always appear to be noticed by their carer or staff. Observations showed that each was able to:

- locate themselves in relation to me by showing a preference for what we did

- show emotional characteristics about themselves by expressing pride, pleasure or annoyance to varying degrees

- relate to other people.

An example of Self 1 (self-awareness) was seen when Anna continued to associate my visits with looking at pictures, right through until the end of her life.

Self 2 (insight into emotional characteristics) was evident by all three individuals showing positive or negative characteristics about themselves. For example, Clara took pleasure in exploring the handbag, Brian in showing off his college certificates and Anna in 'getting it right'.

Self 3 (how people see themselves publicly and socially) was less evident as it relied on the cooperation of others. By not responding to opportunities for interaction or socialisation, those providing support were not acknowledging each person's sense of self and individuality.

Anna was observed taking pride in showing the other residents that she had a visitor. Similarly, Clara's 'conversations' used appropriate tone, body language and expression, albeit without words. If staff do not realise that someone is presenting themselves in a particular way, or respond appropriately, then the social identity of that person is weakened. Continued positioning of the person as incapable means that the opportunity to take meaning from experience and interaction is lost.

Location of care

The question originally raised by Hubert and Hollins (2000) still requires investigation – whether shared accommodation with a small number of others with an intellectual disability or with an intellectual disability and dementia, is more or less favourable than moving to a care home with residents who have dementia but not an intellectual disability and are significantly older. In my research, although staff in intellectual disability settings were well intentioned, there appeared a lack of knowledge of how dementia affected people, including the lack of realisation that it was a condition that would ultimately lead to the person's death. In the generic care home the opposite applied, with little awareness of what it meant to have an intellectual disability. This includes recognition of the importance of knowing the person, person-centred approaches relating to both dementia care and to intellectual disability, acknowledging the importance of maintaining previous friendships and relationships and supporting meaningful activities. Priority should be given to not introducing a potentially younger person with an intellectual disability to an older person's service, where staff have little or no knowledge or training in intellectual disability – or even at times knowledge or training in dementia care, which is not mandatory for care home staff in the UK.

Independence should not be viewed as a long-term goal for people with an intellectual disability syndrome and dementia, even if this is the lifestyle that the person may have been used to, although it should be supported for as long as is possible. If the person lives alone, then ageing in place is only appropriate if the support level continues to increase on an individual basis, including at night-time. A dementia specific or dementia capable environment does not necessarily involve a move. This may be the person's existing home with appropriate supports and adaptations. People with an intellectual disability often choose to live with others in a shared setting. This should not be ruled out as inappropriate after a diagnosis of dementia. Instead, it requires different support and input for the person with dementia, other residents and staff.

Intellectual disability services seem to be in the best position to lead the coordination of future care, due to the fundamental basis of their work being across the lifespan of the person. Such services are more likely to have had contact with the person before diagnosis. In place progression, dementia specific accommodation for people with intellectual disabilities, was not represented among the accommodation settings in my research, although it is increasingly being developed or considered as an appropriate model among service providers. In the UK, this has not yet extended to incorporate the original in place progression model which suggested that a range of intellectual disability and dementia specific settings should be considered within the same service, each accommodating people at different stages of dementia. Perhaps in time, as the in place progression model is increasingly seen and evaluated, it will become apparent that issues still exist in dementia specific or dementia capable settings if residents are at different stages in terms of mobility, health needs and social supports. Further research is also needed on the timing of transition to such settings to maximise the experience of the person with an intellectual disability.

Importance of adapted communication

The extent to which each person's experience was influenced by non-verbal communication was apparent. It also became obvious how far traditional research methods were a barrier to including people with any form of complex needs in research. Most methods rely on verbal interaction and a level of cognitive ability that remains relatively intact for the duration of the research period. Whilst any communication has the potential to be temporary due to the nature of dementia, relationships were built up with Anna, Brian and Clara over a considerable period of time. These relationships were not temporary as personality and temperament remained constant throughout, even as dementia progressed.

Communication and identity have been shown to be constructed together. Both are shaped by where people live and how they are supported. Research with people who have an intellectual disability has undoubtedly made strides towards greater inclusion and understanding experiences from the perspective of the person. This is largely as a result of an active human rights agenda within intellectual disability services and is under the commendable umbrella of promoting choice and reducing inclusion. However, it is still a developing area of research for those with more complex disabilities, and with dementia, for whom communication methods may not be verbal.

Care settings in both intellectual disability and dementia services should give consideration to identifying staff members to be trained as specialists or local experts in intellectual disability and dementia. This will ensure that adapted, and increasingly non-verbal, communication is seen as a priority rather than implemented retrospectively when the person has already become non-verbal. Intellectual disability training should be incorporated into training for carers in dementia settings and, similarly, dementia care should be incorporated into training for carers in intellectual disability settings. All training should begin with an assets-based focus on retaining and consolidating skills, meaningful activities and an individualised approach.

Conclusion

A case study approach proved suitable as it supported the exploration of individual experiences. The observed experiences cannot be said to be of dementia, as although participants had a diagnosis they were not aware of it; as a result it did not frame their lives or experiences in the way that knowledge of their intellectual disability may have done. The progressive nature of dementia, plus an early requirement for a palliative approach and an increased emphasis on medical intervention and end of life planning, means that social care and medical intervention cannot be kept separate. At the same time, this cannot be discussed in a meaningful way if the person with an intellectual disability does not know that they are ill.

Even with deteriorating speech and a degenerative cognitive condition, participants with an intellectual disability and dementia were able to communicate with me, although meaningful communication with staff was less evident, possibly due to the length of time required for a response. This supports Williams' statement that research should not only focus on those with a literal voice (Williams, 2013). People with an intellectual disability actively participate in society and research, as do people with dementia. Paradoxically, in terms of both representation and inclusion in research, individuals with both an intellectual disability and dementia are far less visible, leading to their experience being one of isolation and further marginalisation.

Overall, the study was largely a poor reflection of the care provided for people with an intellectual disability and dementia from the point of diagnosis through to end of life. Staff interactions, although at times positive, were also limited and at times neglectful. Despite knowledge of the association between intellectual disability and dementia for decades, the combination continues to create a situation beyond the understanding of most carers, professionals and commissioners of services. Strategic understanding is needed of the demographics of people with intellectual disabilities and their trajectory of housing, health and support needs.

References

Barrientos, A. and Hulme, D. (2008) *Social Protection for the Poor and the Poorest: Concepts, Policies and Politics*. Basingstoke and New York: Palgrave.

Brewster, SJ. (2004) Putting words into their mouths? Interviewing people with learning disabilities and little/no speech. *British Journal of Learning Disabilities 32*, 166–169.

Devereux, S., Allister McGregor, J. and Sabates-Wheeler, R. (2011) Introduction: Social protection for social justice. *IDS Bulletin Special Issue: Social Protection for Social Justice 42*, 6, 1–9.

Hubert, J. and Hollins, S. (2000) Working with elderly carers of people with learning disabilities and planning for the future. *Advances in Psychiatric Treatment 6*, 6, 41–48.

Janicki, M., McCallion, P. and Dalton, A. (2003) Dementia-related care decision-making in group homes for persons with intellectual disabilities. *Journal of Gerontological Social Work 38*, 1/2, 179–195.

Kelly, F. (2010) Recognising and supporting self in dementia: A new way to facilitate a person-centred approach to dementia care. *Ageing and Society 30*, 1, 103–124.

Kitwood, T. (1997) *Dementia Reconsidered.* Buckingham: Open University Press.

MacDonald, A. (2005) Care homes and dementia. *Aging and Mental Health 9*, 2, 91–92.

Nolan, MR., Brown, J., Davies, S., Nolan, J. and Keady, J. (2006) *The Senses Framework: Improving Care for Older People through a Relationship-Centred Approach. Getting Research into Practice (GRiP) Report No 2.* Project Report: University of Sheffield.

Oswin, M. (1973) *The Empty Hours: Weekend Life of Handicapped Children in Institutions.* London: Pelican.

Sabat, S. (2002) *The Experience of Alzheimer's Disease: Life through a Tangled Veil.* Oxford: Blackwell.

Sabat, S. and Harre, R. (1992) The construction and deconstruction of self in Alzheimer's disease, *Ageing and Society 12*, 12, 443–461.

Scottish Government (2013) *Scotland's National Dementia Strategy 2013–2016.* Edinburgh: Scottish Government.

Watchman, K. (2007) Dementia and Down's syndrome: The diagnosis and support needed. *Learning Disability Practice 10*, 2, 10–14.

Watchman, K. (2008) Changes in accommodation experienced by people with Down's syndrome and dementia in the first five years after their diagnosis. *Journal of Policy and Practice in Intellectual Disability 5*, 1, 61–63.

Williams, V. (2013) *Learning Disability Policy and Practice: Changing Lives?* London: Palgrave MacMillan.

9

Family Experiences of Supporting a Person with Down Syndrome and Dementia in Australia

Rachel Carling-Jenkins, Christine Bigby, Teresa Iacono

Introduction

The path to diagnosis and support for people with Down syndrome and dementia who live with their family can be convoluted and unnecessarily complex. The journey is particularly fraught for families who have little or no contact with intellectual disability services at the time of diagnosis. This chapter describes the experiences of four families who participated in research funded by Alzheimer's Australia that examined potential service models for people with an intellectual disability diagnosed with dementia. This snapshot of family experiences illustrates the diversity of family constellations and cultural backgrounds in Australia, the anxiety associated with diagnosis of early onset dementia, and the difficulties encountered in gaining access to skilled support and appropriate services.

Most people with Down syndrome diagnosed with dementia in Australia live in a family environment with their parents or siblings, or in small group homes of between four and six people, which form the backbone of the intellectual disability service system. A minority live in residential aged care, either in large nursing homes or smaller hostel setting; others live in their own homes in the community with drop-in support from disability services or generic home care services. Despite various initiatives to trial services for people aging with an intellectual disability, a clear policy framework has yet to be developed, and services remain largely unprepared to respond to the needs of people with an intellectual disability diagnosed with dementia or to support their families (Bigby, 2008, 2010). The four accounts of family experiences encapsulate the breadth of issues that require attention from the perspective of policy, programme design and frontline practice in both the disability and aged care system in Australia.

Paula

Paula was the youngest daughter of Italian immigrants who spoke little English. She was born with Down syndrome, and doctors told her parents she would not live beyond the age of 16. Paula's mother had always regarded Paula as her 'baby' and attached little importance to encouraging her to develop independence skills. Paula attended a special school for two years, but after one day refusing to get on the bus, her mother decided she could stay at home. School was the only contact Paula or her family had with intellectual disability services during her childhood. When Paula lived beyond the age of 16, her mother began to lose confidence in what she was told by doctors. She struggled to care for Paula; nagged by thoughts that she was responsible for Paula's disability. Despite being eligible for a Disability Support pension from the age of 16, no claim was made on Paula's behalf and her parents continued to support Paula with all aspects of her life as she entered adulthood.

When they left home, Paula's two sisters and brother settled near the family home, and this close-knit family often socialised together. Paula's family described her as 'the life of the party' – always wanting to dance at weddings and go out for coffee. She was her mother's favourite and her siblings did jobs for her, drove her around as she did not like to walk, and acceded to her demands for attention. Paula loved to read books, and to eat her favourite food. She was a fussy eater and her mother often cooked separate meals for her. Generous servings and a lack of exercise combined to cause her gradually to become obese.

Things changed for Paula when she reached her late 40s. Her social skills deteriorated and she made increasingly vocal demands for food and attention. At first, her family thought it might be related to her mother's recent cancer treatment and changes to the household. Her widowed eldest sister Mara had moved back to the family home to help her father provide care for both Paula and her mother. Increasingly, Mara became the primary carer for Paula as well as for her mother. However, while her mother recovered well from cancer treatment, Paula did not improve. Instead she became more and more demanding and increasingly aggressive.

Mara took Paula to the GP to get some help. Apart from a prescription for anti-depressants for herself, the doctor had little to suggest. Mara began to think the change in Paula's behaviour might be related to her intellectual disability, and searched out disability organisations for help. After numerous phone calls that offered little, a worker from an intellectual disability organisation suggested she call the tertiary university clinic that worked exclusively with people with intellectual disabilities.

By the time Mara got this information she felt unable to cope. Paula had become unsettled at night and Mara moved into her room. Paula refused to go grocery shopping anymore and Mara was afraid to leave her at home with her frail mother. Mara finally secured Paula an appointment with a psychiatrist specialising in intellectual disabilities and dementia at the university clinic. Over the course of two visits, the psychiatrist diagnosed Paula with dementia.

The family were very upset with the diagnosis. Paula's mother denied that there was anything wrong with her daughter – after all, the doctors had been wrong when Paula was born, so they were probably wrong again. Paula's father and siblings were relieved by the diagnosis as it helped to explain what had been happening to Paula. They had been wondering whether it was their fault and if their actions had been triggering Paula's behaviour.

Paula's health and capacity gradually declined over the following two years. The family received very little help. An occupational therapist gave advice on supporting Paula to exercise and take part in meaningful activities, but the family struggled to act on this. The local council organised an aged care package to provide some in-home respite for Mara and her mother. The package was in her mother's name, as it was considered 'too hard' to get one for Paula as she was only 49, below the age-related eligibility criteria of 65. The family had little experience of services or workers coming into their home, and although the in-home respite was designed to give Mara a break, her mother preferred Mara to stay when the carers were in the house.

By the time of her 50th birthday, Paula was in mid stage dementia. A reassessment of the support package enabled funding for a personal care worker to assist Paula to shower three days a week. Mara, now aged in her 60s, provided most of Paula's care. Her brother and other sister helped, but had responsibilities to their own children and partners that had to be met. The family were adamant that they would always look after Paula at home, insisting she would never be moved to an aged care facility. Mara did ask the researcher, 'How long do you think she will live?' on several occasions. She felt guilty about asking and always reiterated her commitment to look after Paula and her mother for as long as it was necessary.

Jana

Jana was the eldest daughter of Australian-born parents. Her parents were told she would be best cared for in an institution, and they should not have any more children due to the high risk of another with Down syndrome. Her parents kept Jana at home and when they decided to adopt another child were told it would only be approved if Jana was in an institution. They refused and eventually conceived another biological child, a daughter without an intellectual disability.

Jana's parents were determined that she would live as normal a life as possible. They became adept at creative solutions to overcome some of the difficulties she confronted. In the 1960s, when she was a toddler, her father bought a large doll's pram because there were no walkers for children; he weighted it with bricks to make it stable and Jana learnt to walk by pushing it around. Her sister taught her to read and write. When Jana left special school, she began work at the sheltered workshop affiliated with the school. She proved to be a good worker and was 'promoted' to work in an opportunity shop where she sorted clothes and talked with the customers.

Jana loved clothes and always dressed impeccably, carefully matching her jewellery, shoes and handbag. She had a wide circle of friends, some from school and some from work. Her father often drove her to a friend's house, or Jana entertained people at home. Jana loved to shop, often spending hours in the shopping centre where shop owners greeted her by name and helped her make choices. Jana had her own money (from her employment and the Disability Support pension) and her parents helped her to manage her bank account and budget.

When Jana's father retired, she travelled extensively with her parents, both around Australia and internationally. Jana particularly loved the family's caravan, and had her own set of self-allocated jobs when they travelled. She took care of her own suitcase, packed and unpacked the caravan to a set routine. When she was home from travelling she returned to work in the opportunity shop.

Jana travelled independently to and from work in a taxi, benefitting from the government subsidised fares for people with disability. On the way to work one day, Jana was sexually assaulted by the taxi driver. The trauma that followed this incident eventually led to her giving up work. For a period she received individualised support from a direct care worker for a few hours a day, several days a week to rebuild her confidence. Together they went on day trips, shopping or visited her friends.

One day when Jana was in her late 40s, she began to make loud noises at the dinner table. At first her parents thought she was doing this on purpose and sent her to her room as punishment, something they said they later regretted. Over the next several weeks, she began shouting at various times during the day as well. Jana's parents took her to the general practitioner (GP) concerned that something may be wrong. The GP said he could find nothing and her shouting seemed to settle down.

Not long after, however, Jana was refusing to get out of bed except to go to the toilet and shower. This continued for several weeks. Her parents could not coax her up, and the support worker began to do craft activities with Jana while she was in bed. Now and again, Jana could be coaxed to go out, and on one occasion went to a restaurant, but froze on the doorstep unable to go into the foyer. The tiles inside were black and white, and she refused to walk on them until the support worker persuaded her to close her eyes and let herself be guided over them. Shaken by this incident, Jana didn't leave the house for some weeks.

When her parents decided on another caravan holiday to cheer her up, Jana seemed enthusiastic. She had difficulty, however, following her usual routine of packing. She put her clothes in the case without the usual care and chose combinations that did not match. She left her camera at home, and barely noticed it was missing, despite the fact that on previous holidays she had been an avid photographer.

Her parents found it difficult to cope with Jana's uncharacteristic behaviour, and her father's heart condition meant more of the household activities fell on her mother. A private psychiatrist diagnosed Jana with dementia, but her parents would not accept this diagnosis and did not make any follow-up appointments. Jana continued to 'not be herself', becoming disinterested in her many previous interests and forgetting who some of her friends were. Her parents eventually took her to a GP who made a referral to another psychiatrist. Jana was again diagnosed with dementia but her parents still refused to accept it.

Her mother found it difficult to look after both Jana and her father, and eventually, an acute health episode meant she landed in hospital. The hospital social worker suggested that Jana move to a residential aged care facility to give her parents a break. Jana's parents reluctantly agreed and, to afford the fees, sold their home and moved into a small unit. Things did not go well for Jana in the aged care facility: she was accused of disturbing the other residents; wandered through the building's corridors; became very possessive of the piano; screamed when people walked into her room; and refused to go outside. Nursing staff complained they were not trained to look after someone with an intellectual disability, and family members of other residents complained to the management that the facility was not suitable for her. Finally, when the management discovered Jana's diagnosis of dementia had not been disclosed, they asked her parents to find somewhere else for her.

Jana's sister found a place in a specialist dementia care facility close to her parent's home. The staff talked compassionately with Jana's parents about her dementia. They organised a senior staff member from her former disability service to meet with them to discuss Down syndrome in general and Jana in particular. This discussion helped the facility staff to focus on Jana as a person rather than on her intellectual disability, and begin to problem-solve. Jana's parents were welcomed at the facility, and allocated the job of running 'happy hour' on Fridays, which they enjoyed immensely. Whilst staff often said it was like taking on three people, they did so with a smile, and genuinely liked the family. When she progressed to end stage dementia, staff helped the family to prepare for her death, and provided palliative care to Jana. Jana's parents spoke highly of the time she had spent in this facility.

Rowan

Rowan was the younger of two boys and had Down syndrome. He lived in the suburbs with his parents. After attending a special school, he began to work in sheltered employment. Around this time, Rowan's father passed away and his brother moved interstate. Rowan and his mother continued to live in the family home, now alone, and developed a very close relationship. Rowan did the 'men's jobs' such as lawn mowing and taking out the rubbish, while his mother shopped, cooked and cleaned for them both. On weekends, they attended church together and occasionally visited friends. Generally, they kept to themselves, playing board games or watching the television together in the evenings. Rowan was an easy-going man, always quick to smile and offer sympathy to people around him. He prided himself on being helpful. While Rowan needed prompting to complete personal care tasks, he was quite independent.

When his mother became ill, Rowan looked after her. But it became difficult for him to manage the household and look after her, and eventually his mother agreed to consider moving. She was also worried how Rowan would manage without her. The Aged Care Assessment Service assessed her as eligible for residential aged care and, having evaluated her relationship with Rowan as 'co-dependent', recommended they should not be separated. Rowan moved into an aged care hostel with his mother, despite being in his late 40s, and not eligible in his own right for a place. Rowan wanted to stay with his mother even though this meant he had to give up work. Rowan's brother, who still lived interstate, was supportive and promised his mother he would ensure Rowan could stay at the hostel after her death. Rowan and his mother settled well into the hostel. Rowan was very congenial to staff, helped with the laundry and attended to his mother's needs whenever he could. He became a 'mascot' within the service, and staff and residents alike smiled at his attempts to be helpful.

Rowan's mother died when he was in his early 50s. The hostel agreed to let Rowan stay, and the arrangement worked well for several years during which he continued to help staff with the laundry, and get on well with everyone. He received very few visitors, and the hostel staff and fellow residents became his surrogate family.

The first signs of change came when Rowan began to resist staff prompts to shower, and to stand in the doorway of his room for hours at a time. He stopped helping with the laundry and could not be persuaded to sit down to eat. Staff became impatient with Rowan's behaviour and eventually called in a specialist geriatric behaviour team to assist. They told the team they felt they could no longer provide a home for him and wanted Rowan to be moved.

A nurse in the geriatric behaviour team understood the association between Down syndrome and dementia, and suspected that this might explain what had been happening to Rowan. An assessment confirmed her suspicion that Rowan had dementia and the nurse took on short-term case management for him. She assessed the hostel as no longer a suitable environment for Rowan. The staff were unsupportive, the staff to resident ratio was too low to ensure his needs could be met adequately, and he had difficulty navigating its open plan design. Although Rowan's brother was bitterly opposed to a move to a residential aged care facility, wanting to keep the promise to his mother, there was no alternative. Rowan moved into a modern residential aged care facility and some of his changed behaviour, such as standing in doorways and refusing to eat diminished. He enjoyed walking the wide, spacious circular hallways and seemed comfortable sitting in the large dining room for lunch. Staff wondered if it reminded him of the dining room at the workshop he used to attend. His brother continued to visit occasionally. Sometimes Rowan did not appear to recognise his brother, but always did so at Christmas when he brought in a Christmas stocking to share with him, a family tradition since childhood. Rowan continued to live at the facility until his death, in the end stages of dementia.

Connor

Connor was the youngest in the family, and had an older brother and sister; he had Down syndrome. Connor's father died when he was young, resulting in his mother returning to work full-time. Connor needed a lot of supervision and never really learned to do things for himself, such as showering. When Connor left special school, he worked with his mother doing odd jobs in a number of pubs. Connor travelled with her in their van, helping out where he could, and chatting to the bar staff. Everyone knew Connor as a friendly, likeable chap, always ready to laugh at their jokes. On weekends, he spent time with his brother and sister's families, and quickly became a favourite uncle when the nieces and nephews arrived. Often, he went out for a beer with his brother, or they would share a drink on the back veranda at home. Connor cherished the times he spent with his brother. Connor's family loved to go out to restaurants and to the theatre, and Connor enjoyed getting dressed up to go out with them.

Connor was in his late 30s when his mother died. As well as losing his mother he also lost his job, his daily routine and his home when he moved in with his sister. He began going to a day programme for people with intellectual disabilities. Connor seemed unhappy at his sister's and when things hadn't improved after a couple of years, the family decided he should try living with his brother instead. He was familiar with his brother's home, having spent weekends there on a regular basis, and continued at the same day programme.

Connor initially seemed to love living with his brother, his wife, and their high-school age children. They lived on acreage outside of town in an architect designed open-plan house with multiple levels and many steps. Connor settled into a routine of going to the day programme during the week, out with his brother on weekends, shopping with his sister-in-law and spending some holiday time with his sister. Connor was often the first to arrive home. He usually let himself in and sat in his favourite chair to wait for the family to arrive home from work or school.

Gradually, Connor's behaviour changed. He no longer wanted to go out on weekends; he started stumbling over the many stairs, and favoured staying on the downstairs level of the house. It became difficult to encourage him to go upstairs to bed at night. Connor took less care of himself, refusing to step into the shower, and required more supervision with personal care from his brother or sister-in-law. Once when the family went out to a restaurant, Connor couldn't seem to make himself step over the threshold. Restaurant staff eventually found a mat which Connor was able to walk over to exit the building. Visits to restaurants and theatres became increasingly difficult. He found it difficult to cope with the fast-paced schedule at the day programme, and was moved to a slower-paced programme within the same organisation. Fortunately, this meant that the bus driver stayed the same, so Connor continued to be happy to leave for day placement each day.

Over the course of a few months, things progressively worsened for Connor and his family. Determined to do their best by Connor, they decided to sell their house and move into a more traditional dwelling where Connor could have a bedroom on the ground floor. His sister-in-law gave up her job to be home with him more, now that it was clear that Connor needed supervision at all times. The family bought a new lounge suite, but Connor seemed upset at his missing chair, so they put his old chair in the lounge. This is where he could often be found, sitting contentedly. Connor no longer went shopping, or out on weekends, but the family seemed to cope – especially with his sister-in-law at home. She simply did the shopping during the day while Connor was out, and they made sure someone was always home with him. The children were older now, starting university and jobs, so they were able to help supervise him more as well.

After 12 months, Connor began to hit his head and claim that 'something was wrong'. He asked for beer at all times of the day, but seemed content when he was given a beer mug with water in it, and was occasionally incontinent. His sister-in-law decided it was time to have Connor assessed by a specialist, although the GP had assured her nothing was wrong. She phoned a community health centre, amongst other places, and was referred to a psychiatrist, who diagnosed Connor with dementia. Suddenly, so many of Connor's behaviours made sense to his brother. But Connor's sister refused to believe the diagnosis, and tried to have Connor move back in with her. This caused family tension and, for a brief period of time, looked set to end in a guardianship hearing.

Connor's brother and his family were determined to care for him at home as long as possible. When his dementia progressed to later stages and the physical care he required became too much for his sister-in-law, he moved into a residential aged care facility. Connor's brother had visited a number of facilities close to their home 'just in case' so when the need arose, the move did not have to be rushed.

Implications

These four vignettes have in common with previous research the long-term commitment by families to care for a member with an intellectual disability, often with little assistance from external support services (Janicki *et al.*, 2010). In some respects, these parents represent the generation whose children with an intellectual disability were born in the 1950s and 60s who, rather than placing their child in institutional care, chose to keep their child at home, relying on their own resources to cope (Bigby and Atkinson, 2010). In light of the short lifespan of people with intellectual disabilities at that time, these families had little way of knowing the potential issues they would face as their family member aged.

In fact, these parents did not expect their child to live to adulthood, much less to outlive them, as was the case with Rowan and Connor. Parents and siblings alike cared deeply for their family member with an intellectual disability and struggled to understand the changes in personality and behaviour that occurred in middle-age.

These family members had no forewarning that they might have to support the person through the early onset of a progressive terminal condition, such as dementia. Families coped with a sense of guilt as they struggled to get good information, advice or support from health, disability and community services. Three of the four families found their way, somewhat serendipitously, to an aged care system that had an unpredictable and inconsistent capacity to provide care to people with intellectual disabilities and dementia, or support to their families. Left essentially on their own to navigate the early stages of dementia, the quality of care these families provided, their resilience and depth of commitment demonstrate the enduring role that families play in the quality of life for people with intellectual disabilities. Family care can seldom be replicated by formal services (Bigby, 1997; Litwak, 1985) but as these vignettes illustrate there is ample room for it to be complemented by more coherent and informed responses by health, aged and disability systems.

Lack of knowledge about dementia and risks of early onset among some groups

The vignettes point to a lack of knowledge by families about the higher risks of dementia faced by people with Down syndrome. For these families, as has been found in other studies, this causes unnecessary anxiety as they ponder explanations for changes or come to terms with an unexpected diagnosis (Carling-Jenkins *et al.*, 2012). For example, the refusal of Connor's sister to accept that he had dementia caused friction with her brother that came close to involving lawyers and a guardianship board hearing. Had she been aware of the link between Down syndrome and early onset dementia, this diversion of energy and the additional stress and anxiety in the family could have been avoided. Denial or unpreparedness for the possibility of early onset dementia may add to the delay in gaining access to appropriate services (Auty and Scior, 2008). The denial by Jana's parents, for instance, and their failure to disclose the diagnosis to the residential aged care facility where she was placed initially possibly meant that the placement was inappropriate, but also that staff were not fully aware of her needs.

The families in this study experienced a sense of guilt, reflecting that reported for other families in which a member without an underlying disability of intellectual disability has been diagnosed with dementia. As Buijssen (2005, p. 11) found, for example, 'when one talks with relatives of people with dementia about their worries and their problems, sooner or later the question of guilt will rise to the surface. "Am I doing it properly?", "Am I doing enough?", "If only I had not".' A greater understanding of the trajectory of dementia can potentially lessen this sense of guilt. For example, if Rowan's brother had understood better the implications of leaving Rowan within an unsuitable environment, he may have felt easier about going against his mother's wishes that Rowan stay in the hostel. Similarly, Mara's guilt over wanting to know how long Paula would live was assuaged through a discussion on the progression of dementia that helped her to prepare for what she would be facing in the future.

Families, including both parents and siblings of people with intellectual disabilities, need access to knowledge about risks of early onset dementia, the nature of the condition and potential sources of expertise and help. Some may benefit too from mutual support groups as they confront their reactions to and the implications of this very difficult diagnosis of their family member. In Australia, where families have been marginalised in the move to an individualised service system, it is not clear where responsibility for this type of education and knowledge dissemination might lie. There are national bodies with state branches that reach out to families and other informal carers of people with disabilities, such as the Carers Association or Down Syndrome Australia, which might be well placed to take on this task. While mainstream organisations, such as Alzheimer's Australia, have a role in community education, families of middle-aged people who are not usually considered at risk of dementia are unlikely to look to this source of information.

The vignettes reported here also demonstrate that difficulties that seemed to arise from the lack of knowledge among families were exacerbated by a similar unawareness among professionals. Although modules about intellectual disability are now integral to some medical undergraduate training in Australia, the study demonstrates that the medical profession has a long way to go in equipping general practitioners with sufficient knowledge to identify and respond appropriately to symptoms of first stage dementia in people with intellectual disabilities. This may be due also to the tendency for other symptoms to be overshadowed by intellectual disability. In Australia, there are at best only one or two specialist health services for people with intellectual disabilities in each state (Koritsas et al., 2012), which aim mostly to provide secondary consultation to health professionals, rather than primary care services. Neither is there a specialist cadre of psychiatrists, similar to that in the UK on which mainstream services can call for knowledge about health needs of people with intellectual disabilities (Jess *et al.*, 2007). The heavy reliance of people with intellectual disabilities on mainstream health professionals to meet their needs in Australia suggests the ongoing need for continuing professional education in this area among general practitioners and others in the medical profession.

The vignettes highlight that some families have, for various reasons, remained distant from disability support services and are unfamiliar with potential supports, such as respite care or in-home support. As was the case with Paula and her family, their hesitancy, the need to introduce services gradually and not make assumptions about a family's capacity to follow through in care plans must be taken into account by professionals. Allied health professionals and social workers can provide a role in assisting families if they have an understanding about a family's history, and the nature of disability support services that can be provided over time, as well as knowledge of intellectual disability and ageing. Hence, content on intellectual disability has relevance in the undergraduate curricula and training of these professionals.

Previous research has pointed to the limited knowledge about age associated issues of staff in intellectual disability services (Bigby, 2004; Webber *et al.*, 2010). This, together with the lack of an agreed identifiable pathway to diagnosis of dementia and early support for people with an intellectual disability contributed to the delay in gaining assistance.

No clear pathways to diagnosis and support

The State of Victoria, where the study was conducted, has made very few programmatic responses to people who are ageing with intellectual disabilities in general, or those with early onset dementia, in particular, reflecting the situation across Australia. Unlike in Ireland, for example, neither disability nor aged care services have developed expertise in this area, and reliance is placed on access to the same diagnostic, assessment and support services available to all older people. In Victoria, Aged Care Assessment Services (ACAS) and Cognitive, Dementia and Memory Services (CDAMS) provide gateway assessments into aged care services. However, the age-related eligibility criteria of 65 years (or thereabouts) create a major impediment to access by people aged 50–65 years. Some evidence suggests that neither ACAS nor CDAMS have the necessary confidence or expertise in regard to people with intellectual disabilities (Bigby and Torr, 2011).

Similar to the experiences of the families discussed earlier, clinical experience and research has identified the absence of dementia care pathways for people with an intellectual disability, leading to diagnostic overshadowing, carer stress and poor quality care (Carling-Jenkins *et al.*, 2012; Runge *et al.*, 2009; Bigby and Torr, 2011). Each of the four families whose stories are presented here experienced an ad hoc pathway to diagnosis, largely dependent on coming across a professional who understood the changes seen in these adults as potential indicators of cognitive decline associated with dementia. It is difficult to predict how their journeys may have differed had there been a clearly mapped and more direct pathway to diagnosis. Would Connor's family have avoided having to sell their home, or Rowan's hostel staff been more willing to engage in a constructive process to ease transition into a dementia care facility, and thereby reduced the potential for emotional, physical and financial stress (Auty and Scior, 2008; Janicki and Dalton, 2000)?

Whilst each of the families was initially determined for their loved one to age in place, this can be very difficult to achieve within the family home (Carling-Jenkins *et al.*, 2012; Janicki *et al.*, 2010). There is evidence that support can be provided within the person's home during the early stage of dementia (Hales *et al.*, 2006), but increasing care needs, especially in relation to deteriorating medical conditions associated with late stage dementia, can mean a tipping point is reached where specialist care, whether dementia specific or palliative, becomes necessary (Janicki, 2011). The deteriorating health of Jana, for example, meant that her ageing parents could no longer care for Jana at home. It would seem that provision of support to families to provide the care that is within their capacities and to prepare for transition to external care has the potential to both improve the quality of life for the person with an intellectual disability and dementia, and reduce the experience of burden on families (Janicki, 2011). There is a need, however, for policy to drive the provision of in-home support and planned transition to avoid the experience of a system that reacts to crisis.

In Australia, there is a need for recognition in health and aged care policies of the early onset of age-related disorders, such as dementia, in people with intellectual disabilities and in particular the increased risk associated with Down syndrome (Bigby and Torr, 2011). It is necessary to remove the barriers to health, assessment, diagnostic and care services for age-related conditions. Australian disability services are in the early stages of a major reform, a National Disability Insurance Scheme (2013), which will double the funding to services and introduce a consumer-driven individualised system of funding. The reformed disability system will only fund 'reasonable and necessary support' and not those considered to be the responsibility of other services systems. It is likely to act as a catalyst for improved access and responsiveness of mainstream services, such as ACAS and CDAMS services. The reforms will also help to ensure the type of coordination and case management functions are in place that were missing for the families in our study.

Conclusion

On a final note, this study, like others, has identified the role of siblings as well as parents in the lives of people with intellectual disabilities as they age (Bigby, 2004; Heller and Arnold, 2010), suggesting the need to move away from simply talking about parents and carers and return to thinking more broadly about families. There is a long way to go in Australia to hone the health, disability and aged care service systems to respond well to people with an intellectual disability and dementia, but reforms hold significant promise for the future. Despite the difficulties experienced by families in our study who have struggled to cope with the progression of dementia in their son/daughter, brother/sister, their determination can lead to good quality care: Paula is living out her days in a close-knit family committed to keeping her at home; Jana died peacefully in an aged care facility surrounded by her family; Rowan lived well in a similar facility surrounded by supportive staff who seemed genuinely to care for him; and Connor made a planned and smoothly executed move to an aged care facility when, in later stages, the physical requirements of care became too much for his family to manage.

References

Auty, E. and Scior, K. (2008) Psychologists' clinical practices in assessing dementia in individuals with Down's syndrome. *Journal of Policy and Practice in Intellectual Disabilities 5*, 4, 259–268. doi:10.1111/j.1741-1130.2008.00187.x.

Bigby, C. (1997) When parents relinquish care. The informal support networks of older people with intellectual disability. *Journal of Applied Intellectual Disability Research 10*, 4, 333–344.

Bigby, C. (2004) *Ageing with a Lifelong Disability: A Guide To Practice, Program and Policy Issues for Human Services Professionals.* London: Jessica Kingsley Publishers.

Bigby, C. (2008) Beset by obstacles: A review of Australian policy development to support aging in place for people with intellectual disability. *Journal of Intellectual and Developmental Disabilities 33*, 1, 1–11.

Bigby, C. (2010) A five-country comparative review of accommodation support policies for older people with intellectual disability. *Journal of Policy and Practice in Intellectual Disabilities 7*, 1, 3–15.

Bigby, C. and Atkinson, D. (2010) Written out of history: Invisible women in intellectual disability social work. *Australian Social Work 63*, 1, 4–17.

Bigby, C. and Torr, J. (2011) Aging with an intellectual disability: Issues, evidence and solutions. In C. Bigby and C. Fyffe (eds) *State Disability Policy for the Next Ten Years – What Should it Look Like? Proceedings of the Fifth Roundtable on Intellectual Disability Policy.* Bundoora: La Trobe University.

Buijssen, H. (2005) *The Simplicity of Dementia: A Guide for Family and Carers.* London: Jessica Kingsley Publishers.

Carling-Jenkins, R., Torr, J., Iacona, T. and Bigby, C. (2012) Experiences of supporting people with Down's syndrome and Alzheimer's disease in aged care and family environments. *Journal of Intellectual and Developmental Disability 37*, 1, 54–60.

Hales, C., Ross, L. and Ryan, C. (2006) *National Evaluation of the Aged Care Innovative Pool Disability Aged Care Interface Pilot: Final Report.* Canberra: Australian Institute of Health and Welfare.

Heller, T. and Arnold, C. (2010) Siblings of adults with developmental disabilities: Psychosocial outcomes, relationships and future planning. *Journal of Policy and Practice in Intellectual Disabilities 7*, 1, 16–25.

Janicki, M. (2011) Quality outcomes in group home dementia care for adults with intellectual disabilities. *Journal of Intellectual Disability Research 55*, 8, 763–776.

Janicki, MP. and Dalton, AJ. (2000) Prevalence of dementia and impact on disability services. *Mental Retardation 38*, 3, 276–288.

Janicki, MP., Zendell, A. and DeHaven, K. (2010) Coping with dementia and older families of adults with Down's syndrome. *Dementia 9*, 3, 391–407.

Jess, G., Torr, J., Cooper, S-A. *et al.* (2007) Specialist versus generic models of psychiatry training and service provision for people with intellectual disabilities. *Journal of Applied Research in Intellectual Disabilities 21*, 2, 183–193.

Koritsas, S., Iacono, T. and Davis, R. (2012) Australian general practitioner uptake of a remunerated medicare health assessment for people with intellectual disability. *Journal of Intellectual and Developmental Disability 37*, 2, 151–154.

Litwak, E. (1985) *Helping the Elderly.* New York, NY: Guilford Press.

National Disability Insurance Scheme Act (2013) Commonwealth of Australia.

Runge, C., Gilham, J. and Peut, A. (2009) *Transitions in Care of People with Dementia: A Systematic Review of the Literature.* Canberra: Australian Institute of Health and Welfare.

Webber, R., Bowers, B. and Bigby, C. (2010) Hospital experiences of older people with intellectual disability. *Journal of Intellectual and Developmental Disability 35*, 3, 155–164.

10

Planning Ahead
Supporting Families to Shape the Future after a Diagnosis of Dementia

Christine Towers, Heather Wilkinson

Introduction

A diagnosis of dementia has major implications for a person with an intellectual disability and their family. As growing numbers of people with intellectual disabilities live to an older age and develop this and other age-related illnesses and conditions, it is important to find strategies to help families cope.

Family carers often find it difficult to think about and plan for the future when they have a son or daughter with intellectual disabilities, especially when they themselves are older. Their perception of the need to plan ahead is likely to change as they will have to think about, and come to terms with, a different future. The immediate focus is more likely to be on the diagnosis and coping with day-to-day matters. Families may feel that practitioners and service providers have more expertise regarding the long-term needs of people with intellectual disabilities and dementia and can lose sight of the wealth of knowledge and understanding they themselves have of their relative and what is important in their life.

Families in this situation need to have opportunities to think ahead, consider options and to have information written down. This will improve the likelihood of their relative being well supported and having a secure and contented future whilst living with dementia. Planning will help to get the right supports in place for the immediate future and also to consider options for the longer term as their relative's needs change. The person with an intellectual disability needs to be involved in this planning as far as possible, especially before their dementia makes any input more difficult. Planning in this way should help to reduce stress and anxiety for both the person with dementia and their family carers. It is also an opportunity to make arrangements for the possibility that the person with intellectual disabilities and dementia outlives their family carers.

This chapter looks at the ways in which practitioners can support families to carry out this planning. Practitioners may have experience of working with people with intellectual disabilities or people with dementia, or they may have supported family carers, but they are unlikely to have worked in an environment where they bring together practices from all three areas.

The key approaches and thinking underlying this chapter are that the individual with an intellectual disability should be involved as much as possible in discussions, about how best to support them and to ensure they receive appropriate healthcare treatments. Families usually know the person best and their knowledge and understanding is central to finding the right solutions. Using person-centred tools and bringing together a group of people who know and care about the person, will gather different perspectives and lead to creative ways of supporting the person. Practitioners may bring their own expertise, for example around good practice in dementia care or arranging individualised support. Planning will be most effective when all of this expertise is combined in the assessment and support planning processes. The contribution of families was essential to the planning and development of the Thinking Ahead research.

Whilst the focus here is on supporting families after their relative has received a diagnosis of dementia, the suggestions and our learning could be used to help any family with an adult relative with an intellectual disability to be prepared for other unexpected future events.

Coping with dementia and planning for the future

The increased and increasing number of people living with intellectual disabilities and dementia poses significant new challenges, not just for those experiencing the symptoms, but also for their family carers, and health and social services (Llewellyn, 2011). Yet, existing research mainly focuses on the experiences of staff in intellectual disability services, with much less known about the experiences of caregiving in the family context (Courtenay et al., 2010).

Family carers of people with Down syndrome aged over 35 years old and living at home have been identified as 'adaptive copers'. This group are settled in their long-term caring role and do not show the extent of health-related issues typically identified among carers in the general population of people with dementia (Janicki *et al.*, 2010). However, less is known about how these respond to the onset of dementia symptoms, or about their own needs when supporting someone with intellectual disabilities and dementia, either at home or elsewhere. A recent study of family carers of adults with Down syndrome and dementia (Furniss *et al.*, 2011) found that they felt a huge sense of responsibility and commitment towards caring for their family member at home, were willing to sacrifice their own needs, and showed signs of emotional and physical strain.

McLaughlin and Jones (2011) undertook a qualitative study to determine the information and support needs of carers of adults who had Down syndrome and dementia. They found that carers' information and support needs were seen to change at the stages of pre-diagnosis, diagnosis and post-diagnosis. Supporting carers to manage the changing and progressive nature of dementia is considered to be an essential part of the health professional's role (McLaughlin and Jones, 2011).

Much of the research about families planning for the future has focused on older family carers (usually defined as aged 60 and over). This is typically relevant to the experience of parents whose son or daughter is diagnosed with dementia as they are likely to fall within this age category. Research with older family carers indicates that whilst the majority have not made plans for the future, this does not mean that they are not thinking about it. Older carers are described as living in a state of increasing stress and anxiety about the future or as being fatalistic (Johnston and Martin, 2005), burying their heads in the sand (Davys *et al.*, 2010); and hoping, or assuming, that they will outlive their son or daughter with intellectual disabilities (Bowey and McGlaughlin, 2007; Hubert and Hollins, 2000; Johnston and Martin, 2005; Stafford, 2010).

Research literature also shows that there are many practical and emotional barriers that have prevented older carers from planning for the future. Older carers may feel guilty for thinking of the prospect of letting go of their caring responsibilities (Bowey and McGlaughlin, 2007). They may have had a negative experience seeking help from statutory services in the past, they may worry that a request for help is interpreted as not being able to cope, and they may worry that their son or daughter would be taken away from them if they seek help (Hubert and Hollins, 2000). Parents have to be supported to prepare themselves for the idea of relinquishing their role as primary carer (Freedman et al., 1997), which can be a stressful transition for any family to make (Dillenburger and McKerr, 2009).

Other barriers to future planning for older carers is a historical mistrust of services (Davys and Haigh, 2008); and dissatisfaction with the range and quality of care available (Bowey and McGlaughlin, 2007; Dillenburger and McKerr, 2009). Older carers are worried that future carers of their family member will not offer continuity of care or will not be reliable (Johnston and Martin, 2005). Services are perceived as changeable and unstable (Mansell and Wilson, 2010), a concern that has become even more prevalent in the current economic climate.

In addition to emotional and psychological challenges, older carers also face practical barriers in future planning. Gilbert et al. (2008) suggested that the majority of older carers are unaware of the different options for future housing and that many do not have access to the internet to research this information themselves. Siblings are commonly seen as next of kin when older parents die or become unable to continue their caring role (Davys et al., 2010). However, many older parents say that they would prefer siblings to be involved in a supervisory or advisory role or as an advocate, rather than take on the caring responsibilities themselves (Davys and Haigh, 2008; Johnston and Martin, 2005).

Gilbert et al. (2008) noted that some older carers acknowledged the need to make plans, but expressed concern about the impact on their dependent relative. This included questioning whether their son or daughter either would be able to understand why such planning was necessary with the potential for them to become distressed, or perceive this as rejection (Bowey and McGlaughlin, 2007).

Thinking Ahead research

The Thinking Ahead research was carried out by the Foundation for People with Learning Disabilities in the UK. It was developed as a result of increased concern raised by families about what would happen when they were no longer able to care for their son or daughter, along with a perceived lack of support from services to make plans that could help to reduce this worry. A planning guide was produced for families based on the research findings (Towers, 2013).

Qualitative and quantitative data was collected from people with intellectual disabilities and their parents and siblings. Workshops were held with people with intellectual disabilities to gain their perspective at the start of the project, and to ensure that their voice was heard. Resulting key messages were that people with intellectual disabilities need to be listened to and that those taking part felt better able to cope when they were involved in discussions and decision-making. The findings from these workshops helped to shape the questions that family carers were subsequently asked.

The workshops for parents and siblings were carried out in the same geographical areas and were attended by over 40 parents. They explored what each thought the barriers were to planning, and what would help to overcome these barriers. These workshops highlighted families' need for ongoing emotional and practical support in order to use their knowledge and expertise to make decisions for the future.

A national survey was also conducted to gather quantitative and qualitative information, exploring parents' experiences and what they would find most helpful. Publicity was sent out widely through intellectual disability forums and organisations supporting family carers. The data was gathered using an online survey and hard copies were provided on request for family carers without access to the internet. The results were generated from a sample size of over 300 parents with a son or daughter with intellectual disabilities aged 18 and over. The survey asked about three key areas:

- the level of worry that parents experienced about the future

- how much help they felt that they had received with planning for a future when they are no longer here to care for their son or daughter

- what would help them to plan for the future.

In relation to the first area, parents were asked to rank the level of worry they had against a number of statements. The data below shows the percentage of carers who were either worried or very worried about this aspect of their son or daughter's life:

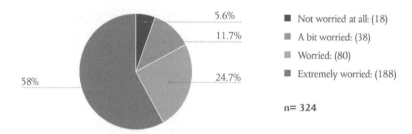

5.6%
11.7%
24.7%
58%

■ Not worried at all: (18)
■ A bit worried: (38)
■ Worried: (80)
■ Extremely worried: (188)

n= 324

Figure 10.1: Will my son or daughter have a place to live where he/she is happy?

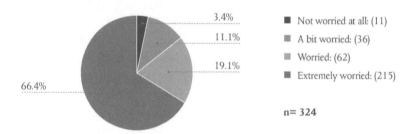

3.4%
11.1%
19.1%
66.4%

■ Not worried at all: (11)
■ A bit worried: (36)
■ Worried: (62)
■ Extremely worried: (215)

n= 324

Figure 10.2: Will my son or daughter get the support he/she needs?

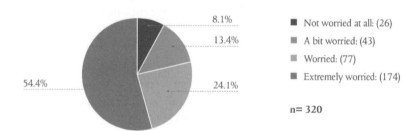

8.1%
13.4%
24.1%
54.4%

■ Not worried at all: (26)
■ A bit worried: (43)
■ Worried: (77)
■ Extremely worried: (174)

n= 320

Figure 10.3: Will anyone help my son or daughter to make decisions that are in his/her best interest?

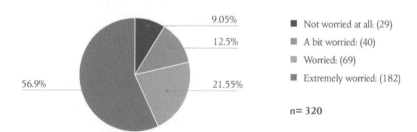

9.05%
12.5%
21.55%
56.9%

■ Not worried at all: (29)
■ A bit worried: (40)
■ Worried: (69)
■ Extremely worried: (182)

n= 320

Figure 10.4: Will anyone make sure my son or daughter is safe and well?
Source: Foundation for People with Learning Disabilities

Survey participants were also asked whether they had been spoken to or supported to look at these issues. In relation to each question, the majority said that either nobody had spoken to them, or that a conversation had taken place but nothing had subsequently happened. Yet, these questions are all central to planning a good life and will contribute to the development of sustainable and cost-effective solutions in the longer term. The survey also included open-ended questions for parents to comment on what would help them. The responses were predominantly about the provision of information in a comprehensible format and at an appropriate time, workshops with other family carers to obtain peer support, and access to practitioners who understood the emotional journey of parents when planning with their relative. A survey published in the UK by the Carers Trust (2013) supports these findings, with carers of people with dementia also emphasising their need for quality and timely information throughout their caring journey, something that was often not provided.

A planning model for families

From the research, a model of planning was developed to be used by families independent of services and organisations. This was in the knowledge that there are currently limited resources in care management and family support services to help families to be proactive about planning for the future. The model has been piloted with carers groups and care management teams, in addition to individual family carers. It lends itself to adaptation by practitioners across intellectual disability, dementia and family support organisations involved in the lives of people with intellectual disabilities and dementia.

Making plans for the future in a person-centred way

Person-centred planning involves gathering information about a person to solve problems and develop ideas, to ensure that they have the best possible life. In this context, it means keeping a focus on the individual rather than on their intellectual disability and dementia. Families may feel able to lead on this or practitioners may need to find ways to support families through the process and facilitate discussions.

The involvement of parents and other relatives in planning is paramount as it is usually families who have the most detailed knowledge about the person and it is important this does not get lost or ignored. Sometimes small details make a huge difference in the quality of a person's life. This well of knowledge is particularly important as an individual may seem to change with the onset of dementia and the person they were may be forgotten. Person-centred approaches can help to keep a focus on issues that have always been important in the person's life, a sense of continuity that is invaluable especially if formal carers or accommodation change over time. Family involvement needs to be combined with information from trained practitioners who have detailed knowledge about the signs, symptoms and progression of the different types of dementia and can offer timely advice and support.

A key point about planning in a person-centred way is that it starts with the person rather than the services that are available, producing ideas and solutions that fit the person, in order to keep them safer and maintain quality of life. Families should be encouraged to make a written record of the information they gather, so that it can be shared with others who may be involved in the support of their relative. The information can be used to develop a person-centred plan that can be adapted as their relative's needs change.

This does not need to be complicated – a few simple tools can be used to collect information. Families who have an understanding of some of the tools that help with this type of planning should find it easier to make sure their relative gets the support they need. Examples of tools that would be particularly useful in this situation will be introduced:

- Build a history/story of their life.

- Work out what is important to, and important for, the person with an intellectual disability.

- Work out what constitutes a good day, and bad day, for them.

- Make a 'people in my life' map (a map of relationships that can use photographs in addition to written names).

- Develop a profile of the ideal person they would like to be supported by.

Build a history/story of the person's life

Putting together a person's history or life story can sometimes be the easiest place to start and is especially important when someone has dementia and is losing their short-term memory and communication skills. Sharing life stories and memories can help a person with dementia to develop and affirm their sense of identity. Family members can facilitate this by supporting their relative to remember important life events, significant people and everyday memories. With permission, a life story can also be shown to people who spend time with the person socially or as a paid worker; it enables others to learn about the person before they developed dementia and aids conversations. Individualised memory boxes, which may also be multi-sensory, can also be created. Written information can be added, which others can use to support the person to reminisce.

Important to/important for

Making a list of what is important for a person helps to keep them safe, healthy and well. The list is likely to include medication, diet, meaningful activities, home adaptations and information about their daily routine. Things that are important to a person frequently get overlooked, especially when there are medical needs, but they can help to maintain wellbeing and to reduce stress. Families often have detailed knowledge of what is important to, and for, a person – a person may say what is important to them or they may show this through their actions and behaviour; for example, having a specific duvet cover on their bed, meeting up with a group of friends, eating certain foods and avoiding others, being spoken to in a certain way. Identifying what is important to and for a person helps to prioritise what needs to be put in place to make things work. This can then be used by staff supporting the person to provide support in a way that is responsive to their personality and preferences. Equally important is that it reduces the focus on the label of dementia and intellectual disabilities.

Good day/bad day

Daily routine may become more important after a diagnosis, and providing details about what makes a good day and a bad day will help establish what needs to be built in to a person's day and what needs to be avoided.

'People in my life' map

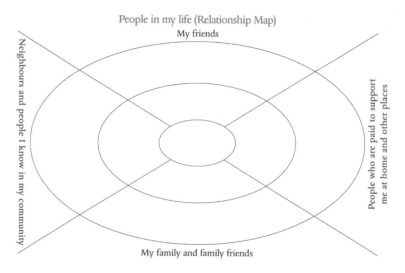

Figure 10.5: 'People in my life' relationships map

Mapping the people in a person's life can identify who could be involved in planning, making decisions, helping out in emergencies or providing social contact.

Profile of ideal support worker

Family carers and the person with an intellectual disability should be encouraged to describe the kind of people they like to be supported by. This can be used in the future to create a profile to recruit support workers who have a compatible personality, share interests, or have specific skills that the person needs or wants. Suggestions to make sure the person with intellectual disabilities and dementia is at the centre of discussions include:

- supporting individuals to be as involved as possible and finding ways for the person to take the lead, choosing who they would like to plan with, and where and when that planning should take place

- making sure any discussions are directed to the person rather than around them, not talking about them in the third person

- making sure discussions are carried out at a speed that works for each individual, giving space for them to think through their ideas about the future and support to say or indicate what they think (this may be different from what other family members are saying)

- using drawings, pictures, objects, photographs or any other resources or media that is meaningful for the individual.

For a person who finds it difficult to communicate their needs and wishes, it is even more important that there are people who can speak up for them and act as an advocate. It is best to have a number of people involved so that they can support each other and keep things going between them – some may need to take a back seat when they have pressures in their own lives. A network of support is particularly beneficial if the person's parents are frail or family no longer live nearby. Developing an informal support network, that is not paid people, is not a substitute for services and paid support, but rather a complement. The two should work together to improve the person's life and keep them safe.

Parents often need encouragement to accept that it is all right to ask other people to become involved in the life of their son or daughter. They may need to hear that people like the chance to contribute to the lives of others, but may feel reluctant to offer as they do not know how to. As decisions will need to be made on a wide range of issues, it may be a good idea to help families to actively develop a Circle of Support (also known as a Circle of Friends). A Circle of Support is a group of people with a commitment to the person with an intellectual disability, who meet together on a regular basis to help the person to accomplish their personal goals in life (Foundation for People with Learning Disabilities, 2014). For a person with an intellectual disability and dementia it would be helpful if the group met regularly, contributed to person-centred planning and made sure the necessary approaches or interventions were being put into place. Families can be supported to think about who they would like to invite, so that they include people with the right mix of knowledge; for example, both intellectual disability and dementia. A family may get to know other families in the same situation and they may want to consider being part of each other's Circles to share their learning. A personal budget could be used to pay for someone with this expertise or for someone to facilitate the circle meetings. A Circle can:

- provide friendship and a sense of security at a time that may be frightening and unsettling for the person

- gather stories and bring memories of the past to share with the person

- help with planning changes, particularly significant ones such as moving home

- act as advocates, trustees or executors

- keep an eye on progression and developments, particularly when someone leaves the family home.

Making decisions

Following a diagnosis of dementia, many decisions about a person's current life or the things they would like to happen in the future may need to be taken. These may include medical treatments, the best ways of providing support and where to live. Families will require support to understand the legislation and practice that relate to decision-making, so that they feel empowered to influence decisions where possible and understand why some choices have been made.

Some people with intellectual disabilities will have the capacity to make many decisions about their life at the point of diagnosis, but may lose this with the progression of dementia. Whatever their ability, it is usually the case that the best decisions are made when it is a partnership between the person, their family and friends, and people who are paid to support them. Families may need guidance to see how their son or daughter can be involved in decisions. Suggestions to help the decision-making process include the following:

- Break down big decisions into smaller ones, which the person might be more able to make.

- If the person does not already have a communication passport, or similar, a referral could be made to a speech and language therapy service to develop one. A passport describes a person's most effective means of communication and enables others to involve the person in discussions, help them to make sense of events and contribute their thoughts as much as possible. The passport can describe how they can be best supported to make decisions and explain how emotions are expressed such as pleasure or pain.

- It may be helpful to make a written record of what has been learnt from observing specific activities and using this to inform future decisions. This log can be used by family and paid carers to look at what worked well, what did not and gauge how well any changes have gone. A written record helps to build on success and avoid repeating things that have not worked well.

Family carers may also need support to think about ways in which their relative can arrange for other people to make decisions for them in the future. Legislation in different parts of the UK includes lasting powers of attorney (LPAs) and advance decisions to refuse treatment (ADRTs). An LPA is set up to make decisions about property and financial affairs (a property and affairs power of attorney) or personal welfare, including medical treatment (a health and welfare power of attorney). An ADRT, also sometimes referred to as a living will, enables a person to stipulate which medical treatments they would not want to receive in the future. An LPA and an ADRT need to be made whilst the person has the capacity to do so, and it is therefore important that people with intellectual disabilities have the opportunity to create one before their dementia progresses. However, in order for this to happen there needs to be an explanation of why it is necessary.

Date	What was the person doing?	Who was there?	What did you learn about what worked well?	What did you learn about what didn't work?

What have we learnt that we need to do differently:

What have we learnt that we need to keep doing the same way:

Figure 10.6: Learning log

Talking about difficult subjects

Family carers are often reluctant to talk about difficult subjects with their relative with an intellectual disability as they feel protective or do not know how to broach sensitive or complex matters. They may avoid talking to their relative about dementia as they think they would be worried or would not understand. However, the research with people with intellectual disabilities in the Thinking Ahead workshops showed that people felt a greater level of anxiety when they were excluded from conversations and discussions (Towers, 2013). A person with dementia may be worried about the changes they are experiencing if they do not understand the reasons for them. Parents and other family carers are likely to need support to find ways of talking about dementia, even if the word 'dementia' is not used, and to ensure consistency in how the discussion takes place.

In the early stages of dementia (if this has not already taken place at a much earlier stage, even before the person is ill, as part of ongoing care planning) it is helpful to find ways for a family to talk about end of life planning and funeral arrangements with their relative. People with intellectual disabilities have produced resources about end of life planning, such as *We're Living Well but Dying Matters* (Change, 2011). With support, people are often able to think about how they would like to be cared for. If the person lacks the capacity to talk about these matters, their family, friends and paid supporters can discuss and make a plan together. The following are some suggestions to help families talk about difficult subjects:

- Support family carers to have conversations with their relative about other family members or friends who have/had dementia.

- Support family carers to have conversations with their relative about other family members or friends who may be ill, or be reaching the end of their life.

- Give the family a copy of *Ann has Dementia* (Hollins *et al.*, 2012) or *What is Dementia?* (Kerr and Innes, 2001) to introduce difficult topics, such as dementia.

- Suggest family carers discuss story lines about illness and death from television programmes with their relative.

- Share accessible palliative and end of life planning resources with family carers to provide a guide to this sensitive topic, such as those complied by the Palliative Care for People with Learning Disabilities Network (PCPLD Network, 2013). Palliative needs should be addressed early and not left until end of life.

Housing and support

Understanding the options for housing and support can be a challenge for family carers of people with intellectual disabilities. If their relative develops dementia, they face the additional issue of getting the right living arrangements and support as their needs change and the condition progresses. It may be difficult for families to think ahead about these issues, but if they have information in advance about the way housing and support services work and are accessed, then they can develop their ideas and may feel more prepared for the future.

Parents and other family carers of people with intellectual disabilities often worry about whether people outside the family can support their relative as well as they do. The provision of information enables them not only to make a reasoned choice, but also to realise that they do not have to cope on their own. The following key points can help family carers to understand that there are a number of choices available:

- There are alternatives to residential and nursing care including supporting people to live and age in place in their own familiar environment.

- Levels of care can be increased as the person's dementia advances, whether they are living in the family home or in supported living.

- If personal budgets are available this can provide a flexible way of arranging support that can be designed around the person and their family.

- Families can be involved in choosing support providers and/ or the people providing support.

- Additional resources can be sourced, such as adaptations to the person's current home or use of assistive technology.

If planning has not begun and a change of accommodation becomes necessary, the starting point may be when there is an available place, an approach that can lead to a person having to 'fit into' something that may not be suitable. When a person has dementia, choices are more limited and this can result in them having to move away from the area where they are known, increasing the sense of isolation and stress following a move. Family carers are likely to feel more confident about other people providing care if they have shared the information that they have gathered specifying the best ways to make sure the person is safe and well. The involvement of members of the extended family, as well as friends, to keep an eye on the quality of care and support will also provide reassurance.

Making an emergency plan

When a person is living at home with their parents or another family member it is helpful to have a plan in place for an emergency situation. The existence of such a plan helps to ensure continuity of care should a person's main carer(s) become ill or experience another form of emergency.

In the UK, carers who provide a substantial amount of care have the right to request a carer's assessment, and the local authority has a duty to respond to that request. As part of this assessment, carers should be asked about emergencies and offered help with planning them. However, this is not always carried out in enough depth, particularly when the person's support needs are complex. Suggestions are offered for developing an emergency plan:

- A good place to start is to think about the emergencies that might arise; there may be some events that are more likely to happen because of the family's situation, such as having other caring responsibilities or their own health needs.

- Families can then be supported to think about what can be put in place to mitigate the impact of an emergency: Do the right people have the right telephone numbers? Is essential information about the person easily available? Do people have spare keys?

- The response in an emergency is often to move the person to a place where they can receive support, but it may be more appropriate to consider support coming to the place where the person normally lives. The 'people in my life' map can be used to identify who might be able to help, whether by coming to stay, helping out at certain times of the day, offering reassurance over the phone or holding a spare set of keys.

Those who provide support can be family, friends and other unpaid people and/or paid supporters who already know the person. If the person has a personal budget, a request could be made for this to be increased should an emergency arise. A template for making a plan is available in the Thinking Ahead planning guide (Towers, 2013).

Summary checklist to use when supporting families
Early planning

- Make sure that plans are person-centred and developed around, and including, the individual.

- Support the family to gather relevant information using questions such as 'What is important to/for?' and 'Who are the important people in their life?'

- Look at how the person can be involved in gathering information and making plans; identify what would help them to communicate their thoughts.

- Support the family to create a life story and/or memory box.

- Provide the family with information about the symptoms, stages and likely progression of their relative's type of dementia, so that this information can inform their planning including palliative approaches.

Building friendships and relationships

- Use a 'people in my life' map to identify who is part of the person's life and who the family think could make a contribution in the future.

- Support parents, or the main family carer, to talk with other relatives (siblings, cousins, nieces and nephews) and friends about how they might help to make decisions, plan or spend time with the person.

- Look proactively at how the person's friends can continue to be part of their life and supported to understand what is happening.

- Encourage the setting-up of a Circle of Support that regularly meets to discuss ideas and put things in place; this may involve looking for a paid facilitator.

Making decisions

- Provide family carers with easy-to-understand information about relevant national legislation or best interests decisions where applicable.

- Support the family to find ways to involve their relative in making decisions about their current life and the future as much as possible.

- Ensure the person has a detailed communication passport and that there are arrangements for it to be updated should their dementia affect their ability to communicate.

- Encourage parents to involve other family members, particularly siblings, and other people important in the person's life in making decisions.

- If relevant legislation is in place, look at whether the person could set up a lasting power of attorney, either for property and affairs or health and welfare.

- Look at whether the person could make an advance decision to refuse treatment.

Talking about difficult subjects

- Provide family carers and friends with easy-to-understand information about dementia. This is in order to explain the changes being experienced at a level that can be understood by the person, and ensure consistency in this.

- Support the family to think about end of life planning and how to involve their relative.

Housing and support

- Provide family carers with detailed information about the housing and support options, including those for end of life care.

- Help families to think about the best way for personal support to be provided.

- Involve the family in putting together information that helps other people to support the person to keep safe and well.

- Encourage the involvement of extended family members and friends who are willing to help parents to keep an eye on the quality of care and carry on this role when the parents are no longer able to.

Making an emergency plan

- Find out how emergency plans are being put in place locally, who will coordinate this and whether the responsible service will draw up a plan with the family.

- Look at what 'cushions' the family could put in place to mitigate the impact of an emergency before it occurs.

- Support the family to think about who could help in an emergency.

- Ensure a plan is written down and given to the relevant people so that it is implemented when an emergency arises.

Conclusion

Families supporting a relative with an intellectual disability and dementia face many challenges when thinking about and planning for their future, yet little research is available that specifically looks at the needs of this group of carers. The Thinking Ahead model provides practitioners with a way of working alongside parents, siblings and other family carers to consider different options and to ensure individualised, person-centred information gets written down. The model is in its early days and further research is required to find out how the Thinking Ahead model could be adapted for carers of people with intellectual disabilities and dementia. However, families we support are already suggesting that it helps them to see a way of using their knowledge and understanding to shape their relatives' future for the better.

References

Bowey, L. and McGlaughlin, A. (2007) Older carers of adults with a learning disability confront the future: Issues and preferences in planning. *British Journal of Social Work 37*, 1, 39–54.

Carers Trust (2013) *A Road Less Rocky – Supporting Carers of People with Dementia.* Available at www.carers.org/sites/default/files/dementia_executive_summary_english_only_final_use_this_one.pdf, accessed on 7 December 2013.

Change (2011) *We're Living Well but Dying Matters.* Available at http://dyingmatters.org/page/were-living-well-dying-matters, accessed on 7 December 2013.

Courtenay, K., Jokinen, N. and Strydom, A. (2010) Caregiving and adults with intellectual disabilities affected by dementia. *Journal of Policy and Practice in Intellectual Disabilities 7*, 1, 26–33.

Davys, D. and Haigh, C. (2008) Older parents of people who have a learning disability: Perceptions of future accommodation needs. *British Journal of Learning Disabilities 36*, 1, 66–72.

Davys, D., Mitchell, D. and Haigh, C. (2010) Futures planning, parental expectations and sibling concern for people who have a learning disability. *Journal of Intellectual Disabilities 14*, 3, 167–183.

Dillenburger, K. and McKerr, L. (2009) *What the Future Holds: Older People Caring for Adult Sons and Daughters with Disabilities.* Report for the Changing Ageing Partnership. Belfast: Institute of Governance, School of Law, Queen's University Belfast.

Freedman, RI., Krauss, MW. and Seltzer, MM. (1997) Aging parents' residential plans for adult children with mental retardation, *Mental Retardation 35*, 2, 114–123.

Foundation for People with Learning Disabilities (2014) *Circles of Support and Circles of Friends.* Available at www.learningdisabilities.org.uk/help-information/information-for-teachers/transition-to-adulthood/building-circles-of-support, accessed on 18 December 2013.

Furniss, K., Loverseed, A., Dodd, K. and Lippold, T. (2011) The views of people who care for adults with Down's syndrome and dementia: A service evaluation. *British Journal of Learning Disabilities 40*, 12, 318–327.

Gilbert, A., Lankshear, G. and Petersen, A. (2008) Older family-carers' views on the future accommodation needs of relatives who have an intellectual disability. *International Journal of Social Welfare 17*, 1, 54–64.

Hollins, S., Blackman, N. and Eley, R. (2012) *Ann has Dementia.* London: Royal College of Psychiatrists Publications/St George's, University of London.

Hubert, J. and Hollins, S. (2000) Working with elderly carers of people with learning disabilities and planning for the future. *Advances in Psychiatric Treatment 6*, 1, 41–48.

Janicki, M., Zendell, A. and DeHaven, K. (2010) Coping with dementia and older families of adults with Down's syndrome. *Dementia 9*, 3, 391–407.

Johnston, L. and Martin, M. (2005) *Older Family Carers and Learning Disabled Adults Cared for at Home: Their Views, Thoughts and Experiences of Future Care.* South Lanarkshire: South Lanarkshire Council.

Kerr, D. and Innes, M. (2001) *What is Dementia?* Edinburgh: Down's Syndrome Scotland.

Llewellyn, P. (2011) The needs of people with learning disabilities who develop dementia: A literature review. *Dementia 10*, 2, 235–247.

McLaughlin, K. and Jones, A. (2011) It's all changed: Carers' experiences of caring for adults who have Down's syndrome and dementia. *British Journal of Learning Disabilities 39*, 1, 57–63.

Mansell, I and Wilson, C. (2010) 'It terrifies me the thought of the future': Listening to current concerns of informal carers of people with a learning disability. *Journal of Intellectual Disability 14*, 1, 21–31.

Palliative Care for People with Learning Disabilities Network (PCPLD) (2013) *Resources and Academic Articles.* Available at www.pcpld.org/links-and-resources, accessed on 7 December 2013.

Stafford, PB. (2010) 'The Age Wave: What It Means for Families' in Institute on Community Integration (UCEDD) & Research and Training Center on Community Living (ed.) *Impact Feature Issue on Aging and People with Intellectual and Developmental Disabilities 23*, 1, Winter 2010. Available at http://ici.umn.edu/products/impact/231/default.html, accessed on 21 March 2014.

Towers, C. (2013) *Thinking Ahead: A Planning Guide for Families.* London: Foundation for People with Learning Disabilities.

PART 3

Service Planning

What Are We Going to Do?

11

Sharing the Diagnosis of Dementia

Breaking Bad News to People with an Intellectual Disability

Irene Tuffrey-Wijne, Karen Watchman

Introduction

Should people with an intellectual disability be told that they have dementia? If so, what is the best way to communicate and share this type of bad news; will it even be perceived as bad news by someone who may not have an understanding of what it means to have dementia? These questions are not easy to answer when they concern people who may have always found it difficult to understand new information, and who are now in the process of losing further skills, including cognitive awareness. Staff and family members worry about how to talk to a person with an intellectual disability about dementia and how to cope with the possible response. This leads to a situation where many choose not to say anything because it is easier not to, or there may be a perception that the person will not understand. It can be tempting to break bad news quickly and move on without providing additional information or checking understanding.

We will introduce the issues around breaking bad news to people with intellectual disabilities developed by Tuffrey-Wijne (2013) following a programme of research in this field. Research offers evidence for the use of the guidelines when breaking bad news about cancer to people with intellectual disabilities. Similarly, there is evidence for the value of post-diagnostic support to older people generally when their diagnosis of dementia is known. Yet, there is far less evidence for sharing the diagnosis of dementia with a person with intellectual disabilities or how this impacts on the person, their family and friends.

After presenting an overview of the guidelines for breaking bad news, we consider their application as a model of practice when sharing a diagnosis of dementia with people with intellectual disabilities. In doing so, suggestions are made for how the guidelines could be used to help people to make sense of their changing situation. We look at the case of Tom and discuss how the consequences of not knowing his diagnosis affected him, both socially and emotionally. The application of the breaking bad news model highlights how those supporting Tom may have been able to maximise their existing and previous knowledge of Tom and how information can be communicated in 'chunks' based on his understanding. This differs from a previously seen linear, 'stepped' approach. Until now, the development of a framework or practice guidelines for giving a diagnosis of dementia to a person with an intellectual disability has not been addressed in literature. It is important to review the experiences of dementia from people with intellectual disabilities themselves, but these experiences pose difficulties for researchers if participants are not aware of their diagnosis.

Should bad news be broken?

There has been a huge shift in attitudes around disclosure of a poor prognosis to patients and their families. Whereas in the 1960s most doctors did not tell cancer patients their diagnosis (Oken, 1961), it is now widely accepted among health care professionals in Western societies that realistic and truthful disclosure is preferred to withholding information (Novack et al., 1971; Seale, 1991). Patients themselves share this view and are overwhelmingly in favour of honesty and openness (Fujimori and Uchitomi, 2009; Innes and Payne, 2009).

With a diagnosis of dementia, there is now a consensus that early disclosure is beneficial to the patient (Werner et al., 2013). Disclosure of the diagnosis is seen as the starting point for other interventions, both medical and social. The dementia strategies across the UK in England and Wales (Department of Health, 2009), Scotland (Scottish Government, 2013) and Northern Ireland (Department of Health, Social Services and Public Safety, 2011) state that everyone should be given their diagnosis. The National Institute for Health and Clinical Excellence (NICE) guidelines (2006) state that only in exceptional circumstances should information about a diagnosis of dementia be withheld from someone. Instead, discussion should take place early after diagnosis to enable the person to be involved with future planning in advance of changes in their capacity and ability to communicate.

Yet, research opinion regarding the disclosure of a diagnosis of dementia to an older person (without an intellectual disability) continues to be divided. Debate includes a consequentialist argument that diagnosis should be given only if it will be of more benefit to the patient than not sharing the information (Brodaty *et al.*, 2003). This includes the notion that sharing the diagnosis may increase the feeling of stigma experienced, especially in the early stages when people will be aware of the implications (Marzanski, 2000). It is perhaps less surprising that there is reluctance to share a diagnosis of dementia as there is not the same outlook, or prospect of positive treatment available with other conditions (Keightley and Mitchell, 2004).

Shamail *et al.* (2010) found that general practitioners were not always convinced of the importance of an early diagnosis due to the lack of follow-up specialist support. Studies with older people suggest that the diagnosis of dementia is not always given effectively and that carers often do not want their family member to be told (Pucci *et al.*, 2003). Woods and Pratt (2005) noted that when a diagnosis was given to the person with dementia it was more likely to be in the form of a euphemism, such as 'memory loss'. Hubbard *et al.* (2009) found that the most common reason for giving a dementia diagnosis was quite simply that the person had indicated that they wanted to know. Most were aware that changes were being experienced and wanted to know why. Patients often considered the fear of not knowing to be worse than having an honest explanation.

Issues around a reluctance to disclose a dementia diagnosis are compounded when the person has an intellectual disability and it will not always be apparent how much information has been retained or understood. Despite the strong move towards openness around a life-changing diagnosis among the general population, attitudes and practices around disclosing this kind of bad news to someone with intellectual disabilities have not changed accordingly (Bernal and Tuffrey-Wijne, 2008; McEnhill, 2008; Tuffrey-Wijne *et al.*, 2013). There are many reasons heard as to why people with intellectual disabilities are protected from bad news:

She couldn't possibly understand it.

It will upset him. What's the point of upsetting him?

We don't know how she will react. She is quite an emotional person.

If he knows what is going to happen, things will get worse. He will just give up.

I think she should know, but I don't think I will be able to cope with her distress.

I don't have the skills. I think someone else should tell him.

His family don't want him to be told anything.

However, not telling someone about bad news doesn't make the bad news disappear. If we don't help people to understand the changes in their lives, we may make it more difficult for them to cope. The same happens if someone has not anticipated the death of someone close to them. They will experience it as sudden and unexpected, and this is usually much more difficult to come to terms with than a death for which there has been some preparation (Blackman, 2003). Many people cope best with bad news if they are helped to understand the changes they experience. Denying that there is bad news, or pretending that changes are not being experienced, can be very confusing; the person's emotions don't match with what they are being told. There is often a culture of people with intellectual disabilities being 'jollied along', expected to smile even when they have every reason to be sad. Families, carers and professionals may be tempted to gloss over the bad news situation. Thus, someone who is distressed because they can no longer manage to have a shower independently may be told cheerfully:

Never mind! Look, I've come to give you a hand in the shower! Aren't you lucky today!

instead of:

You can't manage by yourself in the shower anymore. That is sad because you like having a shower by yourself. I am here to help you today.

The argument that it may cause further distress to the person if they are given their diagnosis of dementia has been refuted in the general population. For example, Carpenter *et al.* (2008) found no increase in depression and instead identified a reduction in anxiety after an explanation had been given for the change being experienced.

This also applies to people with an intellectual disability, albeit in a different context. The explanation that a family member was not able to speak or move the right-hand side of their body because of a medical condition (stroke) provided enormous relief for a woman with intellectual disabilities who had not been told about her mother's illness (Watchman, 2013). This clarification resulted in an immediate change in her body language, a visible expression of relief and her immediate change in conversation to talk in a relaxed manner about a current television programme. Another woman with intellectual disabilities regretted all her life that she was never told that her mother had a brain tumour. As a result, she was confused and upset as she didn't understand why her mother's behaviour towards her had changed (Cresswell and Tuffrey-Wijne, 2008).

Adapting existing guidelines for breaking bad news

Even if there is a general willingness to help people with intellectual disabilities to understand a life-limiting diagnosis, there are complications around the actual process of breaking bad news. Blackman and Todd (2005) maintain that this is related to the difficulty in adapting existing general models for breaking bad news to the specific needs of people with intellectual disabilities. These models, which have been developed for and by healthcare professionals (Baile *et al.*, 2005; Buckman, 1992; Fallowfield and Jenkins, 2004; Kaye, 1996) are linear models consisting of a set of distinct steps. They begin with 'preparation': planning for an appropriate setting, finding out how much the patient knows and finding out how much the patient wants to know. This is followed by giving the patient a 'warning shot' before breaking the bad news in small pieces. The underlying assumption is that patients are given as much information as they want and can cope with. Finally, there are steps around 'follow up' planning for support and subsequent meetings.

The problem with a general model such as this is that it can be very difficult to elicit the information needs and preferences of people with intellectual disabilities, particularly those with limitations in communication. 'Warning shots', such as 'I'm afraid the results of the test are not as good as we have hoped,' are often lost on people with intellectual disabilities; this may lead health care professionals to believe that they do not wish to know more (Tuffrey-Wijne *et al.*, 2010).

Once someone's information needs have been established, professionals and carers need to be ready to give the bad news in the appropriate format. This does not always happen and is complicated by the fact that, unlike the general population, people with intellectual disabilities are often given bad news about their own health by carers rather than medical staff, most of whom are not trained or prepared for the task and many of whom will need to cope with the bad news themselves (McEnhill, 2008; Tuffrey-Wijne, 2010).

General guidelines for breaking bad news to people with intellectual disabilities need to also incorporate the awareness that whilst most people in the general population want to know the truth about illness and death, some people do not. It is important to respect their wishes and allow them to utilise the important coping mechanism of denial. The challenge, therefore, is to develop a framework for assessing exactly what and how much someone with intellectual disabilities should be helped to understand at any one time. It is crucial to understand people's own preferences and concerns, as well as the reasons why families, carers and professionals may wish to withhold the truth from them: are they protecting the person with intellectual disabilities from the genuine possibility of harm, or are they protecting themselves from a difficult and distressing situation?

How is bad news understood and processed?

Many people worry about having to explain difficult news. It may help to know that verbal explanations are only one way in which people begin to understand bad news. Indeed, for people with limited verbal capacity or significant cognitive impairment, verbal explanations may be of no use at all. For most people, not just those with intellectual disabilities, 'experience' is a much more powerful and influential way of gaining knowledge than an explanation of facts. A simple and honest acknowledgement of someone's current experience that they are no longer able to make a cup of tea, as well as some gentle support with the tea-making, may be much more effective in helping to understand dementia than an explanation of the expected process.

There are no 'one size fits all' guidelines for breaking bad news; everyone is different, and individual needs must always take precedence. However, it can be very helpful to think about how people with intellectual disabilities (and all of us, for that matter) understand and process bad news. As a starting point, it is important to think very carefully about the nature of the bad news, and consider whether it is actually bad news! Bad news has been described as 'any news that drastically and negatively alters the patient's view of his or her future' (Buckman, 1984, p. 1597). The first question to ask, therefore, is how this person sees the future, and what his or her capacity is for abstract thinking. We cannot be sure that what we see as bad news will be experienced as such by someone else.

Just imagine someone who has a limited capacity for abstract thinking, who has never heard of dementia, and who has a limited concept of time and future. Telling this person that they have dementia, and will gradually lose the ability to do things, is unlikely to be experienced as 'bad news'! It is also possible that what we think is perfectly ordinary information will be experienced as very bad news indeed. This same person, who shrugged his shoulders and remained unaffected by the news that he has dementia, may be devastated by the news that his favourite television programme has been replaced by coverage of a sporting event.

This brings us to the central point of the application of the breaking bad news model to sharing the diagnosis of dementia: any new information needs to make sense to the person and fit in with their current experience of life. We need to build on an individual's existing 'framework of knowledge'. This is a fluid process, rather than a linear step-by-step process that can be planned. It is likely to involve a wide range of people, including not only professionals with breaking bad news skills, but also families and carers in the person's own social setting.

Building a framework of knowledge

'Breaking bad news' is actually a misnomer. Rather than bad news being broken, and understood, in one instant, we need to help people cope with a reality that is changed and changing. In order to do so, we need to break new information down into singular, distinct, small chunks of information. We then need to try to establish which of these chunks the person already possesses, which will make sense now, which may not make sense until later and which are unlikely ever to be retained or make sense at all. It is helpful to try to see these chunks from the person's own perspective.

Table 11.1: Understanding the importance of chunks of knowledge

Background: foundation of knowledge	Present: framework of knowledge	Future
Doctors make ill people better	I don't want to get out of my chair	I won't get better
When people get old they get forgetful	I am confused	I won't be able to go back to work anymore
My mum had dementia and she died	I like looking at my photographs	I am going to hospital tomorrow
I used to live with my dad before I got my own flat	I am scared walking across the floor	I don't want to go to the day centre next week

Some of these chunks of knowledge are related to the person's background knowledge. This includes people's view of the world and their life experience, for example the left-hand column in Table 11.1:

Doctors make ill people better.

When people get old they get forgetful.

My mum had dementia and she died.

I used to live with my dad before I got my own flat.

Others, in the middle column, are related to what people experience in the present moment. These are easiest to explain and easiest to understand. Even for someone whose framework of knowledge is very small and limited, there will be some chunks of knowledge related to what is happening right now:

I don't want to get out of my chair.

I am confused.

I like looking at my photographs.

I am scared walking across the floor.

A third category of knowledge chunks is related to the future. Whether people can understand information about the future depends on their intellectual capacity, their capacity for abstract thinking, and their concept of time:

I won't get better.

I won't be able to go back to work anymore.

I am going to hospital tomorrow.

I don't want to go to the day centre next week.

Trying to understand someone's current framework of knowledge will help us to decide which chunks of new information to add. There is little use in explaining to someone what will happen in the future if there are very few (if any) chunks about the future already present. It is only useful to explain to someone that they have dementia if their background knowledge includes an understanding or experience of dementia. If these background or future chunks of knowledge are absent, it may be best to stick with information about the present moment. This is particularly relevant for people with complex and profound intellectual disabilities, who often live life completely in the present moment, and find it hard to link previous experiences to current situations or to anticipate the future.

Deciding how to build on someone's 'framework of knowledge' is a team effort. Without a fairly detailed knowledge of someone's experience and 'foundation of knowledge', it will be difficult to know whether, and how, new information will be understood and processed. It is useful to gather information about the person's foundation of knowledge from as many people as possible; the insights of families and carers are of particular importance. Together, they can try to answer the following questions:

- How large or small is this person's 'foundation of knowledge'? How much insight and understanding does he or she have of the past, present and future?

- What is this person's experience of life? What is their view of the world?

- How does the person usually process new information? Do they benefit from verbal explanations, pictures, experiences, lots of repetition?

- Does the person like to think about what is going to happen tomorrow or next week, or does he or she live day to day?

Collectively, the team can then begin to consider what the nature is of the bad news that needs to be communicated. How much should someone be helped to understand, and why? Usually, people need enough support to understand the current changes in their life. Many people benefit from being able to anticipate these changes in some way, but there are also people who find such anticipation too difficult. It makes them so anxious that they find it difficult to cope, for example they may be better off not knowing that they need to go to hospital until the morning of the appointment.

How does dementia affect someone's framework of knowledge?

Usually, someone's framework of knowledge grows over time. People build up their background knowledge through life experience and education. It is possible to plan for this by carefully selecting experiences that will help someone build an understanding of bad news situations. For example, we know that at some point most people will experience a parental or family bereavement. Building their background knowledge of death, not only the physical side but also the emotions involved, will help them to cope when this happens. This could include talking about deaths that occur in television programmes, attending funerals, or remembering other people who have died.

When someone's mother is terminally ill, experiencing the current changes will help to build the 'what is happening right now' section of their knowledge framework: helping to look after the ill mother, visiting her in hospital, acknowledging confused emotions as their mother is no longer the person she once was. If, sometime in the future, their father reaches the end of life, this person will be better prepared. Their framework of knowledge has been built to include an understanding of what is happening. This may include a better understanding of what will happen in the future.

When people have dementia, there is a significant difference in the way their framework of knowledge changes. Rather than the framework growing over time, it is shrinking, and the chunks of knowledge that are present are gradually shifting. The boundaries between background knowledge and 'what is happening right now' may become blurred, so that what used to be seen as a memory or past experience can become part of today's experience. Any knowledge and understanding about the future may begin to disappear. The consequence of this can be that a person's individual needs or concerns at that time are not addressed. Kitwood (1997) found that when a person with dementia did not have their individual basic needs met, whether in terms of information, attachment or inclusion the result was depersonalisation. This is a process that placed each participant in a negative position, creating withdrawal and social isolation. Whilst it has been most commonly written about in connection with dementia in older people generally, Watchman (2012) showed that this process of depersonalisation was evident among people with an intellectual disability and dementia, resulting in their further marginalisation.

Background framework of knowledge

Knowledge that consists of memories ('My mum had dementia and she died') can begin to disappear, especially memories that are more recent. Older memories may emerge more strongly. A particular feature of dementia is that these older memories can begin to shift and become an experience of the present day. Thus, the background knowledge that 'Mum always waited for me when I got off the bus' can become an experience of what is happening right now: 'Mum is waiting for me.' Correcting this, trying to turn this back into a memory of the past, may be of little benefit and can cause unnecessary confusion or distress.

Background knowledge that consists of the person's world view, or an understanding of how the world works, may also change. Values and behaviour learnt in recent decades may gradually disappear, leaving the person with an understanding that is related to a much earlier time in their life. For some, who grew and spent both formative and adult years in a long-stay hospital or institution, this may not be a time that evokes pleasant memories. Additionally, knowledge that is expressed through life skills may also disintegrate over time.

Knowledge of what is happening right now

Over time, the ability of someone with dementia to understand or even experience what is happening right now will be reduced to an ever-decreasing window. Perhaps someone used to experience a mealtime in its entirety: understanding the process of setting the table, sitting down, eating potatoes before dessert, clearing up; but now experiences the meal a mouthful at a time, and cannot understand why they cannot eat the dessert that is just out of reach.

When we introduce new experiences or new information, it needs to make sense in relation to someone's experience of life as it is happening right now. For example, leave the dessert out of sight until it is time to eat it. If someone's past has shifted into their present, it can help to present current experiences in a way that makes sense, using familiar words, sounds, smells and tastes.

Knowledge of the future

Knowledge and understanding of what is going to happen in the future, whether that is next year or tomorrow, will gradually disappear. Sometimes, this can mean that the person becomes less distressed or worried about their situation. The ability to worry about what is happening to us depends, to some extent, on our ability to anticipate the future.

How much should someone with dementia be helped to understand?

Assessing what and how much someone with dementia should be told, or helped to understand their diagnosis, needs a constant re-evaluation of their framework of knowledge. Any new chunks of information need to relate to their current framework. If someone's current experience and understanding is that their mother is alive and present today, it is not helpful to insist on repeated explanations that their mother is dead. Such explanations will result in unnecessary distress: it does not fit with the person's current experience, and it is a devastating chunk of bad news to be processed again and again.

During the earlier stages of dementia, people are likely to notice that things are changing for them. Perhaps they get things wrong that they used to get right. This can be worrying; they may need help to understand that this is part of an illness. Those around them, in particular their peers, need help to understand this too. There are some useful resources available including pictorial books (Hollins and Sireling, 1994; Hollins and Tuffrey-Wijne, 2009; Hollins *et al.*, 2012; Kerr and Innes, 2001; Watchman, 2004).

An assessment of what someone with dementia can be helped to understand should include a consideration of future changes. People with intellectual disabilities have as much right to be involved in decisions around their future as the rest of the population. The changes in someone's framework of knowledge mean that people may lose the capacity to make certain decisions. They become less able to retain and balance the information and to understand implications for the future. Any involvement in decision-making should therefore take place as early as possible, before such capacity is lost. Even if it is too early to make firm decisions around future care, it is important that the person's views and preferences are established before they lose the capacity to express or even consider them.

Case study: Tom

Tom is 55 years old and has lived at home with his parents all his life. Tom has Down syndrome. Although he only speaks in single words or short sentences, his verbal understanding is good. Tom's father died suddenly of a heart attack eight years ago and since then he has been living with his mother. The two are not only very close but have also become dependent on each other for mutual care. She cooks simple meals; he makes the cups of tea. He is well known in his local community, as he usually does the daily shopping, an important task that makes him feel proud and valued, and also attends church on Sundays. There has been limited involvement from health and social care services over the years. Tom used to attend a day centre, but it has now closed. Tom has a sister who is married with children, and a brother who lives alone. Both live in a different part of the country. He is close to them but doesn't see them often, although he has noticed that they have been visiting more often during the past few months.

Tom's behaviour started changed six months ago, he started to get confused about the money for his shopping, and he has been getting lost on his way home. He was diagnosed with Alzheimer's disease. Once or twice, he has commented on his situation ('My head is wrong') but these comments were not picked up on by his family who only later understood the relevance.

Tom's mother has recently been diagnosed with advanced lung cancer and has gone into hospital; she is waiting for a place in a hospice. Temporary accommodation has been found for Tom: a residential group home that offers respite care, shared with three other people with intellectual disabilities and staffed by a team of carers.

Tom has never received any explanations about his dementia symptoms. In addition, he has not been told what is happening to his mother and he has not visited her in hospital, as his siblings thought that would be too upsetting for him. In his current home, he appears isolated. He usually sits away from the other residents, doesn't take part in any of the activities that are offered, and has stopped speaking altogether. The carers at the home don't know how to engage with him and usually leave him alone. They assume that Tom's lack of verbal communication is normal for him. However, his brother, sister and a nurse from the community intellectual disability team, who has got to know him over the past months, have noticed a marked difference. Not only has he withdrawn from interaction, but his daily living skills have deteriorated significantly. He now needs help with personal care. The nurse suspects that he is in a state of shock and distress.

There are a number of significant changes in Tom's life, all of which amount to bad news. He doesn't understand why these changes have happened, and he has not been helped to cope with them.

- He has lost skills that were important to him.

- His mother has disappeared (he has been told she is in hospital).

- He has moved into a strange new environment with people he doesn't know.

There are likely to be further changes ahead:

- His mother will die.

- He may move into another care setting.

- He will lose more skills and need more care.

Without help to understand these changes, Tom is likely to be increasingly confused and distressed. He will be unprepared for new changes and as a result these changes, including the death of his mother, will be unexpected.

Using the framework for breaking bad news in Tom's situation

In order to help Tom, the carers at the group home will need advice and support from a range of professionals. It would also be highly beneficial to involve his siblings and talk to them about how Tom has coped with life and changes in the past, and how they think he experiences the world around him. It is useful to build up a picture of his life and fill in the chunks in his framework of knowledge as early as possible. It might help to use a life story book or other pictures and mementoes of Tom's life, in order to elicit his memories and prompt discussion. Tom's background knowledge might include the following chunks shown in Figure 11.1.

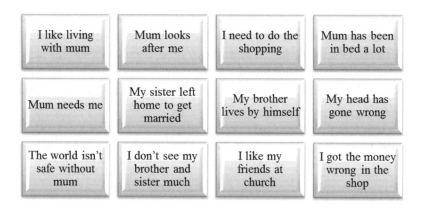

Figure 11.1: Tom's chunks of background knowledge

Tom's knowledge about what is happening right now might be shown as in Figure 11.2.

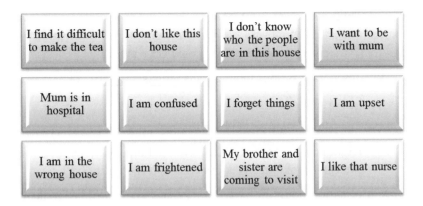

Figure 11.2: Tom's chunks of present knowledge

Tom's understanding of the future may be more limited as suggested in Figure 11.3.

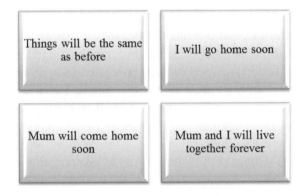

Figure 11.3: Tom's understanding of the future

In order to help Tom understand both his present and future situation, it is probably most important that he understands what is happening with his mum and his home. His current understanding of the future is erroneous and needs to be rectified. First of all, it is important to establish the facts: is Tom indeed unable to go back home, or is it possible for him to live at home with the support of a team of paid carers? Until this is clear, it is probably best to keep explanations to known facts: your mother is ill; she will not get better; she will die; you will stay in the respite care home for now. Tom's siblings and his mother may disagree that Tom needs to be told about his mother's illness. They will need a lot of support in understanding that not knowing is adding to Tom's distress. New chunks of information to add to Tom's current framework of knowledge are:

- Yes, you miss your mum because she is not with you.

- She is very ill.

- She is not going to get better.

- Right now, it is not possible to live at home with her (because she can't look after you and you can't look after her).

This information does not have to be given only in words. Frequent visits to the hospital are particularly important. Tom will need to be given the news that his mother is going to die, but before that information can be taken on board, Tom needs to understand how serious her illness is. It is also necessary to assess how much Tom understands about death and dying, and whether cancer and death feature in his background foundation of knowledge. Furthermore, it is important to assess his concept of time.

The next important piece of information for Tom is that he has dementia. This needs a simple explanation in words that he can relate to. If he knows what dementia is, perhaps because he has relatives or friends with the condition, it is easiest simply to name it, and relate his symptoms to this. Otherwise, it might be helpful to explain to him that his head has gone wrong, since he has used this terminology himself, because there is an illness in his head. It makes him forget things and get things wrong, such as not using the correct money and getting lost on his way home. This can be accompanied by a reassurance that others are willing to help him when things go wrong, and that he isn't to blame.

Tom's understanding of the future, and his ability to anticipate it, will reduce. Knowing this, it is important to begin to help him think about the changes ahead. His head will get worse; he will need more help. If there are options for Tom's future situation, they need to be spelled out, so he can express an opinion about them.

Being able to help and do something for his mother is an important part of Tom's sense of self. This will continue to be the case as she progressively worsens, and even after she dies. In time, as Tom's dementia gets more advanced, he is likely to forget that his mother has died, and his sense that he needs to do the shopping and make a cup of tea for her may remain. Tom can, and should, be supported in this. In the immediate future, he could be helped to buy things for her whilst she is in hospital, such as flowers or tea bags. Once she has moved into a hospice, he may be able to actually make her a cup of tea himself, with support if he needs it. In the more distant future, when he has forgotten that his mother has died, the information about his mother's death does not need to be repeated as he will not retain it. It will be crucial, though, that his carers understand his current framework of knowledge, so that he can be given sensitive support in the way he experiences the world.

Tom is currently in a state of deep distress, and he will need intensive and coordinated support to cope with his situation. This should involve not only the professionals from his community team, but also all his care staff and, ideally, if possible, his family and friends, to ensure that everyone gives him the same messages.

Conclusion

A challenge in dementia care generally is to provide appropriate post-diagnostic support recognising that everyone is entitled to know of their diagnosis. This challenge also applies to people with intellectual disabilities. Sharing the diagnosis in an appropriate format, and within an appropriate framework of understanding, is just the start of this process. Breaking bad news to people with intellectual disabilities is complex. The difficulties are compounded when there is a diagnosis of dementia in a person who already has reduced cognitive awareness and requires adapted communication. The model for breaking bad news to people with intellectual disabilities has been reviewed, with the recommendation that this is applied to sharing information about a diagnosis of dementia. This is new territory, and further evidence is needed to refine the model and to understand how it can be best used in practice. To answer the question posed at the start of this chapter: yes, people with intellectual disabilities should have information about a diagnosis of dementia shared with them, but in a way that takes cognisance of each individual's previous experience and their current framework of understanding, in order to decide how far to meaningfully discuss the future.

References

Baile, W., Buckman, R., Lenzi, R., Glober, G., Beale, E. and Kudelka, A. (2005) SPIKES – a six-step protocol for delivering bad news: Application to the patient with cancer. *The Oncologist 5*, 4, 302–311.

Bernal, J. and Tuffrey-Wijne, I. (2008) Telling the truth – or not: Disclosure and information for people with intellectual disabilities who have cancer. *International Journal on Disability and Human Development 7*, 4, 365–370.

Blackman, N. (2003) *Loss and Learning Disability.* London: Worth Publishing.

Blackman, N. and Todd, S. (2005) *Caring for People with Learning Disabilities who are Dying: A Practical Guide for Carers.* London: Worth Publishing.

Brodaty, H., Green, A. and Koshera, A. (2003) Meta-analysis of psychosocial interventions for caregivers of people with dementia. *Journal of the American Geriatric Society 5*, 5, 657–664.

Buckman, R. (1984) Breaking bad news – why is it still so difficult? *British Medical Journal 288*, 6430, 1597–1599.

Buckman, R. (1992) *How to Break Bad News: A Guide for Health Care Professionals.* Baltimore, MD: The Johns Hopkins University Press.

Carpenter, BD., Xiong, C., Porensky, EK. *et al.* (2008) Reaction to a dementia diagnosis in individuals with Alzheimer's disease and mild cognitive impairment. *Journal of American Geriatric Society 56*, 3, 405–412.

Cresswell, A. and Tuffrey-Wijne, I. (2008) The come back kid: I had cancer, but I got through it. *British Journal of Learning Disabilities 36*, 3, 152–156.

Department of Health (2009) *Living Well With Dementia: A National Dementia Strategy.* London: The Stationery Office.

Department of Health, Social Services and Public Safety (2011) *Improving Dementia Services in Northern Ireland.* Available at www.dhsspsni.gov.uk/improving-dementia-services-in-northern-ireland-a-regional-strategy-november-2011.pdf, accessed on 7 December 2013.

Fallowfield, L. and Jenkins, V. (2004) Communicating sad, bad, and difficult news in medicine. *Lancet 24*, 363, 312–319.

Fujimori, M. and Uchitomi, Y. (2009) Preferences of cancer patients regarding communication of bad news: A systematic literature review. *Japanese Journal of Clinical Oncology 39*, 4, 201–216.

Hollins, S. and Sireling, L. (1994) *When Mum Died.* 2nd edition. London: Gaskell/St George's Hospital Medical School.

Hollins, S. and Tuffrey-Wijne, I. (2009) *Am I Going to Die?* London: Royal College of Psychiatrists Publications/St George's, Unversity of London.

Hollins, S., Blackman, N. and Eley, R. (2012) *Ann has Dementia.* London: Royal College of Psychiatrists Publications/St George's, University of London.

Hubbard, RE., O'Mahony, MS. and Woodehouse, KW. (2009) Characterising frailty in the clinical settings – a comparison of different approaches. *Age and Ageing 38*, 1, 115–119.

Innes, S. and Payne, S. (2009) Advanced cancer patients' prognostic information preferences: A review. *Palliative Medicine 23*, 1, 29–39.

Kaye, P. (1996) *Breaking Bad News: A 10 Step Approach.* Northampton: EPL Publications.

Keightley, J. and Mitchell, A. (2004) What factors influence mental health professionals when deciding whether or not to share a diagnosis of dementia with the person? *Aging and Mental Health 8*, 1, 13–20.

Kerr, D. and Innes, M. (2001) *What is Dementia?* Edinburgh: Down's Syndrome Scotland.

Kitwood, T. (1997) *Dementia Reconsidered.* Buckingham: Open University Press.

McEnhill, L. (2008) Breaking bad news of cancer to people with learning disabilities. *British Journal of Learning Disabilities 36*, 3, 157–164.

Marzanski, M. (2000) Would you like to know what is wrong with you? On telling the truth to patients with dementia. *Journal of Medical Ethics 26*, 2, 108–113.

NICE (2006) *Supporting People with Dementia and their Carers in Health and Social Care, Clinical Guideline 32.* London: National Institute for Clinical Excellence and Social Care Institute for Excellence.

Novack, D., Plumer, R., Smith, R., Ochitill, H., Morrow, G. and Bennett, J. (1971) Changes in physicians' attitudes toward telling the cancer patient. *Journal of the American Medical Association 241,* 9, 897–900.

Oken, D. (1961) What to tell cancer patients: A study of medical attitudes. *Journal of the American Medical Association 175,* 13, 1120–1128.

Pucci, E., Belardinelli, N., Borsetti, G. and Guiliani, G. (2003) Relatives' attitudes towards informing patients about the diagnosis of Alzheimer's disease, *Journal of Medical Ethics 29,* 1, 51–55.

Scottish Government (2013) *Scotland's National Dementia Strategy 2013–2016.* Edinburgh: Scottish Government. Available at: www.scotland.gov.uk/Topics/Health/Services/Mental-Health/Dementia, accessed on 1 November 2013.

Seale, C. (1991) Communication and awareness about death: A study of a random sample of dying people. *Social Sciences and Medicine 32,* 8, 943–952.

Shamail, A., Orrell, M., Iliffe, S. and Gracie, A. (2010) GPs' attitudes, awareness, and practice regarding early diagnosis of dementia, *British Journal of General Practice 60,* 578, 360–365.

Tuffrey-Wijne, I. (2010) *Living with Learning Disabilities, Dying with Cancer: Thirteen Personal Stories.* London: Jessica Kingsley Publishers.

Tuffrey-Wijne, I. (2013) A new model for breaking bad news to people with intellectual disabilities. *Palliative Medicine 27,* 1, 5–12.

Tuffrey-Wijne, I., Bernal, J. and Hollins, S. (2010) Disclosure and understanding of cancer diagnosis and prognosis for people with intellectual disabilities: Findings from an ethnographic study. *European Journal of Cancer Nursing 14,* 3, 224–230.

Tuffrey-Wijne, I., Giatras, N., Butler, G., Cresswell, A., Manners, P. and Bernal, J. (2013) Developing guidelines for disclosure or non-disclosure of bad news around life-limiting illness and death to people with intellectual disabilities. *Journal of Applied Research in Intellectual Disabilities 26,* 3, 231–242.

Watchman, K. (2004) *Let's Talk About Death.* Edinburgh: Down's Syndrome Scotland.

Watchman, K. (2012) Reducing marginalisation in people with learning disability and dementia. *Journal of Dementia Care 20,* 5, 35–39.

Watchman, K. (2013) *At a Crossroads in Care: The Experience of Individuals with Down's Syndrome and Dementia.* PhD thesis, University of Edinburgh.

Woods, B. and Pratt, R. (2005) Understanding awareness: Ethical and legal issues in relation to people with dementia. *Aging and Mental Health 9,* 5, 423–429.

Werner, P., Karnieli-Miller, O. and Eidelman, S. (2013) Current knowledge and future directions about the disclosure of dementia: A systematic review of the first decade of the 21st century. *Alzheimers Dementia 9,* 2, 74–88.

12

Staff Knowledge and Training

Karen Dodd

Introduction

Staff in all settings are a key component in ensuring that people who live with any form of dementia continue to experience wellbeing through all stages. The dementia guidance from the National Institute for Health and Care Excellence (NICE, 2006) states that: 'Health and social care managers should ensure that all staff working with older people in the health, social care and voluntary sectors have access to dementia care training and skill development that is consistent with their roles and responsibilities' (pp. 292–3). The need for effective training and leadership were also key issues in the Commission for Social Care Inspection (2008) report *See Me, Not Just the Dementia* in England.

The State of Care report from the Care Quality Commission in England (2003) showed that those services that maintain people's dignity and treat them with respect all have a number of things in common: they recognise the individuality of each person in their care, and help them to retain their sense of identity and self-worth; take time to listen to what people say; are alert to people's emotional needs as much as their physical needs; and give them control over their care and the environment around them. These attributes can only be achieved by ensuring that staff are well trained and supported.

Putting the person at the centre of their care has been a key issue for people with intellectual disabilities since the work of O'Brien (1989) and has been embedded in policy and guidance in the UK since the turn of the century (Department of Health, 2001; Scottish Government, 2013). Person-centred care is a more recent phenomenon within mainstream dementia services and has been referred to as the 'gold-standard' for residential services (Evardsson *et al.*, 2011). Ballard *et al.* (2001) emphasised that staff training is unanimously seen as one of the key factors in ensuring that the gold standard of care is achieved.

This is confirmed by the British Commission for Social Care Inspection – now part of the Care Quality Commission – which reported that all the services that they rated most highly for social care had consistently invested in training in dementia awareness and person-centred care (Commission for Social Care Inspection, 2008). They also found a statistically significant relationship between the quality of the staff training and wellbeing of the people who lived in the home. Consideration will be given to the evidence base for staff training in dementia care generally, and then in relation to intellectual disability and dementia.

Research into staff knowledge and training for people in the general population with dementia

There is an increasing evidence base on many aspects of staff training with regard to people with dementia, covering such issues as the value of training, delivery of training, evaluation of training, content of training and the organisational context. This section will highlight some of these key areas. It is clear that staff are the most important resource within care settings, and this was recognised long before the publication of national guidance. Wills *et al.* (1997) recognised the vital role played by staff in the experience of people who have dementia. For example, they found that the use of medication was directly related to attitudes and practices of staff, rather than to the diagnosis of dementia or to symptoms and behaviour.

Organisational context and support

Organisational context and support are the key issues in determining whether staff training is successful in meeting the intended aims of changing or enhancing practice. Kuske *et al.* (2007) undertook a systematic review of evaluated programmes of staff training for nursing home staff. They identified 21 studies, mostly from the USA. Their conclusions were that although almost all studies reported positive effects of staff training, the majority of studies had poor methodological quality. The most successful programmes of training which demonstrated sustained implementation of new knowledge were those that had extensive interventions and additional ongoing support.

In a review of 382 articles published between 1995 and 2009, Beeber *et al.* (2010) found 25 articles meeting their criteria for inclusion on challenges and strategies for implementing and evaluation training in long-term care settings. Their findings show that training is challenged by a number of features including low staff attendance, lack of organisational support and financial limitations. Kaasalainen (2002) had demonstrated that organisations need to have committed management and supervisory staff to ensure changes in practice in long-term care settings. The organisational context that may enhance or inhibit improvement through training was examined by Corazzini *et al.* (2010) who identified the importance of the administrative climate of the organisation, which they said refers to the baseline staff knowledge about communication, pain and task orientation; communication patterns; and the perceived need for training. Clearly, staff need to be ready to participate in training to benefit from it. This is emphasised in the studies by Brane *et al.* (1989) and Schonfield *et al.* (1999) who both concluded that change in practice and outcomes for people with dementia were evident when all staff received the training and then applied their new skills consistently. McCabe *et al.* (2007) found that there were indications that training may lead to greater staff satisfaction and also have an impact on staff turnover rates. However, they also found that continuing refresher courses may be required to sustain change.

Evaluation of staff knowledge and training

The literature on the evaluation of staff knowledge and training is characterised by many studies that have a range of methodological weaknesses. These include lack of control groups, reliance on self-report measures and outdated measures. Many studies also focus on measuring knowledge of symptoms or behaviour rather than taking a person-centred approach. McCabe *et al.* (2007) reviewed studies on staff training programmes for behavioural issues. They found that very few training programmes included a control group in their design, and that most studies relied on self-report from staff which makes results more questionable. However, they still concluded that skills training for nursing staff increases the knowledge and skill base of staff and reduces the number of behavioural problems among residents, although the gains were frequently short-lived.

Measures of knowledge in dementia were identified in a literature search undertaken by Spector *et al.* (2012). Five measures were identified but all had limitations with weaknesses in psychometric properties, being outdated with regard to a contemporary understanding of dementia and having limited scope. Existing measures tend to concentrate on biomedical and cognitive domains. They concluded that more robust, contemporary measures of knowledge are needed which incorporate biopsychosocial and person-centred models of care.

A number of studies have looked at the effects of a variety of training approaches. Zimmerman *et al.* (2010) demonstrated only minimal positive effects of a Foundations of Dementia Care course. This was a national training curriculum for nursing home and residential care and assisted living staff developed by the Alzheimer's Association in the USA. Evaluation focused on three modules taught through six sessions of one hour each – Learning to Lead (3 sessions); Improving Communication (1 session) and Reducing Pain (2 sessions). They used a range of tools and found that only Improving Communication showed improvement both immediately after training and at three-month follow-up.

Lee *et al.* (2013) examined, in a large sample of over a thousand staff, the attitudes of frontline residential care staff towards their residents with dementia and how specialist programmes or units affected staff attitude. They concluded that the majority of long-term care staff found dementia care difficult, yet held positive attitudes towards further training and were committed to stay in dementia care. Having a specialised dementia care unit or programme in the workplace was associated with commitment to stay in dementia care and was marginally associated with positive attitude towards further training.

Hughes *et al.* (2008) used a questionnaire design to look at the knowledge and confidence of 254 staff across 30 homes with regard to dementia. This was an interesting study that used a mixed approach within the questionnaire. Overall there were 12 items looking at knowledge. Seven related to which symptoms are a sign of dementia, one question on the perception of the relationship between dementia and ageing, and four questions which asked for a response to four different care scenarios. Confidence was measured by rating staff's expressed confidence in managing five hypothetical situations involving the care of people with dementia, using a scale that ranged from feeling 'very confident' to 'call for help'. The results showed that the majority of staff recognised some characteristic symptoms of dementia. However, one in ten staff thought that headaches and joint pain were each a symptom of dementia. Additionally, between 10 per cent and 28 per cent of staff were unsure about other symptoms. Of more concern was that just under a half of the staff thought that dementia was part of the ageing process. Staff confidence was found to be lower than knowledge. There was greater confidence in dealing with repeated questioning and 'wandering' behaviour, but lower levels of confidence were noted by staff if the person with dementia was angry or agitated.

Content and delivery of training

Most of the studies and programmes described here used traditional methods of delivering training. Many studies did not clearly specify the actual content of the training or the message that they wanted to get across to those attending. Ballard et al. (2001), Innes (2001) and Nolan et al. (2008) all concluded that traditional 'chalk and talk' didactic methods of instruction are unlikely to be effective in instilling the type of conceptual shift that is needed in staff, yet this is still a common approach in practice. This is supported by the Department of Health and Ageing in Australia (Department of Health and Ageing, 2006) who conducted a survey of educational provision in Australia. They criticised much of the workforce education for dementia care for its continued reliance on teacher-centred delivery methods using knowledge-based materials, and the poor integration of practical experience and real life context.

A study by Hobday et al. (2010) evaluated an internet-based training module. The CARES model has five elements: Connect with the resident, Assess behaviour, Respond appropriately, Evaluate what works and Share with the team. The training was delivered online to 40 nurse assistants with evaluation showing that dementia care knowledge improved significantly. The majority of the staff agreed or strongly agreed that CARES improved mastery, care competency and reduced stress related to dementia care. Hobday et al. (2010) concluded that online programmes represent a time and cost efficient method in the delivery of dementia care training in long-term care settings.

It is clear that training needs to be able to give staff a thorough understanding of what it means to have dementia and the importance of person-centred care. The aim of person-centred education is not about simply imparting knowledge, but encourages a paradigm shift for staff in moving from simply acquiring knowledge to changing their attitudes and practice in order to deliver person-centred care. To achieve this, training methods must also move beyond traditional didactic methods to student-centred adult learning, integrating reflection and experience (Gee *et al.*, 2012). What is required is to have reflective practitioners who can respond in creative person-centred ways to each unique individual and situation (Innes, 2001; Loveday, 2011). The literature on staff knowledge and training within the population of older people with dementia therefore demonstrates the shift from traditional symptom-based training and evaluation, to ensuring and implementing person-centred dementia care where staff can use their skills to respond individually to the needs of each person with dementia.

Training models for people with intellectual disabilities

Evaluation of training models used with staff who are supporting people with intellectual disabilities and challenging behaviour suggest that the best outcomes occur when three conditions are met. These are: when there is interactive training which involves the development of care plans (Gentry *et al.*, 2007; Tierney *et al.*, 2007), there is follow-up consultation and support for implementing care plans and where the training is conducted in conjunction with allied changes in the organisational system (Lowe *et al.*, 2007). Within intellectual disability and dementia literature, there are only a limited number of studies that have investigated staff knowledge and training. However, the emphasis from the start has always been underpinned by a person-centred approach. This section will consider what these studies have shown, and then look at how guidance documents have advanced in their thinking about staff knowledge and training over the last two decades.

Research in intellectual disability and dementia

Early studies with intellectual disability staff with regard to their knowledge about dementia all demonstrate a lack of knowledge. This is unsurprising as dementia was still a relatively new condition within the field of intellectual disabilities. The first published study in this area was conducted by Whitehouse *et al.* (2000). They investigated the knowledge and attributions of dementia held by 21 care staff who supported older people with intellectual disabilities and dementia. They demonstrated that staff had comparable level of knowledge to that of college students. The staff indicated that forgetfulness was the most prominent indicator of dementia, however normal forgetting needs to be distinguished from memory problems which occur with dementia (Alzheimer's Society, 2011). There was a lack of awareness of early changes other than memory loss that are associated with Down syndrome and dementia. Other changes identified were those that are normally seen in mid stage dementia such as confusion, agitation, frustration and incontinence. Staff also saw behaviour change as stable, global and not under the person's control. This meant that when the behaviour occurred it would always be seen as a result of 'the dementia' with a belief that it would be apparent in all situations.

Wilkinson *et al.* (2005) interviewed staff working with people with intellectual disabilities and dementia across six case study sites, and found a sense expressed by staff of 'floundering'. Lack of knowledge and uncertainty about what was needed to give the best support to people with dementia was commonly expressed across all sites. Lack of knowledge was specifically identified in two key areas: the impact of the built environment, and detection and management of pain. Within this study, few intellectual disability staff had received prior training in supporting people with dementia.

A specific study was undertaken by McCarron *et al.* (2010) into the end of life needs of people with intellectual disabilities and dementia. This study involved 57 participants who were seen in 13 focus groups. Staff came from six services for people with intellectual disabilities and one specialist palliative care provider. Three themes emerged from the analysis of the focus groups. These were: readiness to respond to end of life needs, fear of swallowing difficulties, environmental concerns and ageing in place. This shows that staff were ready to engage with people at the late stage of dementia but had unrealistic thoughts about the issues that they faced. These were further described with four main issues of concern: there were differences in staff preparation associated with different settings, lack of understanding and collaboration with palliative care, uncertainties about the ability to transfer existing palliative care models to people with intellectual disabilities and dementia, and the need to develop training in end stage dementia with related care approaches.

Many of these issues have been addressed by Levitan *et al.* (2012a, 2012b) who undertook a project to bring together professionals and staff working with people with intellectual disabilities with staff from a range of palliative care services in a think-tank day to share knowledge, approaches and understanding. A further study used a vignette approach to look at support workers' knowledge about dementia (Herron and Priest, 2013). Each of the three vignettes depicted the same hypothetical person with intellectual disabilities, with each vignette moving from early indicators of dementia through to middle and then more advanced indicators. The study was conducted with 14 support workers, working for two organisations. Each member of staff was asked to write their responses to 'What do you think is happening here?' and 'What action would you take?' for each vignette. Thematic analysis of the responses resulted in four themes: explanations, actions, obstacles and experiences.

With regard to the first question, none of the staff identified dementia from the first vignette, and only one out of the 14 staff identified dementia in vignette 2. However, most of the staff did recognise dementia in vignette 3 although the number was not specified. In terms of their proposed actions, most staff wanted to refer on to a general practitioner, psychologist or psychiatrist, and it was only in response to vignette 3 that staff would refer for dementia screening. Obstacles that were identified included the level of verbal communication skills of the person and diagnostic overshadowing, whilst the extent of intellectual disabilities and personal knowledge of the person assisted understanding. In terms of experiences, all of the staff had experience of working with people with intellectual disabilities and mental health. Of concern was that the majority of the staff believed that they had an adequate level of training, and only a minority had received any additional specific training. Herron and Priest (2013) concluded that participants' ability to identify signs of dementia was poor, particularly in its early stages. When they did identify dementia in the final vignette they thought that this was the onset, when in reality it was at an advanced stage. However, even when the participants were uncertain about the problem, they still identified that they would take appropriate action. Herron and Priest (2013) stressed the importance of introducing training, in particular the general and specific indicators and expected trajectory of dementia. The results of this study were perhaps disappointing, as dementia in people with intellectual disabilities is now a more common occurrence and has received increasing attention within services for people with intellectual disabilities. However, it emphasises the need for effective staff training for all staff who work with people with intellectual disabilities.

Staff training

There are a small number of studies that have focused on staff training on dementia and people with intellectual disabilities. Watchman (2003) concluded that the timing of training is important. She stressed that this is important so that a service is 'dementia-ready' before their residents begin to develop symptoms of dementia. The effect of staff training was demonstrated in the study by Wilkinson et al. (2005). In this study, they found that where staff had received relevant and targeted training that was practice based and person-centred, they displayed an appreciable difference in confidence, quality of care and support and they also reported reduced stress levels. However, they also stated that inappropriate training was worse than no training at all, as it led staff to have 'false confidence' about some of their practices. Two publications emphasised the need for a focus on specific aspects of dementia care: Kerr et al. (2006) said that recognition and treatment of pain is a critical area for staff training, whilst Watchman (2005) emphasised the need for training in timely palliative approaches and end of life care issues.

Two further studies have looked at whether staff training had increased knowledge in specific areas of support. Kalsy et al. (2007) found that there was a significant increase in knowledge after training, and that training was found to decrease significantly the attribution of controllability. They concluded that training focusing on aspects of change relevant to behaviour can favourably influence care staff's knowledge and attributions of controllability, within the context of people with Down syndrome and dementia.

The study by Fahey-McCarthy *et al.* (2009) described education development and intervention with regard to end of life care for people with intellectual disabilities and dementia. They undertook 14 focus group interviews with staff from six services for people with intellectual disabilities and one specialist palliative care provider. A number of key themes emerged. These were knowledge and skills of: caring for a person with intellectual disabilities, caring for a person with dementia, culturally competent caring, palliative care, addressing nutrition, hydration and pain concerns and facilitating grief and loss. They then progressed to delivering training to a group of 16 staff over two cohorts and refined the educational programme. They evaluated outcomes as significant in increasing knowledge of dementia and palliative care issues, and in beliefs about feeding tubes and palliative care issues. This then formed the development of a 20-session trainer manual which could be delivered over a six to eight week period. Feedback from staff indicated that the educational intervention was highly valued and addressed key training concerns of supporting ageing in place and preparation for a 'good death'.

A final study to be considered is that by Houlton *et al.* (2013). They described two training days held for day care staff. The one day training course covered behavioural and biological effects, the environment, meaningful activities including life story work, effective communication, pain, nutrition and hydration. The trainers used a combination of mediums including didactic teaching, group exercises, discussion and a DVD session. Staff were also asked to think about a specific person with intellectual disabilities and develop an individual care plan. Participants were asked to reflect on the most important things to take into consideration when supporting this person. Responses fell into three themes: environment; interaction and communication; and patient information and background. The most useful components of the training were the psycho-education on signs and symptoms of dementia, the practical example of the DVD, and group work exercises and activities. This study demonstrates how training has moved on to use a mixture of techniques and to help staff focus on the specific needs of individuals that they work with, rather than just thinking about people with intellectual disabilities in general.

The challenge in staff knowledge and training

Examples exist of guidance documents developed over the last two decades, which aim to help staff and services consider best practice in intellectual disability and dementia. Each document has considered staff training to be an issue. In 1995, Janicki *et al.* published the first set of practice guidelines for the clinical assessment and care management for people with intellectual disabilities and dementia. Within the guidelines, Janicki and colleagues stated that training staff in care management techniques is critical. They emphasised that the organising principle should be a focus on the individuality of the adult with dementia and provision of care that promotes personal dignity, autonomy and personal welfare. Further, that staff need to develop skills in working with adults with dementia and an understanding of the process of coping with functional limitations and death.

Further guidance was provided in the document published jointly between the British Psychological Society and the Royal College of Psychiatrists in 2009 (British Psychological Society, 2009). The document states that paid staff will require a basic awareness of dementia in order to provide effective care in the following areas:

- what is dementia?
- types and signs and symptoms of dementia
- working with people in a person-centred way
- using accessible information formats for person-centred plans and health action plans
- life story work
- use of medication in dementia
- communication skills
- roles of different health and social professionals
- safeguarding and protecting adults
- palliative care approaches.

Jokinen *et al.* (2013) took a staged approach when developing guidelines for structuring community care and supports within the USA, which emphasised the need for training at all stages. The challenge is in putting this into practice – a challenge accepted by the National Task Group on Intellectual Disabilities and Dementia

Practice, USA (National Task Group, 2012) who are developing a national training curriculum on dementia and intellectual disabilities.

Staff tend to describe dementia in terms of symptoms and behaviours and view dementia as a negative condition for which little can be achieved. Acton and Kang (2001) suggested that instead of focusing on changing negative experiences, perhaps professionals and services should address positive outcomes such as understanding how the person is feeling, including wellbeing and life satisfaction, whilst acknowledging that the burden remains unchanged. For staff and family carers to achieve this, they need to have a good understanding of what is happening to people who develop dementia and the consequences to the person of these changes within the brain.

Excellence in dementia care for people with intellectual disabilities and dementia is underpinned by the knowledge and skills of the people who support them, and their ability to continuously adapt to the person's changing needs. For this to happen, staff need to have a thorough understanding of the person, of dementia and the consequences of having dementia, and then how to adapt their care as the dementia progresses. This can only be achieved by having a clear framework to underpin the training and support provided to services. Not enough consistent guidance is evident on how to talk to, or communicate with, a person with intellectual disabilities and dementia about their diagnosis or appropriate post-diagnostic support.

Staff training in practice

The importance of developing a shared vision on which to build practice was identified by McCarron (1999) as the requisite of good care. She concluded that without this solid foundation, values, expectations and approaches are likely to differ greatly amongst staff. This will ultimately generate conflict and frustration and will in turn place unnecessary demands on an already confused person.

General dementia awareness training is often delivered to groups of staff from a number of services, often with junior staff attending. This approach may be useful in preparing staff who have no awareness of dementia to begin to engage in the topic prior to caring for people who have dementia. Although this has an advantage in allowing staff to meet with colleagues from other settings and to learn from each other (whether delivered face to face or as part of an online cohort), it needs to lead to change in practice once the person is in their care setting. The trained person returning to their setting has the onus of trying to 'sell' their knowledge and skills to the staff team, often with little commitment from management to implement changes. Improving dementia care for people with intellectual disabilities and dementia requires a whole-system approach within staff teams with some organisations adopting a cascade approach to training and disseminating learning.

Training should not only give people a list of things to do and knowledge about why, it should also give people a real understanding of the lives and experiences of people with intellectual disabilities and dementia. Staff need to understand what dementia is, its specific links to people with intellectual disabilities, and the signs or symptoms that they need to recognise, before diagnosis and at each stage of the condition. However, this needs to be underpinned by a model of dementia that helps staff to really understand what is happening to the person who is developing dementia, and to be able to put themselves in that person's shoes (Gee *et al.*, 2012). An example is Buijssen's two laws of dementia, as a framework to understand and respond to people appropriately: the law of disturbed encoding and the law of roll-back memory (Buijssen, 2005).

Taking such an approach helps staff not only to understand what is happening to the person who has dementia and the consequences of having dementia, but also gives them a framework for delivering person-centred care. This then needs to be followed up with ongoing support, discussions, use of additional resources and further training, and regular review to ensure that excellence in care continues throughout the rest of the person's life. This is vital as it is very easy for staff teams to become proficient at caring for a person in the early stage of dementia, but then to not adapt their care as the person's dementia progresses. This can result in frustration and confusion both for the person and the staff team. Ongoing support in addition to training allows the staff team to focus on their own issues in coming to terms with the emotional labour of supporting the person with dementia and their own bereavement when confronted by the changing abilities of the person.

Training should use a variety of mediums such as didactic, online, cascaded, group work, DVDs, discussions, role plays, case studies, with follow-up tasks. Training can be supplemented by the use of specific resources such as the *Dementia Workbook for Staff* (Dodd *et al.*,

2006), *Dementia Resource Pack* (Dodd *et al.*, 2009) and *Supporting Derek* training pack and DVD (Watchman *et al.*, 2010).

Table 12.1 suggests the types of training, support and outcomes that should be achieved for each stage of dementia. Each stage builds on the information and supports from previous stages and knowledge and ideas can be reiterated and developed with the staff team.

Table 12.1: Suggested training, support and outcome for each stage of dementia

Stage of dementia	Suggested content of formal training	Suggested ongoing support	Outcome required
Pre-diagnosis	• Signs and symptoms of dementia in people with intellectual disabilities • The diagnostic process, how to make a referral and to whom • Life story work • Person-centred care plans including health action plan, communication passport, end of life plans	• Understanding the diagnostic process • Working with the person and their family/friends to develop their life story work • Support to develop end of life plans whilst the person has capacity	• Person is supported through the diagnostic process • Other health issues are identified and treated • Social issues are identified and resolved • Plans are in place
Early stage	• Model of dementia (such as Buijssen, 2005) • Philosophy of care • Physical environments • Importance of picture cues • Medication • Understand a palliative approach	• Helping staff to accept the diagnosis and the changes • Grief and loss • Implementing the philosophy of care • Implementing a palliative approach • Importance of consistency of approach	• Person is supported to maintain their current lifestyle with additional supports and prompts

cont.

Table 12.1: Suggested training, support and outcome for each stage of dementia (*cont.*)

Stage of dementia	Suggested content of formal training	Suggested ongoing support	Outcome required
Mid stage	• Adapting communication • Supporting peers of the person with dementia • Failure-free, meaningful activities • Maintaining health and additional health issues such as epilepsy, mobility, continence • Pain recognition and management • Reminiscence	• Understanding the meaning of behaviours and exploring solutions • Avoidance of confrontation • Understanding and coping with agitation and distress	• Person is supported to live as full a life as possible focusing on preferred activities including reminiscence activities and without unnecessary changes
Late and end stage	• Safe manual handling • Safe eating and drinking • Skin and pressure care • Mobility, falls management, posture and positioning • Meeting spiritual needs	• Support for end of life care for both the staff and their support of the person's peers and family • Support in getting appropriate aids in a timely manner such as a specialist wheelchair, seating, profiling bed, hoist, bathing aids	• Person receives care that allows them to continue to experience activities and support that is familiar to them • Person is supported in all their daily living needs in a dignified and safe manner • Person experiences end of life care that results in a 'good death' in their preferred place

Conclusion

Staff are a key resource for supporting people with intellectual disabilities and dementia. It is imperative that they receive ongoing training and support in order to continuously update their knowledge and skills, so that they in turn can effectively support people through their changing needs. Effective training focuses on giving people a thorough and ongoing understanding of how it feels for the person with an intellectual disability who has dementia; this is an area of emerging research and evidence. It also involves everyone who supports the person. This is essential so that the person with an intellectual disability and dementia experiences care that is consistent and promotes quality outcomes.

References

Acton, GJ. and Kang, J. (2001) Interventions to reduce the burden of caregiving for an adult with dementia: A meta-analysis. *Research in Nursing and Health 24*, 5, 349–360.

Alzheimer's Society (2011) *Factsheet: What is Dementia?* Available at www.alzheimers.org.uk/site/scripts/download_info.php?fileID=1754, accessed on 7 December 2013.

Ballard, CG., O'Brien, J., James, I. and Swann, A. (2001) *Dementia: Management of Behavioural and Psychological Symptoms.* New York, NY: Oxford University Press.

Beeber, AS., Zimmerman, S., Fletcher, S., Mitchell, CM. and Gould, E. (2010) Challenges and strategies for implementing and evaluating dementia care staff training in long-term care settings. *Alzheimer's Care Today 11*, 1, 17–39.

Brane, G., Karlsson, I., Kihlgren, M. and Norberg, A. (1989) Integrity promoting care of demented nursing home patients: Psychological and biochemical changes. *International Journal of Geriatric Psychiatry 4*, 3, 165–172.

British Psychological Society (2009) *Dementia and People with Learning Disabilities. Guidance on the Assessment, Diagnosis, Treatment and Support of People with Learning Disabilities who Develop Dementia.* Leicester: British Psychological Society.

Buijssen, H. (2005) *The Simplicity of Dementia.* London: Jessica Kingsley Publishers.

Care Quality Commission (2012) *The State of Health Care and Adult Social Care in England 2011/12.* London: The Stationery Office. Available at www.cqc.org.uk/sites/default/files/media/documents/cqc__soc_201112_final_tag.pdf, accessed on 23 March 2014.

Commission for Social Care Inspection (2008) *See Me, Not Just the Dementia: Understanding People's Experiences of Living in a Care Home.* Newcastle: Commission for Social Care Inspection.

Corazzini, KN., McConnell, ES., Anderson, RA. *et al.* (2010) The importance of organizational climate to training needs and outcomes in long-term care. *Alzheimer's Care Today 11*, 2, 109–121.

Department of Health (2001) *Valuing People: A New Strategy for Learning Disability for the 21st Century: Implementation.* Available at http://webarchive.nationalarchives.gov.uk/+/www.dh.gov.uk/en/Publicationsandstatistics/Lettersandcirculars/Healthservicecirculars/DH_4004965, accessed on 7 December 2013.

Department of Health and Ageing (2006) *Stocktake of Continence and Dementia Workforce Curricula, Education and Training Project.* Canberra: Department of Health and Ageing.

Dodd, K., Kerr, D. and Fern, S. (2006) *Dementia Workbook for Staff.* Teddington: Down's Syndrome Association.

Dodd, K., Turk. V. and Christmas, M. (2009) *Resource Pack for Carers of Adults with Down's Syndrome and Dementia.* 2nd edition. Kidderminster: BILD Publications.

Evardsson, D., Fetherstonhaugh, D., McAuliffe, L., Nay, R. and Chenco, C. (2011) Job satisfaction amongst aged care staff: Exploring the influence of person-centred care provision. *International Psychogeriatrics 23*, 8, 1205–1212.

Fahey-McCarthy, E., McCarron, M., Connaire, K. and McCallion, P. (2009) Developing an education intervention for staff supporting persons with an intellectual disability and advanced dementia. *Journal of Policy and Practice in Intellectual Disabilities 6*, 4, 267–275.

Gee, S., Scott, M. and Croucher, M. (2012) *Walking in Another's Shoes: Encouraging Person-Centred Care through an Experiential Education Programme.* Canterbury: Canterbury District Health Board, New Zealand. Available at http://akoaotearoa.ac.nz/ako-hub/good-practice-publication-grants-e-book/person-centred-care, accessed on 7 December 2013.

Gentry, M., Iceton, J. and Milne, D. (2007) Managing challenging behaviour in the community: Methods and results of interactive training. *Health and Social Care in the Community 9*, 3, 143–150.

Herron, DL. and Priest, HM. (2013) Support workers' knowledge about dementia: A vignette study. *Advances in Mental Health and Intellectual Disabilities 7*, 1, 2–39.

Hobday, JV., Savik, K., Smith, S. and Gaugler, JE. (2010) Feasibility of internet training for care staff of residents with dementia: The CARES Program. *Journal of Gerontological Nursing 36*, 4, 13–21.

Houlton, P., McNally, P. and Scanlon, M. (2013) Learning disability and dementia: Audit of staff training pilot. *Clinical Psychology and People with Learning Disabilities 11*, 1–2, 28–32.

Hughes, J., Bagley, H., Reilly, S., Burns, A. and Challis, D. (2008) Care staff working with people with dementia: Training, knowledge and confidence. *Dementia 7*, 2, 227–238.

Innes, A. (2001) Student-centred learning and person-centred dementia care. *Education and Ageing 16*, 20, 229–252.

Janicki, MP., Heller, T., Seltzer, G. and Hogg, J. (1995) *Practice Guidelines for the Clinical Assessment and Care Management of Alzheimer and other Dementias among Adults with Mental Retardation.* Washington, DC: American Association on Mental Retardation.

Jokinen, N., Janicki, MP., Keller, SM., McCallion, P., Force, LT. and the National Task Group on Intellectual Disabilities and Dementia Practices (2013) Guidelines for structuring community care and supports for people with intellectual disabilities affected by dementia. *Journal of Policy and Practice in Intellectual Disabilities 10*, 1, 1–24.

Kaasalainen, S. (2002) Staff development and long-term care of patients with dementia. *Journal of Gerontological Nursing 28*, 7, 39–46.

Kalsy, S., Heath, R., Adams, D. and Oliver, C. (2007) Effects of training controllability attributions of behavioural excesses and deficits shown by adults with Down's syndrome and dementia. *Journal of Applied Research in Intellectual Disabilities 20*, 1, 64–68.

Kerr, D., Cunningham, C. and Wilkinson, H. (2006) *Responding to the Pain Experiences of Older People with a Learning Difficulty and Dementia.* York: Joseph Rowntree Foundation.

Kuske, B., Hanns, S., Luck, T., Angermeyer, MC., Behrens, J. and Riedel-Heller, SG. (2007) Nursing home staff training in dementia care: A systematic review of evaluated programs. *International Psychogeriatrics 19*, 5, 818–841.

Lee, J., Hui, E., Kng, C. and Auyeung, TW. (2013) Attitudes of long-term care staff toward dementia and their related factors. *International Psychogeriatrics 25*, 1, 140–147.

Levitan, T., Dodd, K., Boulter, P. and Mackey, E. (2012a) *A Good Death 2: A Guide about End of Life Care for Staff and Carers of People with Learning Disabilities.* Brighton: Pavilion Publishing.

Levitan, T., Dodd, K., Boulter, P. and Mackey, E. (2012b) *A Good Death 3: A Guide for Staff in Acute and Palliative Care Settings on Working with People with Learning Disabilities.* Brighton: Pavilion Publishing.

Loveday, B. (2011) Dementia training in care homes. In T. Dening and A. Milne (eds) *Mental Health and Care Homes.* Oxford: Oxford University Press.

Lowe, K., Jones, E., Allen, D. *et al.* (2007) Staff training in positive behaviour support: Impact on attitudes and knowledge. *Journal of Applied Research in Intellectual Disabilities 20*, 1, 30–40.

McCabe, MP., Davison, TE. and George, K. (2007) Effectiveness of staff training programs for behavioral problems among older people with dementia. *Aging and Mental Health 11*, 5, 505–519.

McCarron, M. (1999) Some issues in caring for people with the dual disability of Down's syndrome and Alzheimer's disease. *Journal of Learning Disabilities for Nursing, Health and Social Care 3*, 3, 123–129.

McCarron, M., McCallion, P., Fahey-McCarthy, E., Connaire, K. and Dunn-Lane, J. (2010) Supporting persons with Down's syndrome and advanced dementia. *Dementia 9*, 2, 285–298.

National Institute of Health and Care Excellence (NICE) (2006) *Dementia: Supporting people with dementia and their carers in health and social care. Clinical guidelines, CG42.* Available at www.nice.org.uk/CG42, accessed on 7 December 2013.

National Task Group on Intellectual Disabilities and Dementia Practice (2012) *'My Thinker's Not Working': A National Strategy for Enabling Adults with Intellectual Disabilities Affected by Dementia to Remain in their Community and Receive Quality Supports.* Available at http://aadmd.org/sites/default/files/NTG_Thinker_Report.pdf, accessed on 7 December 2013.

Nolan, M., Davies, S., Brown, J., Wilkinson, A., Warnes, T. and McKee, K. (2008) The role of education and training in achieving change in care homes: A literature review. *Journal of Research in Nursing 13*, 5, 411–433.

O'Brien, J. (1989) *What's Worth Working For? Leadership for Better Quality Human Services.* Syracuse, NY: The Center on Human Policy, Syracuse University for the Research and Training Center on Community Living of University of Minnesota.

Schonfeld, L., Cairl, R., Cohen, D., Neal, KK., Watson, MA. and Westerhof, C. (1999) The Florida Care College: A training program for long-term care staff working with memory-impaired residents. *Journal of Mental Health and Ageing 5*, 2, 187–199.

Scottish Government (2013) *Keys to Life – Improving Quality of Life for People with Learning Disabilities.* Edinburgh: The Scottish Government.

Spector, A., Orrell, M., Schepers, A. and Shanahan, N. (2012) A systematic review of 'knowledge of dementia' outcome measures. *Ageing Research Reviews 11*, 1, 67–77.

Tierney, E., Quinlan, D. and Hastings, RP. (2007) Impact of a three-day training course on challenging behaviour on staff cognitive and emotional responses. *Journal of Applied Research in Intellectual Disabilities 20*, 1, 58–63.

Watchman, K. (2003) Why wait for dementia? *Journal of Learning Disabilities 7*, 3, 221–230.

Watchman, K. (2005) Practitioner-raised issues and end-of-life care for adults with Down's syndrome and dementia. *Journal of Policy and Practice in Intellectual Disabilities 2*, 2, 156–162.

Watchman, K., Kerr, D. and Wilkinson, H. (2010) *Supporting Derek. A Practice Development Guide to Support Staff Working with People with a Learning Disability and Dementia.* Brighton: Joseph Rowntree/Pavilion Publishing.

Whitehouse, R., Chamberlain, P. and Tunna, K. (2000) Dementia in people with learning disability: A preliminary study into care staff knowledge and attributions. *British Journal of Learning Disabilities 28*, 4, 148–153.

Wilkinson, H., Kerr, D. and Cunningham, C. (2005) Equipping staff to support people with an intellectual disability and dementia in care home settings. *Dementia 4*, 3, 387–400.

Wills, P., Claesson, CB., Fratiglioni, L., Fastborn, J., Thorslund, M. and Winblad, B. (1997) Drug use by demented and non-demented elderly people. *Age and Ageing 26*, 5, 383–391.

Zimmerman, S., Mitchell, M., Reed, D. *et al.* (2010) Outcomes of a dementia care training program for staff in nursing homes and residential care/assisted living settings. *Alzheimer's Care Today 11*, 2, 83–99.

13

Belief in a Place Called Home

Reflections on Twenty Years of Dementia Specific Service Provision

Leslie Udell

Background to the service

Winnserv Inc. is a relatively small non-profit organization in Winnipeg, Manitoba, Canada that has been providing residential supports to people with an intellectual disability for over 35 years. We currently provide support to 78 people with 67 per cent of those individuals being over the age of 50. During the past 20 years, Winnserv has worked with 11 individuals who have had both intellectual disabilities and a diagnosis of dementia. This means that rarely has there been a time when we have not supported at least one resident with dementia. This path began around 1990 with a woman who lived in a house with four other housemates. When she began experiencing changes we had very little information about dementia or its connection to intellectual disabilities. This new, unexpected territory sent us scrambling and our responses were far from perfect, but we learned so much by accompanying her on the difficult journey.

The house this lady lived in was a split-level home, so when she lost the capacity to walk on her own the only way in and out of her house was to carry her; and that is in fact what we did until the licensing authority put a stop to this practice. We were then required to move her into an emergency long-term care placement. The continued presence of Winnserv staff and family members was not enough to prevent a rapid deterioration precipitated by the move and the lack of subsequent quality care. The facility was resentful of our presence and our advocacy and we were resentful of her change in care. It was certainly an emotionally laden experience and led to our decision at Winniserv to commit to whatever changes were necessary to prevent this from happening again, a situation that many other service providers internationally are also increasingly finding themselves in.

Unfortunately, there can sometimes be a gap between intentions and action and that was the case for Winnserv. As we thought about the cost of renovations, another person, in the same house, began to experience eerily familiar changes and rapid decline, often associated with having Down syndrome and a form of dementia. Although the agency had a better understanding of dementia and the supports required, changes had not yet been made to the physical structure of the house. It took almost a year, many heated debates and huge disruption to the lives of the people in the house to install an elevator, widen doorways and build ramps. Two years later, a new challenge arose when the gentleman in question had several bouts of pneumonia. While in hospital, he developed bed sores and was being fed with a syringe when agency staff were not present, so the decision was made by his family, the physician and Winnserv to discontinue antibiotics and bring him home to die. We had no experience whatsoever in the provision of palliative or end of life care, and if it weren't for the commitment and support of the family physician it could have been disastrous. However, it was not, and in the end was seen as a gift given to all involved.

The lessons learned in accommodating the changing needs of these two individuals made a profound change in how supports were offered to people affiliated with Winnserv. The organization has become firmly committed to keeping people in the community, even in the presence of dementia, and to supporting people right through until death. We also recognized that the individuals we work with, their families and the staff all deserved a more planned response to dementia.

Formulating a plan

'A proactive versus reactive response to dementia care requires preparation, strategic planning, redesign, and integration of services' (Jokinen et al., 2013, p. 7). In order to take that proactive approach there needs to be an understanding of the process and progression of dementia and what will be needed at each step along the way. There has been a significant expansion of knowledge and research in the area of intellectual disabilities and dementia in the past 20 years, but when Winnserv first began the journey that was not the case. We started by using two key reports from the American Association on Intellectual and Developmental Disabilities and the International Association for the Scientific Study of Intellectual Disabilities working group to guide the process. We were later influenced by the Preparing Community Agencies for Adults Affected by Dementia (PCAD) project. The project identified five key components to agency planning and the offering of quality dementia supports and services: 'early screening and diagnostics, clinical supports, environmental modifications, programme adaptations, and specialised care' (Janicki et al., 2002, p. 190).

Janicki et al. (2002) found that agencies like Winnserv reacted in one of three ways, when contemplating how they would respond to people who developed dementia. They would either find a way to support that person within their current home – ageing in place, develop a dementia specialized group home – in place progression, or refer the individual to the generic service providers in the community – referral out (Janicki et al., 2002). Winnserv's initial plan was one born of necessity, rather than any debate over best practices, as the first two individuals with dementia lived in the same household and once that house was renovated it became the 'dementia' home by default. What we failed to recognize, in the midst of implementing an aging in place policy, was the impact on the two housemates who remained alive and well. They eventually dealt with seeing three people they cared about go through the stages of dementia, including death. Over the years, the grief overload we were placing on the housemates led the organization to rethink our plan and to consider the development of a dementia specific household.

A three-person dementia specific household was established and Winnserv's support model has become a mixture of in place progression with 'specialised staff and a specialised environment' (Janicki et al., 2002, p. 186) and aging in place. Our aim is to bring the feeling of home to whatever household people are living in. Initially, one dementia friendly home was sufficient to accommodate people who were diagnosed with dementia, but it has become evident that a second house is needed to meet increasing numbers of people with intellectual disabilities and a diagnosis of dementia as our population ages. Currently, with a lack of opportunity to move into the dementia specific household, the organization is also supporting two people with this diagnosis to age in place and those staff teams are now receiving training in dementia care.

There are no easy answers to the timing of the move from an existing home to a dementia capable household and, in our case, the decision is usually driven by availability rather than what is optimal for the individual. Asking anyone to change homes, when they are not choosing that move, is a very difficult decision and a change in environment is often difficult for people with dementia (Jokinen et al., 2013). We have been fortunate that everyone, to date, has adapted to moving regardless of their stage in the condition, and they quickly settle in the place that will be their home for the rest of their life. In Winnserv's experience, staff teams have the capacity to work with people in all stages of the condition, once given appropriate training and support. Household staffing patterns and staff support needs change according to the stage of dementia, but staff can adapt to the multiple skill sets required. The key is to provide the staff training in a timely manner and to ensure environmental adaptations are implemented proactively.

In addition to facilitating group living arrangements, Winnserv also supports individuals who live in their own apartments in the community and the dementia strategy for this group is much more of a challenge with great potential for resorting to crisis management. When someone receives daily support, such as in a group home, there is a greater chance of noting changes at an earlier stage and having the capacity to quickly adapt when needed. Some people who are living on their own only receive a few hours of weekly support from Winnserv in a week and the maximum weekly number of hours is 20. There is a home care program run by the health authority, also with a limit on hours of support, and they can work together with Winnserv until a more suitable living arrangement is found. Years ago, Winniserv supported a lady living in her own apartment who was diagnosed with Alzheimer's disease. Despite enhanced staffing, she was encountering such challenges as overflowing her bathtub, throwing out lunches that had been prepared the previous evening and getting lost on her way to work. Fortunately, that was at the time the dementia friendly household was opened and she was one of the first people to move into that environment where she continued to live for five years.

Currently, no one living in their own apartment has been diagnosed with dementia but there are several older individuals with Down syndrome living independently that have raised a degree of suspicion in the last few years. In response to our concerns, one of them very reluctantly agreed to move into a cluster situation in an apartment block with two other ladies. They each have their own suites but meals are provided in a dining room and staff hours are combined to provide enriched supports. This type of arrangement should buy some time to assist people to plan for alternate arrangements if dementia is diagnosed and noted in the early stage of the condition. Initial conversations with people who are living independently have met with great resistance to the thought of moving into a group living arrangement. Many of the individuals living on their own came from the group home system where they lived with six to eight housemates, and moving out to live more independently was seen as a significant rite of passage and something to strive towards and celebrate. Not unlike some in the general population, who are forced to move out of their homes as dementia progresses, these individuals will see such a move as a significant loss on top of all their other losses.

Assessment and diagnosis

The implementation of a dementia care plan began with assessment and diagnosis (Wilkinson *et al.*, 2004). Early screening and diagnosis is such an important step for a variety of reasons, including the issues of differential diagnosis, future planning and to discuss the appropriateness of medication (Jokinen *et al.*, 2013). Staff turnover at times led to a lack of knowledge of individuals' previous skills and abilities, and thus an inability to note change. In order to attempt to identify changes that might be related to the onset of dementia, Winnserv established screening protocols in 1998. Implementing screening protocols was a reversal of previous philosophical commitments to stop carrying out assessments on people, and was not an easy decision to make or since maintain. The adaptive assessments continue to be done only on people who have Down syndrome, consistent with screening approaches elsewhere (Janicki *et al.*, 2002; Zigman *et al.*, 2004), although we acknowledge that this can lead to dementia being missed in other older adults with intellectual disabilities. Baseline assessments are completed prior to age 35, or earlier whenever possible, and we try to complete them yearly after the age of 40. The first baseline adaptive assessment tool, used for many years, was the Inventory for Client and Agency

Planning (ICAP) and then about ten years ago a switch was made to the AAMR Adaptive Behaviour Scale – Residential and Community Second Edition (Nihira *et al.*, 1993). It has been a challenge to complete screening on a regular basis due to a lack of resources. Initially frontline staff completed the assessments but they were not always carried out correctly, so now they are only completed by staff with the requisite background to ensure they are correct and objective. The new screening tool, the NTG-Early Detection Screen for Dementia, recommended by Jokinen *et al.* (2013), will make this less of a struggle. It has been constructed so it could be easily completed by family caregivers or direct support staff with minimal orientation or training (Jokinen *et al.*, 2013) and will likely become the tool of choice for Winnserv.

Once adaptive assessments indicate changes of concern or of staff, or family bring forward concerns, then the next step is to eliminate other potential causes such as hypothyroidism, depression, pain and side effects of medications (Jokinen *et al.*, 2013; McCarron and Lawlor, 2010). Clinical supports for an accurate diagnosis are limited, as service providers who work with people in the general population with dementia have been reluctant to become involved with people with an intellectual disability, and may not have the necessary skills or experience to do so (McCarron and Lawlor, 2010). Even if they are willing to work with someone with intellectual disabilities, they do not utilize tools specific to this population. There are no clinicians in the province who specialize in this dual diagnosis, indeed many people with intellectual disabilities do not ever receive a confirmed actual diagnosis.

Years ago, there was very little awareness of the connection between growing older with Down syndrome and the risk for acquiring a type of dementia, so the focus was on educating the various professions. Now that information is more widely disseminated, the concern that arises is the tendency to attribute any changes experienced by people with Down syndrome as being related to dementia. Over the years, Winnserv has had people either diagnosed with dementia, or the suspicion of dementia has been heightened, only to find the changes noted had their roots in other causes. An example is a 58-year-old man with Down syndrome who lost the ability to sign his name, stopped cooking, had trouble sleeping at night and was experiencing mood swings and trouble concentrating. It was about six months after his mother had died and once he received support for his grief all of his issues of concern reverted to normal.

Medications

The use of Aricept in the early stage of Alzheimer's disease is common practice in the general population (Prasher, 2004). This is not necessarily the case for people who have an intellectual disability (Prasher, 2004), for a variety of reasons, including difficulty getting an accurate diagnosis. In the province where Winnserv is located, the government medical services cover the cost for the use of Aricept, based on obtaining a certain range of scores on the Mini-Mental State Examination (MMSE). This funding is discontinued once the individual falls below a certain score and so a challenge arises for those who live with intellectual disabilities. Some people who have intellectual disabilities would not have achieved a high enough score to qualify for funding even at their optimum, so the cost of the medication becomes a significant issue. There are instances where physicians can make a case, in writing, for an exception to the guidelines but not all physicians are willing to make this effort.

Courtenay *et al.* (2010) and Prasher (2004) indicate that, in the face of limited research into the use of Aricept for people with Down syndrome, the medication does not always seem to be beneficial. The individuals that Winnserv has supported, who have been prescribed Aricept, with the exception of a couple of people, tolerated the medication well although varying degrees of benefit have been observed and documented. Our approach has been to advocate for a trial of Aricept whenever we feel we have been able to identify possible dementia fairly early on in the process.

When it comes to medication, one concern has arisen for a number of the individuals we have supported. People with Down syndrome often experience a late-onset seizure disorder as part of having dementia (Aylward *et al.*, 1995; Jokinen *et al.*, 2013; Tsiouris *et al.*, 2002). When they arrive at a hospital emergency room they are often given the anti-seizure medication, Dilantin, as it is one of the few medications that can be given intravenously. Unfortunately, people then leave the hospital with an ongoing prescription for the medication and quickly begin experiencing significant side effects. We have seen individuals lose the ability to walk, swallow and even sit upright within 24–48 hours of starting the medication and they again recover these skills and abilities within 24–48 hours of the medication being discontinued. We first observed this in the early nineties and as we spoke with others, both in Canada and the United States, it became apparent that this phenomenon was being observed across North America. Side effects such as a sudden loss of adaptive living skills, cognitive decline, lethargy, loss of ability to walk and bending to one side were noted in a small study conducted with people with Down syndrome and dementia who had been put on Dilantin for late-onset seizures (Tsiouris *et al.*, 2002). That article is now in the personal file of each person we support who has Down syndrome and it goes to the hospital with them. It has made a significant difference in our ability to advocate for the person to be prescribed an alternate anti-seizure medication to take on an ongoing basis.

Environmental changes

A wheelchair accessible environment is a key element to successfully supporting someone to remain in a home in the community. That is not the only environmental adaptation that is required to meet the needs of someone with dementia. It is essential to 'anticipate and plan for environmental modifications that likely support continued independence and reduce stress and demands on the individual as well as the carers' (Jokinen *et al.*, 2013, p. 17). Hard learned lessons led Winniserv to pay much more attention to environmental and physical elements when we decided to open a dementia friendly household. A scan of the houses that Winnserv was operating helped to determine that one of the houses could be renovated to meet the needs of someone with dementia. The house had a sprinkler system, we built a ramp at the front and back, widened doorways and replaced the bathtub with a wheelchair shower. In addition to looking at the accessibility basics, we also tried to create elements within the house that would assist people with the challenges they might encounter when needing to move freely and in understanding environmental stimuli. The home already had a naturally existing open concept and walking route. We have used the evidence base and practice guides to increase low-budget aspects of dementia friendly design such as consistent, non-glare flooring throughout the house, walls in a non-glare contrasting colour, good lighting and a safely enclosed backyard (Mitchell, 2012; Watchman, 2007).

In the past few years, the features of the house have been enhanced by a track system for the Hoyar Lift and the installation of a walk-in tub. Winnserv is fortunate to operate in a province where the government offers the people we support free, relatively quick and easy access to in-home physiotherapy and occupational therapy. The government also funds recommended equipment such as sit-to-stand lifts, mattresses that prevent bed sores, wheelchairs and Hoyar Lifts. This means that accessibility requirements do not become an economic stumbling block to ongoing community support.

Staffing levels and training

Keeping people with both intellectual disabilities and dementia in a home in the community for their lifetime, requires wide-ranging adaptations to the supports offered. The continuum of care that represents the progression of the condition must be recognized and staff training, staff levels and supports offered must be planned in a way that reflects the need for timely changes. Meeting these needs is a challenge within a dementia friendly household but is even more complicated when supporting people within a home where other housemates do not have that dual diagnosis. According to Janicki *et al.* (2005, p. 5), when looking at three particular areas of caregiving, 'personal care, behaviour management, and other supports and care – staff spent notably more time attending to people with dementia than they did with adults who did not have dementia'. This can be a source of stress for both the staff and the other people who live in the house. Winnserv is fortunate to receive funding to provide enriched staffing levels for anyone with intellectual disabilities and dementia, whether they are in the dementia specific household or elsewhere. Even in the early stages of dementia when care is 'not as problematic from a staff management perspective' (Janicki *et al.*, 2005, p. 7), there is still the need to focus on 'engaging residual memories and capabilities, providing social and recreational activities' (Janicki *et al.*, 2005, p. 7). These tasks are not as time intensive as those involved in the provision of personal care assistance that come with the mid to late stages of dementia (McCarron *et al.*, 2002), but the person still requires additional time and attention, translating into more staffing hours. Our goal, in the early stages of the condition, is to provide as much staff support as possible to keep the individual involved in their home and community and to utilize their skills and abilities in order to maintain a good quality of life and to delay a decline in function for as long as possible.

In the dementia friendly household, the staffing patterns change based on a number of factors. It is a three-person home that at any given time can be supporting people with a range of skills and needs, including being ambulatory and non-ambulatory. There can be times when everyone is still able to participate in a day program and times when all three people receive 'in home' support 24 hours a day, seven days a week. There are times, usually when accessing community-based activities, that there may be one-to-one staffing. Within the home, when all three people are present, we maintain a two staff to three people ratio, with the exception of single staffing at night and for two to three hour time slots when staff are comfortable working alone due to decreased care demands.

An awake at night staffing pattern is usually established quite early on in the condition, no matter where the person is living, so that staff can monitor for waking at night and potential exiting of the house. Wilkinson *et al.* (2004) found awake at night staff to be a key factor in keeping someone with dementia in their home, and it was helpful for both the individual and their housemates as it was possible to intervene before behaviour that disrupted others occurred. Staff who are paid to remain awake have less of a tendency to get into power struggles around making the person go to sleep, a more relaxed approach is utilized when addressing the situation and this increases the chance of a successful resolution. Where there has been a delay in implementing awake at night shifts, staff have indicated they do not sleep anyway due to concerns about an individual getting up in the middle of the night.

In addition to staff levels that alleviate high workloads and stress, it is also essential that staff have a good knowledge base about Alzheimer's disease and other forms of dementia, including progression and the impact on people's ability to process and understand their environment. This information allows staff to proactively problem-solve and to try to cope with the many challenges, including changes in behaviour. Winnserv has been able to hire some staff with a background in working with people with dementia, within the health care system. However, few staff have this level of previous training. Winnserv's response to the need for staff training has been to offer a combination of 'in house' seminars on dementia in general, and more specifically how it relates to people with intellectual disabilities. We also access community training resources from other services, particularly around the provision of physical care and addressing medical issues.

An important element of training offered by Winnserv is around supporting someone who is demonstrating 'responsive' behaviours as a result of the impact the condition has on the functioning of the brain, rather than seeing it as an individual issue. Experience and research both reflect the fact that many behaviours observed in people who have intellectual disabilities and dementia mirror what is seen in the general population (Janicki et al., 2002) with the core approaches working for both populations. Staff look at the key elements of Physical, Intellectual, Emotional, Capabilities, Environmental and Social as part of a PIECES framework (Hamilton et al., 2008) to investigate the underlying causes of 'responsive' behaviours. This offers an information-gathering template for identifying precipitating factors and a guideline for exploring potential solutions for the individual.

It has been a challenge to have all staff trained and confident in supporting people with dementia due to the turnover of staff and the somewhat limited availability of the 'in house' trainer. This has become even more difficult now that teams in three different households require training. Having a fully trained residential supervisor in each house is helpful, but it has become apparent that their skill sets lay in supporting the initial training and information, not in providing those essential early building blocks. They do not have the time, on a day-by-day basis, to give all the staff all of the information and training they require. Winnserv has been experimenting with the use of distance education strategies such as webinars and online courses, although our workforce has predominantly indicated a preference for face-to-face training or a more interactive approach, which makes the information more real and applicable.

As people progress into the mid and late stages of dementia, staff teams receive more individualized training from external resources around the provision of personal and physical care. There are no nurses on staff so the agency provides basic body mechanics training to staff and then brings in community nursing services periodically to ensure good practices are being implemented. As indicated, the provincial health and welfare system provides funding for occupational and physiotherapy assessments and those professionals, in turn, provide training in the use of equipment and other recommended procedures.

Swallowing assessments and recommendations are also made available, at no cost to the individual or agency, through provincial programs.

Adapting supports

Residential supports for adults with intellectual disabilities are usually focused on assisting people to increase their independence, acquire new skills and expand their community involvement. Staff working with people who also have dementia can be 'stymied with a philosophically different approach to their previous interactions' (Service, 2002, p. 215). Training helps to change their focus, but they also need ongoing support and guidance to adapt the supports that they offer. In the early stages of the condition 'an adult's support structure needs little modification, save for compensations for individualised losses and problems in orientation and memory, progressive decline in latter stages will involve more specialised care and compensations' (Janicki *et al.*, 2002, p. 192). In Winnserv's experience, staff who are learning to support someone with dementia for the first time struggle in the early stages with such concepts. This includes fully understanding the variability of skills that come with the condition, the need to utilize picture prompts to encourage independence rather than just continually giving verbal prompts and to avoid 'doing for' people when they encounter difficulties. This can also be an issue for staff with years of experience working in the dementia household, with people in the mid to late stages, who begin to support someone with early dementia. There is a tendency to offer a greater degree of assistance than is needed at that stage and this tendency reflects the drawbacks of asking staff to be able to readily adapt to all of the differing support needs from the early to end stage of dementia.

In some instances, day programs and work placements have been unable to continue to support people even in the early stages of dementia, but it is more often the case that such supports are withdrawn in the mid stages. Day services often do not receive the necessary funding to provide sufficient supports to ensure safety and to keep people engaged. Individuals can also find larger, congregated settings too overwhelming, at which point the day program becomes more of a hindrance than a help. When Winnserv steps in to offer 24/7 supports, the daytime staffing is either 1:1 or 2:1 and the focus is on balancing the need for routine and a calm environment with the need for stimulation, engagement and community connection.

Mid to late stage supports shift staff into more of a clinical model of care, something that has been strenuously avoided in community-based services. People begin to lose the capacity to initiate eating and drinking and to tell staff they are thirsty or hungry, so we begin to document their nutrition and hydration. We track bowel movements, so we can assist people in trying to avoid constipation, and seizures so we know when it is time to request adjustments in medications. As people have increased difficulty using utensils, feeding themselves and swallowing there is a movement from the traditional three meals a day to small snacks or meals throughout the day; finger foods are introduced, food is pureed and fluids thickened. It is easy to shift into caretaking mode at this point and there is a need to constantly remind each other of the continued importance of relationships, community access and meaningful activities.

An additional clinical element is the need to monitor and treat pain. Pain is under-recognized and under-treated for both people with dementia in the general population, and people with intellectual disabilities (Oberlander and Symons, 2006; Scherder et al., 2005). An inability to identify the location of the pain, to verbalize pain, or to express it in an easily recognized manner means that staff must have a heightened awareness of the potential for pain (Scherder et al., 2005). When pain is a potential cause of changes in behaviour, Winnserv uses non-verbal pain assessment tools such as the Pain Assessment in Advanced Dementia (PAINAD) scale (Warden et al., 2003) and the Pain Assessment Checklist for Seniors with Limited Ability to Communicate (PASLAC) checklist (Fuchs-Lacelle and Hadjistavropoulos, 2004). The checklist is completed by different staff, on different shifts, over a number of days and that information is given to the health care provider.

The end stage of dementia entails an almost total focus on the physical provision of care and on medical issues (Service, 2002). Individuals require full staff assistance in all aspects of their care including maintaining skin integrity, repositioning in bed or while sitting up, eating and drinking and incontinence care. In addition to providing a high level of physical care, staff offer comfort care through foot rubs, massages and music appropriate to the individual and are reminded that it is still important to talk to, or sing with, the person. Problems with aspiration inevitably lead to a discussion with substitute decision-makers on whether or not to consider tube feeding. Research indicates that tube feeding may not be helpful in providing nutrition or preventing aspiration (Service, 2002). It is an emotionally laden decision to balance potential aspiration pneumonia and inadequate nutrition with tube feeding, but every family Winnserv has worked with has rejected tube feeding. Winnserv, as an organization, has not formally determined what they would do if a family requested the insertion of a feeding tube, but there would be concerns about the ethics of putting someone through such a procedure when there is little or no evidence of efficacy.

Aspiration pneumonia and the complete loss of physical abilities signal the end of life phase for people with dementia. Winnserv is committed to providing a palliative approach from early in the process through to end of life. We have a clear policy around this commitment and staff employed to support people with dementia are told at their interview that the job entails end of life care. Staff training in this area is offered through a program at Hospice and Palliative Care Manitoba, developed specifically for staff supporting people with intellectual disabilities. The course has been extremely helpful in giving staff the skills, information and confidence that they need to provide this care. Staff also must know they have the support of management and that help is only a telephone call away, regardless of the time of day. Death can happen at any given time but when its approach appears inevitable, team meetings are utilized to discuss personal death experiences, fears and concerns and staff are given the option of working elsewhere if they prefer. Over many years of providing end of life care, not one Winnserv staff member has asked to transfer to another location. End of life preparations also include the completion of a Death At Home letter, from a physician, that indicates the presence of a terminal illness and plans for the person to die at home if preferred. This letter is submitted to the coroner's office and a copy is kept at the house; so when the individual dies there is no need for an investigation, the funeral home is called when everyone has had the chance to say their goodbyes and the body is taken away.

Family supports

The first important step in supporting the family members of someone diagnosed with dementia is to provide them with as much information as possible about dementia, to help them understand how to respond to and support their family member and to be available for answering questions. It is also essential to understand that the grief process often begins at diagnosis and can influence the family's responses and coping strategies. In our experience, families are best able to take in information on a step-by-step basis with regular meetings and ongoing communication. Many family members are not able to talk about such issues as Do Not Resuscitate (DNR) orders and end of life care until their family member enters the mid stage of dementia and death seems more of a reality. Families are often able to discuss and take action early on in the area of decision-making, opting first for supported decision-making and then moving to formal substitute decision-making once health issues begin to arise. Discussions around DNR orders and advanced care directives are highly emotional and are not one-time-only events.

Very few families affiliated with Winnserv have taken advantage of family support groups run by the local Alzheimer Society, but they have often reached out to them for information. Overall families have been very engaged with their family member in the early stages, but at times some withdraw as dementia progresses, and interactions become more difficult as unusual or different behaviours arise. At this point, the role of staff becomes one of facilitating and creating successful interactions and supporting the family. One sister, who was heavily involved in supporting her sibling, withdrew shortly after her sister moved into the dementia specific household. She was encouraged to attend some grief seminars, and was subsequently able to become re-engaged until her sister's death. The key element to supporting families is the establishment of a good working relationship with staff, and for families to feel welcome in the home. If family members want to be involved in day-to-day care, it should be facilitated, as long as clear guidelines are set out that respect the fact that the house is home to more than one person, and that staff must be free to meet their job expectations.

Supporting housemates

The need to support housemates arises regardless of whether the person with dementia is living in an aging in place model in a community group home or in the dementia specific household. In a community group home, when a housemate begins to experience the changes that are a part of dementia, both the individual and the housemates question what is happening. Once a diagnosis has been obtained, permission needs to be given to share information with housemates so they can be supported to understand the changes and learn how they can help (Jokinen *et al.*, 2013). Wilkinson *et al.* (2004) noted that where agencies had identified that housemates knew of the diagnosis of dementia they were quite supportive of their roommate. Winnserv utilizes a pictorial booklet (Kerr and Innes, 2001) about dementia for adults who have intellectual disabilities to explain the condition to both the individual and their housemates. People have found it very helpful in trying to understand what is happening to their friend and to not take behaviours personally. Regular house meetings have also assisted in working out the challenges experienced when sharing their home with someone with dementia. Wilkinson *et al.* (2004) found that housemates' responses were influenced by how long they had known the person before they began to experience dementia and that longer term relationships led to a more supportive attitude. This has certainly been Winnserv's experience, as each time someone has been diagnosed with dementia and remained in their home, at least for the initial few years, housemates have known each other for over ten years and have shown incredible tolerance for sometimes difficult behaviour. It should be noted that a dementia specific household does not eliminate housemates creating challenges for each other and behaviours such as yelling at night have an adverse effect on others, with and without dementia. There are no easy answers in balancing what is best for all involved.

The struggles

After more than 20 years of working with people who have both intellectual disabilities and dementia, Winnserv still has a lot of room for improvement and still struggles to find answers that fit the organization and meet the needs of the people we support. We have frequently failed to help people understand they have dementia, either because we did not know how to tell the person or because the diagnosis came at a point where the individual would no longer understand. We do not always get all staff trained in a timely manner and our solutions to challenges sometimes come at a much slower pace than is beneficial for staff and the people we support. Our greatest struggle, however, is in accommodating people who experience changes, prior to demonstrating skill and memory loss associated with dementia, that are indicative of damage to the frontal lobe of the brain. Ball *et al.* (2006) found that some people with Down syndrome seem to experience changes in personality and behaviour prior to the demonstration of characteristics connected to Alzheimer's disease. By the time their research was published, Winnserv had already supported two individuals who had initially experienced behaviours that were extremely difficult to address, followed by an eventual progression to the skill and memory loss associated with Alzheimer's disease.

Winnserv's initial foray into supporting someone with frontal lobe dysfunction was a gentleman with lifelong obsessive-compulsive behaviours that had been well controlled for a number of years. Unfortunately, he became focused on bathroom routines to the point where he spent most of his days and nights in the bathroom, either having a bath or sitting on the toilet. The assumption was that his obsessive-compulsive tendencies had returned with a vengeance and so began the revolving attempts at finding a medication to address the issues. This led to a disastrous array of side effects and it was not until all medications were discontinued and a small amount reintroduced, that he experienced some relief from his obsessive behaviours. Six years later this man can no longer eat on his own, dress himself or remember his sister and is well advanced into the middle stages of Alzheimer's disease. There was a lot of trial and error with approaches and medications and we did not find the magical solution. The focus became about supporting people to deal with their stress and holding on to the mantra 'this too shall pass'.

Despite the struggles, at Winnserv we have never regretted the decision to continue to keep people with intellectual disabilities and dementia in the community until their death. Not all organizations have the resources to follow in our footsteps. However, we believe that the focus, time and effort required to do this work is well worth it, and overall gives a considerably better quality of life and increased sense of wellbeing to the individual and their family, friends and staff who support them.

References

Aylward, EH., Burt, DB., Thorpe, LU., Lai, F. and Dalton, AJ. (1995) *Diagnosis of Dementia in Individuals with Intellectual Disability*. Washington, DC: American Association on Mental Retardation.

Ball, S., Holland, A., Hon, J., Huppert, F., Treppner, P. and Watson, P. (2006) Personality and behaviour changes mark the early stages of Alzheimer's disease in adults with Down's syndrome: Findings from a prospective population-based study. *International Journal of Geriatric Psychiatry 21*, 7, 661–673.

Courtenay, K., Jokinen, N. and Strydom, A. (2010) Caregiving and adults with intellectual disabilities affected by dementia. *Journal of Policy and Practice in Intellectual Disabilities 7*, 1, 26–33.

Fuchs-Lacelle, S. and Hadjistavropoulos, T. (2004) Development and preliminary validation of the pain assessment checklist for seniors with limited ability to communicate (PACSLAC). *Pain Management Nursing 5*, 1, 37–49.

Hamilton, D., Le Clair, JK. and Collins, J. (2008) *Putting the P.I.E.C.E.S. Together*. 6th edition. Canada: Shop for Learning Publishing Services.

Janicki, M., McCallion, P. and Dalton, A. (2002) Dementia-related care decision-making in group homes for persons with intellectual disabilities. *Journal of Gerontological Social Work 38*, 102, 179–195.

Janicki, M., Dalton, A., McCallion, P., Baxley, D. and Zendell, A. (2005) *Providing Group Home Care for Adults with Intellectual Disabilities and Alzheimer's Disease*. Preliminary report prepared for UIC RRTC on Aging and Developmental Disabilities' annual meeting 17–18 February 2005.

Jokinen, N., Janicki, MP., Keller, SM., McCallion, P. and Force, LT. and the National Task Group on Intellectual Disabilities and Dementia Practices (2013) *Guidelines for Structuring Community Care and Supports for People with Intellectual Disabilities Affected by Dementia*. Available at http://aadmd.org/ntg/practiceguidelines, accessed on 7 December 2013.

Kerr, D. and Innes, M. (2001) *What is Dementia?* Edinburgh: Down's Syndrome Scotland.

McCarron, M. and Lawlor, BA. (2010) Responding to the challenges of ageing and dementia in intellectual disability in Ireland. *Aging and Mental Health 7*, 6, 413–417.

McCarron, M., Gill, M., Lawlor, B. and Beagly, C. (2002) A pilot study of the reliability and validity of the Caregiver Activity survey – Intellectual disability (CAS-ID). *Journal of Intellectual Disability Research 46*, 8, 605–612.

Mitchell, L. (2012) *At a Glance: A Checklist for Developing Dementia Friendly Communities*. University of Warwick. Viewpoint No. 25, Housing LIN. Available at www.housinglin. org.uk/_library/Resources/Housing/Support_materials/Viewpoints/Viewpoint25_ AtAGlance.pdf, accessed on 7 December 2013.

Nihira, K., Leland, H. and Lambert, N. (1993) *AAMR – Adaptive Behavior Scale – Residential and Community*. 2nd edition. Austin, Texas: Pro-Ed.

Oberlander, TF. and Symons, FJ. (2006) *Pain in Children and Adults with Developmental Disabilities*. Baltimore, MD: Paul H. Brookes.

Prasher, VP. (2004) Review of donepezil, rivastigmine, galantamine and memantine for the treatment of dementia in Alzheimer's disease in adults with Down's syndrome: Implications for the intellectual disability population. *International Journal of Geriatric Psychiatry 19*, 6, 509–515.

Scherder, E., Oosterman, J., Swaab, D. *et al.* (2005) Recent developments in pain and dementia. *British Medical Journal 330*, 7489, 461–464.

Service, K. (2002) Consideration in care for individuals with intellectual disability with advanced dementia. *Journal of Gerontological Social Work 38*, 1/2, 213–223.

Tsiouris, J., Patti, P., Tipu, O. and Raguthu, S. (2002) Adverse effects of phenytoin given for late-onset seizures in adults with Down's syndrome. *Neurology 59*, 10, 779–780.

Warden, V., Hurley, A.C. and Volicer, L. (2003) Development and psychometric evaluation of the Pain Assessment in Advanced Dementia (PAINAD) Scale. *Journal of American Medical Directors Association 4*, 1, 9–15.

Watchman, K. (2007) *Living with Dementia: Adapting the Home of a Person who has Down's Syndrome and Dementia – a Guide for Carers.* Edinburgh: Down's Syndrome Scotland.

Wilkinson, H., Kerr, D., Cunningham, C. and Rae, C. (2004) *Home for Good? Preparing to Support People with Learning Difficulties in Residential Settings when They Develop Dementia.* Brighton: Pavilion Publishing/Joseph Rowntree Foundation.

Zigman, WB., Schupf, N., Devenny, D. *et al.* (2004) Incidence and prevalence of dementia in elderly adults with MR without Down's syndrome. *American Journal of Mental Retardation 109*, 2, 126–141.

14

Responding to the Challenges of Service Development to Address Dementia Needs for People with an Intellectual Disability and their Caregivers

Mary McCarron, Philip McCallion,
Evelyn Reilly, Niamh Mulryan

Introduction

Shifting profiles in persons with intellectual disabilities in Ireland and elsewhere from a younger to older age has been a great achievement as it has moved individuals with an intellectual disability closer to general population longevity. It has also meant exposure to the chronic conditions of old age, particularly dementia. People with intellectual disabilities are as susceptible to the different types of dementia as other adult populations (Strydom *et al.*, 2007, 2010), with Alzheimer's type most prevalent, but presence of Down syndrome (Cooper, 2006; Prasher, 1995), gait deterioration (Patti *et al.*, 2010), earlier age of onset (Lai and Williams, 1989; Prasher, 1995), more precipitous decline (Visser *et al.*, 1997) and a greater burden of psychiatric symptoms (Wilkosz *et al.*, 2010) together mean its impact is often earlier and greater.

Very different issues present when individuals with intellectual disabilities have symptoms of dementia; issues that challenge traditional intellectual disability service approaches and philosophies. Staffing numbers and patterns, and the training of staff have more usually been focused upon consumer groups who are young and middle-aged, and on supporting and promoting the independence of persons with intellectual disabilities who are in jobs and interested in, and ready for, community participation (McCallion *et al.*, 2012). The inevitable decline associated with dementia challenges this programming philosophy. Similarly, traditional intellectual disability service assumptions of fixed needs are challenged by new needs, such as 24-hour staffing where overnight staff were not previously needed, more frequent hospitalisations and emergency room use as symptoms of both dementia and comorbidities increase. This is in addition to environmental management challenges as falls, apparent 'wandering' and safety concerns occur (Janicki *et al.*, 2002; McCallion *et al.*, 2005). There has been growing evidence that the associated care challenges posed by dementia place increased pressures on families, providers and staff, create additional costs, challenge existing programming approaches in many provider settings and may be perceived as so burdensome that they encourage placement of people with intellectual disabilities and dementia in more restrictive settings (Bigby, *et al.*, 2014; Janicki *et al.*, 2005).

Faced with such concerns, an international workgroup established the Edinburgh Principles (Wilkinson and Janicki, 2002) for the care and support of people with intellectual disabilities and dementia to encourage continued pursuit of person-centred and community-based care. These principles are summarised as:

- promotion of quality of life
- use of person-centred approaches
- need in care and programming to affirm individual strengths, capabilities, skills and wishes
- involvement of the individual, their family and other close supportive persons in all care planning and delivery
- greater access to and availability of appropriate diagnostic, assessment and service resources
- plans and services that effectively support the individual to remain in their chosen home and community
- access to the same services and supports that are available to other persons with dementia in the general population
- proactive strategic planning across policy, provider and advocacy groups.

On the one hand, the need for organisational responses is well established (Bigby *et al.*, 2014; Janicki *et al.*, 2005). On the other, the many barriers experienced and the perceptions that change has to be drastic or resource intensive has meant that such organisational responses are not yet widespread. This may be another example of what Kaskie and Coddington (2004) have argued after looking at organisational responses to dementia generally by healthcare systems. They contended that inaction results when there is a failure to comprehensively understand the increased costs and consequences of poor support of people with dementia, but also from not considering responses that manage within existing resources and may be accommodated within existing organisational structures (Kaluzny and Hernandez, 1983). In concluding their review, Kaskie and Coddington (2004) argue that needs assessment and planning are needed in the areas of public education, professional training, programme development and service integration. This is to support understanding of the extent of challenges, addressing the specific challenges being experienced, improving service access and delivery and better management of costs.

Many of the same issues arise for intellectual disability services and this chapter explains how one Irish services provider, the Daughters of Charity Service, has responded to the challenges of dementia. This involved pursuing the intent of the Edinburgh Principles, whilst undertaking a strategic planning process to develop a more thoughtful response to dementia for the consumers it serves. Information on the process they engaged in, on the tools used and on some of the results of their implementation of the strategic plan are also provided to support other services providers interested in developing their own strategic approach.

The Daughters of Charity

With services in both large urban and rural communities, the Daughters of Charity Service provides a wide range of supports to persons with a moderate, severe and profound intellectual disability, with a commitment to the development of the whole person, the involvement of parents, families and the wider community, the education and development of staff and collaborators and an efficient management structure.

The Service provides a range of day care and residential-type supports, including campus, community, semi-independent and respite care. The consequences of demographic shifts towards an older population and associated increases in dementia, particularly in those with Down syndrome, were recognised by staff and administrators as challenging their ability to realise the mission of the service. These challenges included:

Changing demographics: the realities of both the ageing of existing service users, and the older age of new entrants to the residential portion of the Service (children in Ireland are now rarely referred for residential care).

Ageing population with Down syndrome: the Daughters of Charity Service have traditionally provided supports to a large population with Down syndrome.

Challenges to the current service model: as is true for many services providers, at the Daughters of Charity Service there has been a strong emphasis on supporting service users to gain increasing levels of independence, to participate in work and day programmes and to increase their engagement in the community. As dementia symptoms occur and there is a need to change from adding to maintaining skills, and then to offering greater supports, the prior model of services is less adequate and may frustrate service users, families and staff.

A need to restructure residential and day programmes: advancing symptoms of dementia present additional care, environmental and supervision concerns that are not easily accommodated in existing physical buildings or in programming structures. Nor are funding and regulatory schemes perceived as sufficiently flexible to support needed changes easily.

A need to upskill staff at all levels in the organisation to respond to changing needs: although fortunate to have a stable and educated workforce, the Daughters of Charity Service is nevertheless challenged that staff were often recruited and trained for different support and training needs and in particular may not feel prepared for increased behavioural concerns in mid stage dementia and increased medical concerns in advanced dementia.

End of life care concerns: a service commitment to creating and supporting family-like care means that staff have often spent years working with individuals whom they care about as well as care for. After a diagnosis of dementia they watch, over an extended period, previously independent persons become more frail and ultimately die. There is great concern that such decline and death be as comfortable as possible, and the person's final journey is peaceful and respectful of the individual's wishes. There is also concern about the impact of such experiences on carers.

Early in the preparation for strategic planning, the Service recognised that current incremental responses to dementia were no longer sufficient and that a more fundamental rethinking of services, training and services philosophy was needed including, potentially, a purposeful restructuring of day and residential services and redeployment of staff.

Yet, a realistic and feasible approach was also necessary. A strategic planning group was formed and considered a series of key questions:

- What is the mix of services that is and will be needed and how will they change over time?

- What is the best location for services?

- What are we trying to achieve with the services we provide?

- How will the services that are needed be sustained?

- What is needed to develop dementia specific day and residential programmes?

The planning group was also influenced by a consideration of the literature (McCarron and Lawlor, 2003) on what a dementia-ready service will look like:

- services through specialist multidisciplinary teams offering good clinical support

- early screening and diagnosis using a memory clinic model

- a continuum of residential options to support changing needs of persons at different stages of dementia

- appropriate day programmes

- training and education programmes for staff and families

- research to guide practice and policy.

Why strategic planning?

Strategic planning is recommended when challenges presented and incremental steps already being taken are both not sufficient and probably not well aligned. There is a need for longer-term planning rather than short-term or crisis responses. A more efficient and effective use of resources is required with a desire to ensure that service changes are consistent with agency vision and mission and there is a willingness to set priorities in ways in which achievement will be measureable over time (Allison and Kaye, 2005). Different types of strategic planning may be more suited to specific strategic issues. McNamara (2007) suggests that there are several types of strategic plans including:

Goals-based planning: focused on the organisation's mission (and vision and/or values), goals to work towards the mission, strategies to achieve the goals, and action planning (who will do what and by when).

Issues-based strategic planning: starts by examining issues facing the organisation, strategies to address those issues and action plans.

Strategic planning: articulating the organisation's vision and values, and then action plans to achieve the vision while adhering to those values.

The challenges presented by dementia were such that the Daughters of Charity Service chose to focus their efforts in an issues-based strategic planning process.

Approach

The approach to issues-based strategic planning was also influenced by traditional strategic planning tools (McNamara, 2007):

- assess the current state of the service/organisation
- develop a vision of where to go
- determine the 'gap' between current state and the vision
- set a direction, business plan
- implement the strategic plan
- evaluate the plan.

In a desire to be inclusive of all stakeholders, the initial planning group was also influenced by the strategies in Trochim's (1989) concept mapping phases. This saw the development of a steering committee and workgroups to support strategic planning preparation, the development of focal questions and a process to support generation of ideas, alignment of proposed actions with current science on cognitive concerns and care best practices, and a purposeful and informed selection of action items (Anderson *et al.*, 2011).

Strategic planning implementation: steering committee and workgroups

An initial planning group was formed comprising the chief executive officer, the medical director with the overall process led by the policy and services advisor on dementia. This planning group then recruited a representative steering committee comprising representatives of the Service's executive staff, senior local managers, frontline staff (nursing and care assistants), and clinical team members across a range of disciplines.

In order to ensure that the voices of all stakeholders were included, three workgroups were also formed comprising: service users, families and frontline staff. The steering committee identified and assisted with the recruitment of members to each of the workgroups with the only criterion being all members had to have experiences in supporting persons with dementia.

Strategic planning implementation: preparation and generation of ideas

Phase 1: Preparation

The steering committee guided the entire process of developing and agreeing a set of recommended actions to advance short, medium and long-term approaches to ensuring that the Service was better capable of meeting the needs of service users with dementia.

Phase 2: Generation of ideas

There were three data collection steps to support the generation of ideas. The first was an audit of the dementia-readiness of all residential and day units addressing environmental suitability and readiness to support maintenance of skills and community engagement. This was followed by an assessment of current prevalence of dementia symptoms among consumers and evidence-based projections of five and ten years prevalence and, finally, focus groups to capture stakeholder concerns and ideas.

ENVIRONMENTAL DEMENTIA-READINESS AUDIT

An inventory of the physical environment was completed for every residential and day programming building operated by the Daughters of Charity Service.

Units were given a consensus ranking by the survey team (comprising programme, facilities and administrative staff) in terms of whether they were:

- dementia-ready
- in need of some minor additional dementia-readiness improvement
- in need of some major additional dementia-readiness improvement
- not suitable for dementia care.

In addition, costings were developed for any needed renovations or changes. The feasibility of such expenditures was considered and remaining gaps in the built infrastructure were identified.

Table 14.1: Dementia-readiness inventory

Dementia-ready feature	Currently available	Possible if resources can be redirected (specify resources)	Requires retraining of staff (specify training needed)	Requires renovation (specify type of renovation and cost estimate)	Not possible in current building and/or with current staffing
Preferred environmental features					
Programming areas					
Doorways accommodate walkers, wheelchairs and lifts					
Dementia-ready colours, flooring, way-finding signs and furniture					
Dementia-ready lighting, sound management and small group activity environments					
Kitchen/dining areas					
Cupboards labelled for visual cues (pictorially not with text) and providing safe storage (e.g. using discreet locks)					

cont.

Table 14.1: Dementia-readiness inventory (*cont.*)

Dementia-ready feature	Currently available	Possible if resources can be redirected (specify resources)	Requires retraining of staff (specify training needed)	Requires renovation (specify type of renovation and cost estimate)	Not possible in current building and/or with current staffing
Dementia-ready colours, flooring, way-finding signs and furniture					
Shut-off switches on appliances					
Simplification of meals and use of adaptive utensils and plate guards					
Bathrooms					
Fully accessible for people in wheelchairs					
Ability to regulate water temperature and walk-in shower facilities					
Dementia-ready colours, flooring, way-finding signs					
Outdoor areas					
Walking paths, raised flowerbeds and safe areas					

Programming					
Use of 'failure-free' and personally-valued activities with things already known rather than new learning					
Emphasis on social enjoyment and on things remembered					
Use of adaptive equipment including communication and memory devices, and support for use of glasses and hearing aids					
Capacity for aromatherapy, massage therapy, multi-sensory-room, music, crafts, gardening/horticulture, simple exercise					
Schedules that adapt to the needs and interests of the participant with dementia					
Enhanced staffing where needed					

Source: adapted from Nickle and McCallion, 2005

PREVALENCE

In the Daughters of Charity Service, systematic tracking of symptoms and diagnoses of dementia in persons with Down syndrome began in 1993 when 8.7 per cent were initially diagnosed with dementia. Among a group of 80 services users aged 35 and over detection rates had risen to 74 per cent by 2003.

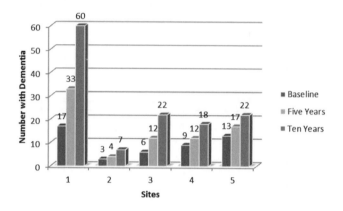

Figure 14.1: Projected number of persons with dementia over ten years

Data gathering also established that all residential settings, campuses, dispersed community housing and group homes at the Daughters of Charity were addressing dementia care issues, with some having done so for more than ten years. A significant number of residential and community group homes had at least one individual with dementia, and some had more than one. There were also concerns that existing dementia assessment strategies may not yet have identified everyone with dementia symptoms. Case reviews were undertaken to determine current prevalence and, using reported age-related prevalence rates for persons with Down syndrome (Lai and Williams, 1989; Prasher, 1995), anticipated prevalence rates after five and ten years were calculated. These yielded estimates of 48 persons with Down syndrome currently with confirmed symptoms of dementia, with an additional 29 at risk of developing dementia in the next five years, and a further 51 in ten years. In examining the data, and in light of other findings (Cosgrave *et al.*, 2000; McCarron *et al.*, 2002) the steering committee agreed that the individuals with dementia tended to fall into three groupings.

Group 1

Some people may experience a relatively slow progression of dementia over five to eight years approximately. While these individuals will require increasing supports, particularly in terms of staffing and some relatively low cost environmental modifications to their living spaces, they can often be maintained within their 'family unit', that is, the home they have lived in throughout their decline. Ageing in place in this way retains contact with familiar environments, family and friends.

Group 2

For some people, while decline may not necessarily be compressed, they present, particularly at mid stage dementia, with behavioural and psychotic features such as night-time waking, apparent wandering, agitation, screaming, and visual and auditory hallucinations. Some behavioural issues may be addressed in existing settings with improved communication approaches and attention to programming and environmental concerns. For other individuals, dementia specific environments with specialist trained staff will be required to respond and address their additional care needs.

Group 3

For some people, decline may be compressed, and the person may progress to a stage of advanced dementia within a relatively short period of time, for example one to two years. It was recognised that persons with end stage dementia will require specialist nursing in addition to ongoing palliative care.

It was agreed that short- and long-term strategies would need to be considered in terms of defining, developing and delivering services to meet the needs of the three groups.

FOCUS GROUPS

To begin the generation of strategic ideas to address the emerging understanding of dementia implications for the Service, the steering committee chose focal questions drawn from Nickols and Ledgerwood (2005). The goals grid considered:

- What do you want that you don't have? (Achieve)

- What do you want that you already have? (Preserve)

- What don't you have that you don't want? (Avoid)

- What do you have now that you don't want? (Eliminate)

The same questions were given to the participants in each workgroup and they had the opportunity to provide written responses and to be interviewed individually or in small groups with notes taken.

Phase 3: Structuring of statements

A full list of responses to each of the four questions was generated and the most frequently occurring items across the groups were identified, as well as the most frequently occurring items in each group. Examples included: ageing in place, a support network and social connectedness, competent care and a suitable environment.

The listings were reviewed with the steering committee and it was agreed that there was room to combine some items, but equally there were items that were not fully understood. In an independent process, two reviewers sought additional information from respondents and, using thematic content analysis, explored opportunities for combining items and developed potential common statements of key issues.

Phase 4: Representation of statements

A final list of items divided into 'Achieve, Preserve, Avoid and Eliminate' categories with proposed definitions was then shared with, and validated by, representative participants from the workgroups, and by the full steering committee.

Table 14.2: Key themes that emerged across groups

What do you want that you don't have? (Achieve)	What do you want that you already have? (Preserve)	What don't you have that you don't want? (Avoid)	What do you have now that you don't want? (Eliminate)
Suitable environment to deal with the progression of dementia	Ageing in place	Restrictive environments	Relocating clients with dementia into non-specific dementia settings
Competent care/ staff education and training	Strong relationships amongst staff and service users	Mini institutions for persons with dementia	Crisis decision-making particularly at end of life
Peer and family education	Competent nursing care	Transfers to generic hospitals and nursing homes	Insufficient staffing levels
Staff consistency across the service	Spiritual care		Fragmented approach to dementia care
Increased family involvement	Policy and service advisor on dementia		Inappropriate environments
A dementia specific day service	Person-centred ethos		Inappropriate day programmes
Clinical nurse specialist/ advanced nurse practitioner in dementia	Care provided within the service		Negative impact on quality of life for other clients in home setting
Memory clinic and dementia screening and assessment	Multidisciplinary support		

Phase 5: Interpretation

The steering committee discussed the items, identified the services and approaches that were to be 'preserved' and where current services represented the 'eliminate' category. They also considered why 'achieve' ideas had not yet occurred and how they would ensure that 'avoid' services would not be initiated. In a final round of deliberations, the steering committee used this listing to help guide them through a process of establishing and refining a vision for dementia-focused services that emerged.

DEVELOPING AN OPERATIONALISED STRATEGIC PLAN

A planning day was convened involving the steering committee and workgroup members and a preliminary plan developed for the implementation of this strategic vision. Four half-day planning sessions with the same group of stakeholders then systematically reviewed the audit and prevalence information, the 'achieve, avoid, preserve and eliminate' issues, agreed next steps and the Service's available resources to arrive at a statement of initial implementation strategies. This comprised six critical strands: screening and assessment, specialist multidisciplinary team for dementia, education and training, residential options, day programmes and research.

SCREENING AND ASSESSMENT

It was recognised that there was a need for timely assessment and diagnosis and the development of appropriate care plans for persons with diagnosed and suspected symptoms of dementia. Given that a mobile memory clinic had been established by the Daughters of Charity Service with key components conceptualised and a number of service users already screened and assessed, it was decided that the most effective use of resources would be to fully operationalise the memory clinic.

The rationale for this was: the growing risk of dementia given the ageing of the population supported, the potential for treatable symptoms of other conditions being mistaken for dementia and, for some individuals, dementia not being recognised until the late stages. It was recognised that all of these concerns would be better addressed if symptoms were identified early, differential diagnosis became routine and screening and diagnostic protocols were implemented within the context of a mobile memory clinic.

Action steps

- Protocols developed for screening and comprehensive diagnostic work-up.

- Clinical nurse specialist hired to assist in the management of the memory clinic.

- Secretary hired to support the memory clinic and the overall dementia service.

- Comprehensive review undertaken of all screening completed to date and status of persons with dementia and suspected dementia documented.

- Annual screening/re-screening of all persons with Down syndrome over the age of 35 years and persons with intellectual disabilities from other aetiologies over 50 years.

- Monthly clinics with an announced schedule of locations for purposes of comprehensive diagnostic work-up.

- Data collected and entered into a minimum dataset to support ongoing evaluation of the operations of the memory clinic.

SPECIALIST MULTIDISCIPLINARY TEAM FOR DEMENTIA

Planned dementia care provision and the operation of a memory clinic were new developments for the Service and it was decided this would require the support of a specialist dementia team with specialised training. Establishing such a team linked to the memory clinic would better prepare the Service to address future as well as current needs but the specialist team would not replace the role of local multidisciplinary teams in day-to-day care. If systematic identification and assessment for dementia symptoms is to become part of routine care, then specialist staff resources are needed to support diagnostic work-up and screening of all persons with an intellectual disability.

Action steps

- Established a core specialist dementia team linked to the memory clinic and available to complete a consensus diagnosis after comprehensive assessment.

- Planned access on a consultant basis to additional team members as needed, including a nutritionist, physiotherapist, speech and language therapist, and palliative care consultant.

- Comprehensive training for team members provided by policy and services advisor.

- Protocols developed for specialist dementia team and post-diagnosis support to develop person-centred plans for day-to-day care and meaningful activities.

TRAINING NEEDS

- Staff need to understand the course and symptoms of dementia, and to be prepared for changing care needs and to offer dementia supportive programming and care.

- Service users, their peers and families need to understand dementia issues, unique problems related to memory and day-to-day functioning and empowering strategies that assist in a meaningful way in caring for their family member or friend.

- As dementia progresses, medical and nursing needs become more complex and maintaining adequate hydration and nutrition, pain management and end of life care decisions are paramount.

- People with dementia and their families require information, guidance and support to make informed decisions which will guide end of life care plans.

Care approaches for persons with dementia are different from care offered to persons with an intellectual disability without dementia. A trained workforce will be better able to maintain quality of life for the person, support ageing in place, support dementia friendly care settings, and reduce or delay the need for a move to a different setting. Staff themselves will experience more competence and less stress in providing care. Similarly, service users, peers and families will be more empowered and better equipped to support dementia care.

Action steps

- Staff on all campuses surveyed about current and desired dementia training and a comprehensive training programme developed in response.

- The training programme comprises:

  o education and resource packs for all relevant residential and community group homes, day services and multidisciplinary departments

  o a comprehensive dementia training programme targeted at nursing and allied health staff

  o a specific education programme designed to support peers

  o a 1–4-day orientation to dementia offered to all staff

  o on a bi-annual basis, an information/education meeting facilitated by the specialist dementia team for family members

  o information/educational packs including easy-read materials developed for persons with dementia, their peers and families

  o support for staff to undertake accredited training and postgraduate courses in ageing and dementia-related care

  o sponsorship of an annual education and research conference.

RESIDENTIAL OPTIONS TO SUPPORT PERSONS
ACROSS THE CONTINUUM OF DEMENTIA

In line with national and international best practices in dementia care and based on consultation and discussions with staff, families and service users, the strategic plan is designed to support the Daughters of Charity Service's commitment to support persons with dementia to remain in their usual home setting, or a home of their choice, throughout the continuum of dementia.

Advancing dementia symptoms have proved challenging. In the strategic planning process it was noted that there were no facilities to support people at mid stage dementia with severe behavioural concerns and/or increasingly complex medical needs. Instead, there had been some instances of persons with mid stage dementia within the Service being moved to houses in the community with higher support nursing staff or to units on one of the campuses. These homes were not ideal, they did not specialise in dementia and were developed and resourced to address the needs of a different population. It emerged from the focus group interviews that, for the people who lived in these higher support houses, having different people admitted on multiple occasions to their home was disruptive and sometimes posed safety concerns for those who were medically frail. Equally, the movement of the person with dementia from 4–5-bedded community residences to larger on-campus settings with others who also presented complex behavioural or medical needs proved traumatic for the person with dementia, their staff and families.

A need was also recognised to offer dementia specific services and supports in some specifically designed units to address behavioural and other concerns for persons with mid stage dementia where they can no longer be supported in their existing placements. This also addressed the more complex nursing and end of life needs of persons with late stage dementia.

Supporting persons with dementia to maintain contact with family/friends and familiar environments is a recognised and fundamental principle underpinning best practice in dementia care. Given the ageing demographics of service users, including a large population who were ageing with Down syndrome, the incidence of dementia was recognised as fast approaching the point where even several specialised units would not be sufficient to address dementia-related care needs. However, the development of these specialist units will ensure that settings, staffing and programming are available that are best able to address the needs of persons with mid stage dementia, plus others with significant complex nursing and palliative care needs.

Action steps

- Local working groups on dementia were formed at each residential campus, and in community-based services. The team comprised the administrator/nursing administration, representatives of nursing and care staff, day programming and a representative of the specialist multidisciplinary team with the following goals:

○ analyse trends, identify needs and project future demands for service users and service delivery in their area

○ identify low cost environmental modifications to be made in homes and units currently supporting persons with dementia.

- Complete renovations recommended by local workgroups to address bathing and personal care needs, safe walking areas, way-finding and safety concerns.

- The specialist dementia team began work with local multidisciplinary teams to identify and address needs for specialist expertise, staffing and the appropriateness of the environment. This will be reviewed on a case-by-case basis by the dementia team.

- The protocol for any new construction or home purchases has been modified. This gives priority to consideration of the suitability of construction or purchases for dementia care, and ensures sustainable housing for all persons with intellectual disabilities.

- A protocol has been developed for situations where the local workgroup, in consultation with the specialist dementia team and central management, determines that additional resources and renovations are not possible, or would be too costly for existing resources. In these circumstances, the protocol would manage the processes involved in transferring an individual to a more appropriate care setting.

- As part of the proposed new developments at two of the campuses, all homes incorporate basic design features to ensure that they are dementia friendly. Several houses will have additional special design features targeted to address additional care challenges of persons with dementia, including behavioural challenges, and the need to address their more complex nursing and palliative needs.

- Use of specialised units is driven by person-centred care needs and concerns, supported by the specialist dementia team.

- Admission and transfer criteria for persons in end stage dementia have been established.

DAY PROGRAMMES

As part of its strategic plan the Daughters of Charity Service decided it was important to ensure there are appropriate day programming options for persons at all stages of dementia.

Traditional day programmes, work settings and activities present levels of stimulation and an absence of environmental supports that make it difficult for persons with dementia to continue to attend and benefit. Yet, with modifications to the environment and to the programming, persons with dementia may continue to enjoy and benefit from valued activities. In addition, the redesign of day programmes will offer opportunities for persons with dementia to leave residences and will increase opportunities for participation in valued activities, maintaining functioning despite decline, and reducing demands upon staff in the residential units.

Action steps

- Local workgroups conducted an environmental audit of day programme sites, identifying concerns with bathroom facilities, way-finding, safe wandering areas and small group programming areas.

- The specialist dementia team work with the local workgroups to identify and schedule low cost renovations likely to support continued participation in day programmes by people with dementia.

- If, after consultation, it is determined that renovations are not possible or too costly, alternative day programme provision will be designed.

- In all new construction and major renovation, principles of dementia appropriate day provision are followed.

- Day programming strategies have been redesigned to incorporate dementia supportive psychotherapeutic approaches to care.

- Staff are redeployed and/or trained to support implementation of dementia specific day programming.

RESEARCH

To support the continued relevance of its strategic plan, and to ensure that action steps are influenced by the latest research, a programme of research has been designed to improve knowledge of dementia, dementia-related programming and outcomes for service users and staff.

Addressing dementia assessment and care issues is a relatively new concern. Although there is a growing research base for approaches, it is not well developed. Services and approaches will be further improved if there is a systematic approach and commitment to research. Active participation in research activities will also offer staff opportunities to evaluate their own practice, develop evidence-based approaches to assessment and care and benefit from high-quality work by others.

Action steps

- All training and education offered is based upon evidence-based practice.

- Collection of a minimum dataset on assessment and care planning activities supports the ongoing evaluation of the operations of the memory clinic.

- With proper safeguards, plan to become a site for testing and developing new assessment instruments and tests.

- The monitoring of quality of life outcomes for consumers, burden levels and training needs for staff, as well as costs associated with ageing in place/dementia friendly, specialist unit, end of life care models and day programme delivery.

BUSINESS PLANNING

A number of the strategic plan recommendations required capital expenditures and a number meant that operational resources would need to be reorganised.

Table 14.3: Business plan inventory template

Strategic area	Objective	Who leads	Performance indicators short term (6 months)	Performance indicators medium term (18 months)	Performance indicators long term (3 years)	Resources available/ required (include potential sources)
Screening and assessment						
Residential/ continuum of care						
Day programming						
Training and education						
Research						

Implementation

Since the development of the strategic plan there have been many achievements.

Specialist mobile memory clinic for people with intellectual disabilities

- A mobile memory clinic has been established and two clinical nurse specialists in dementia have been employed, one a new hire and the second reallocated from existing staffing resources.

- Persons with Down syndrome over the age of 35 years attached to the service have been offered baseline screening for dementia with follow-up annually.

- Comprehensive written report issued within a three-week period.

- All persons identified in the assessment as having possible symptoms of dementia receive a comprehensive diagnostic work-up and a consensus diagnosis established with members of the dementia specific multidisciplinary team.

- Referral process established for persons with intellectual disabilities from other aetiologies with suspected cognitive decline, with approximately 20 referrals received annually and all referrals processed within three weeks.

- Minimum dataset established to support tracking of decline and utility of test instruments.

- Expert advice offered to other services, nationally and internationally.

- Formal undergraduate and postgraduate level dementia-related training for clinicians.

- The memory clinic is now extending its services to other organisations and collaborating with generic dementia services offering specialist advice and supporting dementia assessment and care.

Comprehensive education programme

- A comprehensive staff education programme has been designed and is delivered in courses ranging from a four-day periodic programme to a one-hour programme delivered on a rolling basis. Annual delivery of 100 hours of face-to-face dementia specific education.

- An evidence-based and research-informed resource pack has been supplied to each site (approximately 30) supporting persons with dementia and is updated on an annual basis.

- Dementia specific standards to guide practice have been developed, and all areas supporting persons with dementia have received training on their implementation.

- A peer training curriculum has been developed and annually 40 hours of peer training are delivered.

- Annually two information evenings are facilitated for families, and individual training on dementia is delivered when dementia symptoms are suspected or confirmed.

Person-centred dementia care

- Dementia specific plans are developed for each individual with dementia and the plans are underpinned by the Quality Dementia Care Standards (McCarron and Reilly, 2010).

- Specific end of life plans are developed, discussed and regularly reviewed with family members or the next of kin of persons with advanced terminal dementia.

Ageing in place

- Persons with dementia have been successfully maintained in the community for approximately six years through environmental modifications, staff training and good clinical support.

- All consumers attend a day programme with specialist activities available. This includes a music programme, pottery, art therapy, reflexology and a range of massage therapies, and reminiscence therapy for persons at various stages of dementia.

- On-campus dementia specific respite services are now available and offered to each dispersed housing group home supporting persons with dementia.

A specialist dementia unit

A state-of-the-art specialist dementia unit designed and constructed to support persons at various stages of dementia opened in June 2013. Recognising the different needs at various stages of dementia, the specialist unit incorporates an eight-bed unit to support persons at mid stage dementia and a six-bed unit to support persons with end stage dementia. The facility also offers a respite bed available to support those living in the community. The unit is staffed from existing resources with specialist advice and input from the policy and services advisor in dementia and the two clinical nurse specialists in dementia. Other than the costs of the new construction of the dementia unit, all other improvements have been achieved using existing resources.

Conclusion

There have been concerns in intellectual disability services that when dementia symptoms present this will require increased staffing numbers and patterns, different facilities and a need to completely retrain or replace staff (McCallion et al., 2012). There are also concerns that without a dramatic increase in resources, and a recommitment to person-centred principles, dementia-related pressures will challenge existing programming approaches to the extent that 'home' means referral to a more restrictive setting (Bigby, et al., 2014; Janicki et al., 2005). In an austerity era, it is difficult to see where such additional resources will come from and the quality of life of people with intellectual disabilities and dementia appears tremendously at risk. However, Kaskie and Coddington (2004) have argued for the value of comprehensively considering the implications of dementia, whether for a healthcare system or in this case a service provider, paying attention to understanding the increased costs and consequences of poor support of people with dementia and for developing responses that manage within existing resources and organisational structures. In turn, an issues-based strategic planning approach offers hope of managing such challenges by offering a systematic approach to examining and addressing issues facing an organisation through the development of action plans.

The Daughters of Charity Service's use of Trochim's (1989) concept mapping phases encouraged the development of a steering committee and workgroups to support strategic planning preparation, the development of focal questions and a process to support the generation of ideas. This led to the alignment of proposed actions with current science and a purposeful and informed selection of action items (Anderson *et al.*, 2011). Finally, the experience of implementing the plan has been one of considerable success in achieving goals, a complete transformation of the Service to be dementia-ready and capable, increased likelihood of remaining in a community setting despite dementia, and a readiness to provide specialist care when needed. All of this has been achieved largely with existing financial resources, but more importantly with the genuine engagement of staff, families and people with intellectual disabilities.

A similar approach is likely to be helpful for other services and providers facing increases in the number of persons with dementia; and the tools and processes reviewed here are also likely to assist such providers.

References

Allison, M. and Kaye, J. (2005) *Strategic Planning for Nonprofit Organizations.* San Francisco, CA: CompassPoint.

Anderson, LA., Day, KL. and Vandenburg, AE. (2011) Using a concept map as a tool for strategic planning: The Healthy Brain Initiative. *Preventing Chronic Illness 8*, 5, A117.

Bigby, C., McCallion, P. and McCarron, M. (2014) Serving an elderly population. In M. Agran, F. Brown, C. Hughes, C. Quirk and D. Ryndak (eds) *Equality and Full Participation for Individuals with Severe Disabilities: A Vision for the Future.* Baltimore, MD: Paul H. Brookes.

Cooper, SA. (2006) *Services for Older People with Learning Disabilities.* Presentation given at Conference on Older People with Learning Disabilities, Coventry, UK, 23 March 2006.

Cosgrave, MP., Tyrrell, J., McCarron, M., Gill, M. and Lawlor, BA. (2000) A five year follow up study of dementia in persons with Down's syndrome: Early symptoms and patterns of deterioration. *Irish Journal of Psychological Medicine 17*, 1, 5–11.

Janicki, MP., McCallion, P. and Dalton, AJ. (2002) Dementia-related care decision-making in group homes for persons with intellectual disabilities. *Journal of Gerontological Social Work 38*, 1/2, 179–195.

Janicki, MP., Dalton, AJ., McCallion, P., Davies Baxley, D. and Zendell, A. (2005) Group home care for adults with intellectual disabilities and Alzheimer's disease. *Dementia 4*, 3, 361–385.

Kaluzny, D. and Hernandez, S. (1983) Organizational change and innovation. In S. Shortell and A. Kaluzny (eds) *Healthcare Management.* New York, NY: Wiley.

Kaskie, B. and Coddington, S. (2004) A strategic response to the challenges presented by older patients with Alzheimer's disease and other types of dementia. *Journal of Healthcare Management 49,* 1, 20–30.

Lai, F. and Williams, R.S. (1989) A prospective study of Alzheimer disease in Down's syndrome. *Archives of Neurology 46,* 8, 849–853.

McCallion, P., Nickle, T. and McCarron, M. (2005) A comparison of reports of caregiver burden between foster family care providers and staff caregivers of persons in other settings. *Dementia 4,* 3, 401–412.

McCallion, P., McCarron, M., Fahey-McCarthy, E. and Connaire, K. (2012) Meeting the end of life needs of older adults with intellectual disabilities. In E. Chang and A. Johnson (eds) *Contemporary and Innovative Practice in Palliative Care.* Rijeka, Croatia: Intech.

McCarron, M. and Lawlor, BA. (2003) Responding to the challenges of ageing and dementia in intellectual disability in Ireland. *Aging and Mental Health 7,* 6, 413–417.

McCarron, M. and Reilly, E. (2010) *Supporting Persons with Intellectual Disability and Dementia: Quality Dementia Care Standards. A Guide to Practice.* Dublin, Ireland: Daughters of Charity Service.

McCarron, M., Gill, M., Lawlor, B. and Begley C. (2002) Time spent caregiving for persons with the dual disability of Down's syndrome and Alzheimer's dementia: preliminary findings. *Journal of Learning Disabilities 6,* 3, 263–276.

McNamara, C. (2007) *Field Guide to Non-profit Strategic Planning and Facilitation.* Minneapolis, MN: Authenticity Consulting.

Nickle, T., and McCallion, P. (2005) Redesigning day programmes. *The Frontline of Learning Disability 64,* Winter, 27–28.

Nickols, F. and Ledgerwood, R. (2005) *The Goals Grid: A New Tool for Strategic Planning.* Mount Vernon, OH: Distance Consulting LLC.

Patti, PJ., Galli, M., Ferrario, D., Freeland, R. and Albertini, G. (2010) Movement and dementia in adults with intellectual disabilities. *Journal of Applied Research in Intellectual Disabilities 23,* 5, 410–425.

Prasher, VP. (1995) End-stage dementia in adults with Down's syndrome. *International Journal of Geriatric Psychiatry 10,* 12, 1067–1069.

Strydom, A., Shooshtari, S. and Lee, L. (2010) Dementia in older adults with intellectual disabilities – epidemiology, presentation, and diagnosis. *Journal of Policy and Practice in Intellectual Disabilities 7,* 2, 96–110.

Strydom, A., Livingston, G., King, M. and Hassiotis, A. (2007) Prevalence of dementia in intellectual disability using different diagnostic criteria. *British Journal of Psychiatry 191,* 150–157.

Trochim, W. (1989) An introduction to concept mapping for planning and evaluation. In W. Trochim (ed.) *A Special Issue of Evaluation and Program Planning 12,* 1, 1–16.

Visser, FE., Aldenkamp, AP., Van Huffelen, AC., Kuilman, M., Overweg, J. and Van Wijk, J. (1997) Prospective study of the prevalence of Alzheimer-type dementia in institutionalised individuals with Down's syndrome. *American Journal of Mental Retardation 4,* 101, 400–412.

Wilkinson, H. and Janicki, MP. (2002) The Edinburgh Principles with accompanying guidelines and recommendations. *Journal of Intellectual Disability Research 46,* 3, 279–284.

Wilkosz, PA., Seltman, HJ., Devlin, B. *et al.* (2009) Trajectories of cognitive decline in Alzheimer's disease. *International Psychogeriatrics 28,* 2, 1–10.

15

Intellectual Disability and Dementia Services – Better Together or Apart?

Susan Mary Benbow, Moni Grizzell, Andrew Griffiths

Introduction

Three streams of work are drawn together to understand the service context for people with intellectual disabilities and dementia. First, in 2008–2009, a Royal College of Psychiatrists working group surveyed psychiatrists working in the fields of old age psychiatry and intellectual disability psychiatry to seek their views on services for older people with an intellectual disability and a mental health problem. This included views on services for people with an intellectual disability and a comorbid dementia. The report from that project was published in 2010 (Benbow *et al.*, 2010).

Second, and at about the same time, the Royal College of Psychiatrists (RCPsych) and the British Psychological Society (BPS) jointly published a report subtitled 'guidance on the assessment, diagnosis, treatment and support of people with intellectual disabilities who develop dementia' (Royal College of Psychiatrists/ British Psychological Society, 2009).

The third workstream involved a Wolverhampton-based service improvement project in the UK which identified and screened adults with Down syndrome aged over 30 years. The aim of this locality project was to use a standardised screening instrument and establish a population database in an endeavour to achieve early diagnosis of a dementia, and ensure that people had access to treatment and support at an early stage. Details of the project were published in 2012 (Hobson *et al.*, 2012). Underlying all three of these initiatives were a series of questions that will be of relevance when planning to develop or redevelop services for people with intellectual disabilities and dementia:

- How do services best provide early diagnosis, treatment and support for people with intellectual disabilities who develop a form of dementia?

- Are people with intellectual disabilities who develop dementia better looked after within the intellectual disability psychiatry service, which may already know them, or within an old age psychiatry service, which has expertise in the diagnosis and management of dementia?

- Is there a third way, a way of bringing together the skills of both services in order to better support people with intellectual disabilities and comorbid dementia and their families?

The service context: specialisation versus generalisation

One important service issue is that of specialisation versus generalisation. It is generally accepted that old age psychiatry services (despite the name) will provide services for people with dementia of all ages. Perhaps the name of the specialty of old age psychiatry is unfortunate, as it has been misunderstood to imply an ageist practice of relating service eligibility to a strict age cut-off. Moves to combat age discrimination in mental health arose in response to the perception that people using old age psychiatry services were disadvantaged in terms of resources in comparison with people using services designed for younger adults. However, although sensible things have been said and written about this issue, it has sometimes been taken to imply that old age mental health services are inherently ageist. This has rebounded on the very services which campaigned against age discrimination, in that some people have argued that older people are no different from younger people and have no need for specialist services; an example of inverse ageism (Hill, 2008). As the Royal College of Psychiatrists' position statement on age discrimination in mental health says:

> An arbitrary age is not a satisfactory criterion to determine the service a person receives. Services must recognise the equal value

of all people and be based on need not on age. Age is a continuous variable and there is no point at which populations become discretely separate. A needs-based service will still require the development of comprehensive specialist-based mental health services for older people. (Royal College of Psychiatrists, 2009, p. 2)

It is also true that:

People's needs change as they progress through the life cycle and as people get older those changing needs may be better met by a different service. Failure to recognise that changing need, so that all people attend exactly the same service regardless of need, will serve people badly and amounts to indirect discrimination. (Royal College of Psychiatrists, 2009, p. 3)

A working group of the Royal College of Psychiatrists published a document setting out principles on working at the interface between different services in 2004. Although the work was focused on the boundary between old age psychiatry and general psychiatry, it is equally applicable to other interfaces, and this document clearly stated that: 'The service with the greatest expertise in relation to the care needs of an individual should take responsibility for their care' (Royal College of Psychiatrists Working Group, 2004, p. 2).

For this reason, dementia services operate across the age range, including people with dementia who are of working age and those in so-called later life (Faculty of Old Age Psychiatry, 2006). Few people would find the Working Group statement contentious, but it can become so when services are differently resourced, have very different approaches, or carry with them assumptions and stereotypes.

Thus, the decision on whether someone with intellectual disabilities and comorbid dementia is better supported in an intellectual disability psychiatry service or in an old age psychiatry service may not be straightforward, and may be complicated by the meanings, assumptions and stigma attributed to the different services (Graham *et al.*, 2003), rather than relying on a dispassionate assessment of which service would be best for each individual. Health and social care professionals themselves, often in good faith, can hold conflicting positions on these issues.

One risk is that both services might feel that they lack the expertise to deal with an individual's changing needs. The report on the survey of these two services (Benbow *et al.*, 2010) recommended that clear guidelines on interface working should be developed between the two specialist services; and that joint training initiatives, agreed joint care pathways and interface protocols should be developed. Would these address the dilemma and solve the problem? How services operate on the ground to meet someone's needs may depend more on personal contact and relationships between individual practitioners rather than the paperwork, although this is hardly a blueprint for consistent equitable and high quality services.

Intellectual disability services have established a number of important principles. The Valuing People initiative (Department of Health, 2001) in England and Wales with its emphasis on involving and respecting people using services is a good example. Within intellectual disability services there is a strong lobby for both ageing in place and dying in place (Royal College of Psychiatrists/ British Psychological Society, 2009). These are principles to which old age psychiatry and other services could usefully sign up.

The service context: the challenge of integration

The integration of services has been an issue for a long time in mental health. In old age psychiatry the document *Everybody's Business* highlighted the need for a 'whole systems approach to commissioning integrated services' (Department of Health/Care Services Improvement Partnership, 2005, p. 20) and followed a detailed analysis of the need to integrate community mental health teams for older people (Lingard and Milne, 2004). Despite this, a disconnection between the rhetoric and the reality persists (Tucker *et al.*, 2009), in that the argument for working together is powerful and compelling, but the reality is that services erect boundaries and are adept at finding reasons why it's someone else's job, leading to discontinuities in care. Unfortunately an approach to these discontinuities in dementia care has been to try to introduce a variety of new roles which have created opportunities for increasing confusion and yet more discontinuities in care (Benbow and Kingston, 2010).

Cornwell and colleagues state bluntly that 'continuity is fundamental to high-quality care' (Cornwell *et al.*, 2012, p. 1), particularly for older people with multiple health problems, and that breakdowns in continuity of care put patients at risk. It is not surprising that the Francis inquiry (Francis, 2013) commented on continuity of care in relation to the events at Mid Staffordshire NHS Foundation Trust and acute hospitals:

> A truly caring culture does not stop at the door of the hospital provider. It should never be acceptable for patients to be discharged at any time without knowledge that the patient in need of care will receive it on arrival at their destination. The emphasis should be on continuity of care to include a follow-up as to a patient's well-being after discharge. (Francis, 2013, p. 80)

The boundary in this case was between the hospital and community, but community services in the UK are likewise riddled with boundaries for people to negotiate, between health and social care and the third sector, between different specialist mental health services, for example, old age psychiatry and intellectual disability psychiatry, between different components of a mental health service, for example, community mental health teams and crisis teams.

People with intellectual disabilities who develop a form of dementia are vulnerable to similar discontinuities in their care. The challenge is to find ways of working in partnership (Tait and Shah, 2007). Table 15.1 shows how recommendations from Cornwell *et al.* (2012) might apply to people with dementia and intellectual disabilities being cared for by staff from both specialist services.

Table 15.1: Recommendations applied to the care of people with dementia and an intellectual disability

Recommendation	Implications for old age psychiatry and intellectual disability psychiatry services
Patients and carers receive high-quality appropriate care.	The focus of the care plan should be person-centred and relationship centred care.
Patients and carers always know the name of the person in charge (lead professional) who will deal with their queries and discuss the care plan.	Where people are being looked after by both services a lead professional needs to be identified who takes responsibility for communicating with all those involved, whichever service they are based in.

Patients and carers know how to get hold of the lead professional.	The name and contact details of the lead professional must be made known to the family and if that person is asked something they cannot answer they must take responsibility for dealing with the issue and obtaining an answer.
Patients are asked to name a partner in care who will be closely involved with the care plan.	The person identified as the partner in care should be routinely involved in all aspects of a person's care and the development of their care plan.
Patients and carers complete a 'This is me' document (Alzheimer's Society, 2013) or equivalent.	Community patients will benefit from having personal information available to those caring for them. This might be done using one of the following models: • This is me (or equivalent document) • Life story book model • Patient narrative model
The key people working with the patient change as little as possible.	This enables people to develop relationships over time and is highly valued by patients and carers but needs to be privileged in caseload reviews.
Patients are looked after by people trained to appropriately care for them.	Where staff members from two services are working together joint training initiatives should be developed in the overlap area and will have the added benefit of enabling individual staff to develop links and understand each other's perspective.
Patients and carers are asked to give routine feedback on their experiences, which is properly considered.	Routine feedback should be requested and incorporated into service review systems in order to allow learning from patients and families to influence the shape and operation of services.

Source: modified from Cornwell *et al.*, 2012

The service context: person-centred care

If services focused on providing person-centred care for the patients and families using them, many of the challenges they face would fade into insignificance. Kitwood is credited with developing person-centred care with his work on the experience of living with dementia

(Kitwood, 1997) and his assertion is that: 'Those with dementia have the same value, the same needs and the same rights as everyone else' (p. 55).

The National Institute for Health and Clinical Excellence (NICE) and Social Care Institute for Excellence (SCIE) dementia guidelines assert that there is broad support for applying the principles of person-centred care to the care of people with dementia (NICE/SCIE, 2007). At the same time, the guidelines recognise that to do this in practice can be challenging. The Alzheimer's Society describes person-centred care as follows:

> This approach aims to see the person with dementia as an individual, rather than focusing on their illness or on abilities they may have lost. Person-centred care takes into account each individual's unique qualities, abilities, interests, preferences and needs. (Alzheimer's Society, 2012, p. 4)

We probably still have not made as much progress in this respect in older people's mental health as intellectual disability services have done since *Valuing People* (Department of Health, 2001), and people living with a dementia are still not valued in the way that they should be if we adhere to Kitwood's beliefs in personhood.

Mainstreaming has been a dilemma (Bouras and Holt, 2004). If there is stigma attached to a specialist service, does someone avoid it by being seen in the mainstream or more generic service? Or does this deprive the individual of the specialist care they need? How does that balance of advantages and disadvantages get assessed, and how do the various advantages and disadvantages get weighed against one another? This is a dilemma for older people with mental health problems (do they really want to be seen by an old age psychiatry service?) just as it is for people with an intellectual disability. How does person-centred care come into this? It is easy to say that the service which can best provide for a person's needs should be the one that provides their care, but in practice making this distinction can be difficult and becomes distorted by factors such as stigma and our own beliefs and prejudices. A further complication comes from the recognition that relationships are critically important in dementia care (and elsewhere) and this has led to growing interest in relationship centred care (Davies and Nolan, 2008; Nolan, *et al.*, 2006).

In the survey for the Faculties of Old Age and Learning Disability Psychiatry (Benbow *et al.*, 2010), respondents were asked about the services that existed in their locality for people with intellectual disabilities and a dementia both above and below the age of 65. Twenty-seven per cent of 399 comments were that there were no specific or specialist services. Many comments described gaps in services for this group of people including: perceived lack of staff training, lack of resources, lack of specialist accommodation, absence of a service and, perhaps even more alarming, ignorance on the part of old age psychiatrists and intellectual disability psychiatrists about the other service, so that comments included one old age psychiatrist who suggested, 'Please ask local intellectual disabilities service.' A practical difficulty identified was that the two services might be sited at a distance from one another and/or in different provider organisations: thus exacerbating the fragmentation of care. Obstacles suggested by respondents in providing a service for this group included: service access, capacity, staffing issues, need for a specialist service, and absence of need ('we have had no referrals'). A subtheme underlying staffing and capacity is that of limited resources.

It appears that there is sometimes no clarity on which service should meet the needs of people who have intellectual disabilities and dementia, although the survey did identify some examples of good practice. These examples were varied in design and geography, and included generic old age psychiatry services which provided good access for older people with intellectual disabilities; examples of excellent and close working relationships between primary care and the voluntary (not for profit) sector; and other services which had developed an agreed dementia care pathway. The findings of the survey suggest that there is a long way to go if services are to provide consistent person-centred care for people with comorbid intellectual disabilities and dementia.

Case study: Mr A

Mr A is a 62-year-old man who has Down syndrome, hypothyroidism and epilepsy. He is well known to the local community intellectual disability nursing team, and lives independently in supported accommodation. His only relative is a sister who has little contact with him. His home carers had become increasingly concerned about a decline in his skills over a period of about a year: often he now required prompting with personal care. The carers at the local authority day centre he attended had also noticed deterioration in Mr

A's skills and a need for increasing support. He was initially reviewed by his general practitioner (GP) who arranged some routine blood screens including thyroid function tests. These were all normal.

Following the locally agreed joint care pathway, developed by the intellectual disability and old age psychiatry services, he was subsequently referred to the community intellectual disability nursing team for further assessment. Mr A was initially assessed by the intellectual disability psychiatrist, who thought he might be experiencing a depressive episode, and commenced him on an appropriate anti-depressant drug. Unfortunately, he continued to decline, necessitating closer supervision owing to his decreasing ability to recognise people who were previously familiar to him.

He was screened using the Broad Screen Checklist of Observed Changes (Koenig, 1996). This is an informant-based tool, which measures the abilities and general functioning of a person. It rates change in six domains: health; physical competencies; sensory integration; perceptual/cognitive; social/emotional; and activities of daily living. In addition, it generates a total score and qualitative information can be recorded. Items are scored as follows: no change or always present; change observed within the last six months; change observed more than six months ago but less than three years. Items score higher if change has been observed within the last six months. A numerical score is calculated which indicates the overall level of change and the level of change in each domain (minor, moderate or significant). The Broad Screen Checklist of Observed Changes was used since it is part of the Wolverhampton screening programme (Hobson et al., 2012). It takes about 30–45 minutes to complete, longer if a number of changes are reported. The Dementia Screening Questionnaire for Individuals with Intellectual Disabilities (DSQIID) (Deb et al., 2007), an observer-rated screening instrument consisting of three sections and 43 questions, was also completed: this suggested that Mr A was developing a type of dementia.

Following this assessment, Mr A was referred to the local joint intellectual disability/old age psychiatry memory clinic, where a diagnosis of early onset Alzheimer's disease was confirmed. This involved utilising the expertise of both services: the diagnosis was made by an old age psychiatrist, in liaison with a intellectual disability doctor and nurse. The clinic is normally staffed by one person representing old age psychiatry and one representing the intellectual disability service: either a doctor or nurse might attend on behalf of each service, but one of the two is normally a doctor. Clinical diagnosis focuses on decline in skills rather than decline in memory function. The intellectual disability service took the initial history and organised blood screening tests. At that stage joint assessment commenced. Mr A would not co-operate with a magnetic resonance imaging (MRI) brain scan. An electrocardiogram (ECG) revealed no contraindications to treatment with cholinesterase inhibitors.

Concerns were expressed with regard to Mr A's epilepsy and the potential adverse effects of cholinesterase inhibitors: seizures are increased in people with dementia (Imfeld *et al.*, 2012). With regard to Mr A, no seizures had been witnessed for many years. The community intellectual disability nurse therefore arranged for increased support for him whilst he commenced donepezil. Carers were arranged to call daily in order to supervise medication and monitor any side effects. They started visiting two weeks prior to medication being commenced to obtain a baseline. Carers, both at home and day care, were advised that the medication carried a risk of seizures and that they should be alert to any possible side effects. Any problems were to be recorded and reported back. Mr A was initially started on a dose of 5mg donepezil on alternate days for two weeks and then the dose was increased to 5mg daily. No adverse effects were noted.

The community intellectual disability nurse monitored his progress, supported by the sister from the older adult memory clinic. She facilitated monitoring of side effects and organised the medication to be dispensed via a MediPACK. The home carers monitored his medication concordance. Support was also offered to his fellow resident who was aware of the change in Mr A having known him for many years. Thus, expertise in nursing aspects of dementia care was provided by the memory clinic sister via the intellectual disability nurse. Joint reviews were undertaken in the memory clinic. The intellectual disability nurse would normally visit Mr A at home and then attend the clinic with him in order to inform further assessment and management. The older adult and intellectual disability services jointly organised a training session for both home and day centre carers who supported Mr A. This focused on how to achieve person-centred care, communication and how to promote independence and maintain function. At the meeting a presentation was given by an older adult psychologist, and the memory clinic sister and intellectual disability nurse both attended and took part in discussion. Mr A continued to be followed up by the joint intellectual disability and dementia clinic.

The service context: partnership to achieve person-centred care

Mr A's case study illustrates how two services (in this case old age psychiatry and intellectual disability services) can work in partnership in order to provide person-centred care for individuals with dementia and an intellectual disability. Someone with needs which cross service boundaries benefits from a care plan which identifies the expertise needed from each service. In Mr A's case, the home carers and day centre staff knew of his history, personality and were best placed to recognise and seek help for the changes they observed. The intellectual disability service has expertise in the care and management of people with an intellectual disability, and has services available to this client group. The old age psychiatry service brings expertise in the diagnosis of dementia. (This needs to be supplemented by expertise from intellectual disabilities, as some of the instruments used in routine old age psychiatry practice would not be appropriate for someone like Mr A, since they rely too much on education and verbal skills.) They also bring expertise in the management of dementia and use of anti-dementia drug treatments alongside non-pharmacological treatments. Each service, and staff from that service, needs to recognise and respect the strengths and expertise of the other. At the same time it is important to be clear about contact points and who takes responsibility for what. In Mr A's case, the intellectual disability nurse was the key contact and the memory clinic sister led for the old age psychiatry service, liaising with and drawing in those other members of the old age psychiatry service who could provide additional skills to complement the care plan, including the consultant old age psychiatrist (who was involved in diagnosis and planning anti-dementia drug treatment) and the psychologist who was involved in training Mr A's carers. Two other essential qualities for partnership to work are flexibility and trust. Each service will need to trust the other and individuals must be prepared to respond to requests for help and support.

Cornwell *et al.*'s recommendations are largely met in the description of Mr A's care (Cornwell *et al.*, 2012): there is a clear focus on the individual and their relationships; the lead professional was identified and those involved told who to contact and how; and information and training was made available to all those involved in Mr A's care.

Case study: Ms B

Ms B, a woman with Down syndrome had lived with her mother until she died, then moved to live with her sister (Mrs C) and brother-in-law, and had been living with them for about 18 years. The couple were childless and Mrs C worked as a carer for an older person until 2009 when the person she cared for died. She had promised her mother that she would care for Ms B.

Ms B was known to the local intellectual disability service and attended a local authority day care centre and basic skills training classes. In about 2005, when she was aged 42 years, her family and day centre staff noticed a change in her. She became more agitated and tearful, appeared tired, and her sleep pattern became disturbed over a period of about six months. She was normally interested in, and enjoyed, music, but appeared to lose interest and was described as being 'attention-seeking'. She was seen by an intellectual disability psychiatrist and found to have an underactive thyroid. In addition, the psychiatrist thought that she had a depressive illness and started her on an anti-depressive drug.

Following this, Ms B was followed up by the community intellectual disability nurse, but failed to improve. She became argumentative, forgetful and blamed her sister for all her problems. The observed short-term memory difficulty led to a referral to the joint intellectual disability/old age psychiatry memory clinic in 2006. In the clinic a detailed assessment was carried out, including the Broad Screen Checklist of Observed Changes, and she had blood tests and an ECG, which showed bradycardia but no sign of bundle branch block, a defect of the heart's electrical conduction system. Ms B declined to have a brain scan at this point. Putting all the information together, a diagnosis of probable Alzheimer's disease was made, and she was started cautiously on donepezil at a dose initially of 5mg on alternate days. Over a number of months the dose was gradually increased with close supervision and monitoring by the community intellectual disability nurse and Ms B's sister up to an eventual maintenance dose of 10mg donepezil daily.

Monitoring consisted of two components: visits from the community intellectual disability nurse and telephone counselling from the memory clinic sister for Ms B's sister, who kept a detailed diary of Ms B's physical and emotional state. Mrs C set up an orientation board in the home to help her sister and a pictorial timetable and calendar to remind her of her daily activities. Ms B gradually improved in terms of appearing brighter and more interested, being less repetitive and less accusing or blaming towards Mrs C. Her sleep pattern also improved and she was less incontinent. She engaged with activities and other people more. No side effects were observed from the medication and the healthcare staff concluded that she was showing evidence of a response to the anti-dementia treatment.

In 2009, her sister and the day centre staff noticed that she was developing word-finding problems, and slowing down physically. These changes occurred at the same time as changes at the day care centre, which staff thought might have unsettled her. She had a few episodes of being more confused, which resolved within 24 hours: no cause was found. These episodes were thought to be possible transient ischaemic attacks. She was seen by the intellectual disability psychiatrist in the joint clinic, and found to have more pronounced bradycardia with bundle branch block on ECG. On this occasion she agreed to have a scan of her brain and this showed evidence of vascular damage. Given the ECG changes, the transient ischaemic attacks and the revised diagnosis of a predominantly vascular dementia, it was decided to stop the donepezil treatment and the medication was gradually withdrawn under supervision of both the community intellectual disability nurse and the memory clinic sister.

Unfortunately, Ms B's physical and mental state immediately deteriorated, stabilising again after about three to four weeks, but at a lower level of function. Day care was increased in order to offer more support to Ms B's sister, who continued to care for her at home and eventually accepted a regular respite break. All through this period Mrs C provided thoughtful and person-centred care for her sister, making sure she ate a healthy diet, engaging her in gentle exercise and providing a loving and supportive home for her, aided by her husband. Mrs C took charge of her sister's care, liaised regularly with both services and kept a detailed diary of her sister's progress. After this, follow-up was provided by the intellectual disability service whose staff continued to monitor her progress and to offer her sister ongoing support. Intellectual disability community nurse support was available as necessary.

The service context: learning to work together

Ms B's case study illustrates how two services can work together over a prolonged period to provide flexible care and support tailored to an individual, that individual's family carers and other involved agencies. Negotiating the division of support between staff from two services requires the people concerned to trust and respect the contribution of the collaborating service and to acknowledge that care must be person-centred and built around the individual. Knowledge of what each service can provide and personal links between individual staff members are helpful, but working together helps to nurture and develop these links. In Ms B's case, psychiatrists and senior nursing staff from both services were involved. Ms B's sister drew on support from both services and appeared to be clear what each could contribute, but clarity on behalf of users and carers probably relies on the service personnel themselves being clear about their roles, contributions and routes of communication. One of the risks of involving staff from two services is that care is duplicated, or not provided (if each service relies on the other to take action), or that service users and/or family members are unclear regarding routes of communication and responsibilities. The first few cases shared between services established some of the ground rules, and enabled individual staff members to build up confidence in joint working, making it easier to subsequently work together, reinforcing joint protocols and pathways. It is important, however, that links do not rely solely on particular enthusiastic individuals, as that runs the risk that the partnership relationship will be lost should those individuals move to different jobs. *Everybody's Business* (Department of Health/Care Services Improvement Partnership, 2005) pointed out that effective services for older people with mental health problems and intellectual disabilities will only be achieved through partnership working, and argued that success will require both older people's mental health and intellectual disability services to be prepared to do things differently. It went on to stress that joint protocols should be in place in order to facilitate this, and should cover care pathways, roles and responsibilities, and access and support arrangements.

Conclusion

This chapter started by setting out three questions. First, how do services best provide early diagnosis, treatment and support for people with an intellectual disability who develop dementia? Our experience is that partnership working combined with joint pathways and protocols can work to provide a high-quality diagnostic, treatment and support service that meets the requirements of service users and their families and supports and sustains staff working in both services.

Second, we asked whether people with an intellectual disability who develop dementia are better looked after within the intellectual disability psychiatry service, which may already know them, or within an old age psychiatry service, which has expertise in the diagnosis and management of dementia. The model described here strives to avoid taking an either-or position, and instead to combine the expertise of both services in the interests of people and families who might otherwise fall into the hole between them. However, identification of a lead professional is essential.

Finally, we questioned whether there is a third way, a way of bringing together the skills of both services in order to better care for people with an intellectual disability and comorbid dementia and their families. A third way involves partnership working with the service user and their family at the centre of treatment, care and support, drawing on the expertise that they require when they require it, and with staff contributing and collaborating. Again a word of caution – that family carers are not seen as the coordinator of care, and the situation should be avoided where professionals talk to each other through the family; joint working that includes, rather than relies on, the family is needed.

References

Alzheimer's Society (2012) *Selecting a Care Home.* Available at www.alzheimers.org.uk/site/scripts/download_info.php?fileID=1787, accessed on 24 March 2014.

Alzheimer's Society (2013) *This is Me.* Available at www.alzheimers.org.uk/site/scripts/download_info.php?fileID=1604, accessed on 7 December 2013.

Benbow, SM. and Kingston, P. (2010) Developing the dementia workforce: Numerus turbatio – Total confusion. *Dementia 9*, 3, 307–310.

Benbow, SM., Kingston, P., Bhaumik, S., Black, S., Gangadharan, SK. and Hardy, S. (2010) *Travelling Alone or Travelling Together? The Interface between Learning Disability and Old Age Psychiatry.* Available at www.rcpsych.ac.uk/pdf/Revised_report_FINALinterface.pdf, accessed on 7 December 2013.

Bouras, N. and Holt, G. (2004) Mental health services for adults with learning disabilities. *The British Journal of Psychiatry 184*, 4, 291–292.

Cornwell, J., Levenson, R., Sonola, L. and Poteliakhoff, E. (2012) *Continuity of Care for Older Hospital Patients. A Call for Action.* Available at www.kingsfund.org.uk/sites/files/kf/field/field_publication_file/continuity-of-care-for-older-hospital-patients-mar-2012.pdf, accessed on 7 December 2013.

Davies, S. and Nolan, M. (2008) Attending to relationships in dementia care. In M. Downs and B. Bowers (eds) *Excellence in Dementia Care. Research into Practice.* Maidenhead: Open University Press.

Deb, S., Hare, M., Prior, L. and Bhaumik, S. (2007) The dementia screening questionnaire for individuals with intellectual disabilities. *British Journal of Psychiatry 190,* 5, 440–444.

Department of Health (2001) *Valuing People: A New Strategy for Learning Disability for the 21st Century.* London: Department of Health.

Department of Health/Care Services Improvement Partnership (2005) *Everybody's Business. Integrated Mental Health Services for Older Adults: A Service Development Guide.* Available at www.wales.nhs.uk/sites3/Documents/439/everybodysbusiness.pdf, accessed on 7 December 2013.

Faculty of Old Age Psychiatry (2006) *Raising the Standard. Specialist Services for Older People with Mental Illness.* Available at www.rcpsych.ac.uk/pdf/raisingthestandardoapwebsite.pdf, accessed on 7 December 2013.

Francis, R. (2013) *Report of the Mid Staffordshire NHS Foundation Trust Public Inquiry. Executive Summary.* London: The Stationery Office.

Graham, N., Lindesay, J., Katona, C., Bertolote, JM., Camus, V., Copeland, JRM. and Wancata, J. (2003) Reducing stigma and discrimination against older people with mental disorders: A technical consensus statement. *International Journal of Geriatric Psychiatry 18,* 8, 670–678.

Hill, L. (2008) The dilemma of age integration. *Old Age Psychiatrist 49,* 12.

Hobson, B., Webb, D., Sprague, L., Grizzell, M., Hawkins, C. and Benbow, SM. (2012) Establishing a database for proactive screening of adults with Down's syndrome: When services work together. *Advances in Mental Health and Intellectual Disabilities 6,* 2, 99–105.

Imfeld, P., Bodmer, M., Schuerch, M., Jick, SS. and Meier, CR. (2012) Seizures in patients with Alzheimer's disease or vascular dementia: A population-based nested case-control analysis. *Epilepsia 54,* 4, 700–707.

Kitwood, T. (1997) *Dementia Reconsidered. The Person Comes First.* Buckingham: Open University Press.

Koenig, BR. (1996) *Broad Screen Checklist of Observed Changes.* Brighton, Australia: Minda.

Lingard, J. and Milne, A. (2004) *Integrating Older People's Mental Health Services: Community Mental Health Teams for Older People. A Commentary and Resource Document.* Available at http://nmhdu.org.uk/silo/files/integrating-opmh-services.pdf, accessed on 7 December 2013.

NICE/SCIE (2007) *Dementia. The NICE–SCIE Guideline on Supporting People with Dementia and their Carers in Health and Social Care.* Available at www.nice.org.uk/nicemedia/live/10998/30320/30320.pdf, accessed on 7 December 2013.

Nolan, M., Brown, J., Davies, S., Nolan, J. and Keady, J. (2006) *The Senses Framework: Improving Care for Older People through a Relationship-centred Approach.* Getting Research into Practice (GRiP) Report No 2. Project Report. Sheffield: University of Sheffield.

Royal College of Psychiatrists (2009) *Age Discrimination in Mental Health Services: Making Equality a Reality.* Position Statement PS2/2009. London: Royal College of Psychiatrists.

Royal College of Psychiatrists Working Group (2004) *The Interface between General and Community Psychiatry and Old Age Psychiatry Services: Report of a Working Group.* London: Royal College of Psychiatrists.

Royal College of Psychiatrists/British Psychological Society (2009) *Dementia and People with Learning Disabilities. Guidance on the Assessment, Diagnosis, Treatment and Support of People with Learning Disabilities who Develop Dementia.* CR155. Leicester: British Psychological Society.

Tait, L. and Shah, S. (2007) Partnership working: A policy with promise for mental healthcare. *Advances in Psychiatric Treatment 13,* 4, 261–271.

Tucker, S., Baldwin, R., Hughes, J. *et al.* (2009) Integrating mental health services for older people in England – from rhetoric to reality. *Journal of Interprofessional Care 23,* 4, 341–354.

16

Measuring Outcomes for Services and Individuals

Karen Dodd

Introduction

To understand how far people are being supported to live well with dementia means defining and measuring the outcomes of care; that is, what actually happens to the health of the person as a result of the treatment and care they receive. Measuring outcomes should be about driving up standards of care and ensuring that individuals have the best possible quality in all areas of their life. Outcomes have become a key focus, particularly with the publication of the Francis report in the UK (Francis, 2013) on the widely reported failings at Mid Staffordshire NHS Trust and the Care Quality Commission report on wider hospital failure (Care Quality Commission, 2013) which both concern the neglect, abuse and deaths of predominantly older people. The Francis report concluded that the causes of the failure included: a culture that focused on doing the system's business rather than that of the patients; an institutional culture which ascribed more weight to positive information about the service than to information capable of implying cause for concern; standards and methods of measuring compliance which did not focus on the effect of a service on patients. Clearly these are not the outcomes that are wanted for people receiving care and treatment within health services.

What are we trying to achieve in services for people with intellectual disabilities and dementia?

Within the field of intellectual disabilities there has been a long-standing focus on person-centred care. O'Brien's five accomplishments of respect, choice, participation, relationships and ordinary places (O'Brien, 1989) were the foundation for person-centred planning in the USA. Within services for people with intellectual disabilities a person-centred framework has consistently been applied to people with intellectual disabilities (Carnaby et al., 2011; Robertson et al., 2005).

This approach has gradually become the focus for good dementia care for people within the general population, with an increasing emphasis on what constitutes good person-centred care (Alzheimer's Society, 2013). The Alzheimer's Society states that the key points of person-centred care are: treating the person with dignity and respect; understanding their history, lifestyle, culture and preferences, including their likes, dislikes, hobbies and interests; looking at situations from the point of view of the person with dementia; providing opportunities for the person to have conversations and relationships with other people; and ensuring that the person has the chance to try new things or take part in activities they enjoy.

The Prime Minister's challenge on dementia in the UK (Department of Health, 2012) focuses on three main elements: driving improvements in health and care; creating dementia friendly communities that understand how to help; and better research. Pickup (2012) in her response to the Prime Minister's challenge on dementia concluded that 'we will get the best outcomes if we focus on individuals and their needs in the context of their families and communities, providing treatment or support for specific conditions including dementia, but never losing sight of the person' (p. 13).

What constitutes 'living well with dementia' will change at different stages of the condition. This is a key issue in the measurement of quality outcomes in a condition which is progressive. Guidelines for good dementia care for people with intellectual disabilities have reflected this need to think about the requirements at the different stages (Dodd et al., 2006). Jokinen et al., (2013) have produced guidelines for structuring community care and supports for people with intellectual disabilities affected by dementia which have adopted the staging model for dementia. Within these guidelines they have discussed what the favourable outcomes should be for people with dementia at each stage, although with less clarity over how these outcomes may be measured.

Measuring outcomes for services for people with dementia

The National Institute for Health and Care Excellence (NICE) provides national guidance and advice to improve health and social care in the UK. It has produced two quality standards (QS1, NICE, 2010; QS30, NICE, 2013) which define what constitutes a high standard of care within this area. Each set of standards gives specific, concise quality statements, measures and audience descriptors to provide patients and the public, health and social care professionals, commissioners and service providers with definitions of high-quality care (NICE, 2010).

NICE dementia quality standard QS1 (NICE, 2010) covers care provided by health and social care staff in direct contact with people with dementia in hospital, community, home-based, group care, residential or specialist care settings. This quality standard requires that dementia services should be commissioned from and coordinated across all relevant agencies encompassing the whole dementia care pathway. It states that an integrated approach to provision of services is fundamental to the delivery of high-quality care to people with dementia. According to NICE (2010) this quality standard provides clinicians, managers and service users with a description of what a high-quality dementia service should look like. It describes markers of high-quality, cost-effective care that, when delivered collectively, should contribute to improving the effectiveness, safety, experience and care for adults with dementia.

The quality standard consists of ten quality statements. However, these quality standards have been written as inputs rather than outcomes, and the measures for assessing compliance with these quality standards are purely quantitative in nature; that is the proportion of people with dementia or their carers receiving these inputs.

Quality standards, QS1

- People with dementia receive care from staff appropriately trained in dementia care.

- People with suspected dementia are referred to a memory assessment service specialising in the diagnosis and initial management of dementia.

1.30.

From McDermott
Diana Syria

Hill Dickinson.

EC2A 2EN.

The Broadgate Tower
20 Primrose St

020 7283 9033

Communicate with Service Users who are confused or upset.	<ul><li>Observation of Nurse interacting with Service Users</li><li>Review of management plan</li><li>Awareness of current care plan</li></ul>			
Show understanding of the range of Service Users' feelings, e.g. frustration.	<ul><li>Discussion with Nurse</li><li>Observation of Nurse interacting with Service Users</li></ul>			
Identify factors that may affect the Service Users' ability to retain independence or make informed choices.	<ul><li>Discussion with Nurse</li><li>Care Plans</li><li>Care Plan Evaluations</li></ul>			
Communicate effectively with Service Users with severe deficits, speech difficulties or reality problems, e.g. blindness, deafness, aphasia, dysphasia, CVA, dementia or other mental health problems.	<ul><li>Discussion with Nurse</li><li>Observation of Nurse interacting with Service Users</li></ul>			
Calmly think through stressful situations before communicating.	<ul><li>Discussion with Nurse</li><li>Observation of Nurse interacting with Service Users</li></ul>			

- People newly diagnosed with dementia and/or their carers receive written and verbal information about their condition, treatment and the support options in their local area.

- People with dementia have an assessment and an ongoing personalised care plan, agreed across health and social care, that identifies a named care coordinator and addresses their individual needs.

- People with dementia, while they have capacity, have the opportunity to discuss and make decisions, together with their carer(s), about the use of: advance statements; advance decisions to refuse treatment; lasting power of attorney; preferred priorities of care.

- Carers of people with dementia are offered an assessment of emotional, psychological and social needs and, if accepted, receive tailored interventions identified by a care plan to address those needs.

- People with dementia who develop non-cognitive symptoms that cause them significant distress, or who develop behaviour that challenges, are offered an assessment at an early opportunity to establish generating and aggravating factors. Interventions to improve such behaviour or distress should be recorded in their care plan.

- People with suspected or known dementia using acute and general hospital inpatient services or emergency departments have access to a liaison service that specialises in the diagnosis and management of dementia and older people's mental health.

- People in the later stages of dementia are assessed by primary care teams to identify and plan their end of life care needs.

- Carers of people with dementia have access to a comprehensive range of respite/short-break services that meet the needs of both the carer and the person with dementia.

(NICE, 2010)

This was supplemented in April 2013 by a further set of quality standards, QS30 (NICE, 2013), a quality standard for supporting people to live well with dementia. This set of standards applies to all social care settings and services working with and caring for people with dementia. Again, these standards describe inputs rather than outcomes. Expected levels of achievement for these quality measures are not specified. NICE states that quality standards are intended to drive up the quality of care, so achievement levels of 100 per cent should be aspired to for quantitative measures where numerators and denominators are given. However, NICE (2013) recognises that this may not always be appropriate in practice when taking account of safety, choice and professional judgement and so desired levels of achievement should be defined locally.

Quality standards, QS30

- People worried about possible dementia in themselves or someone they know can discuss their concerns, and the options of seeking a diagnosis, with someone with knowledge and expertise.

- People with dementia, with the involvement of their carers, have choice and control in decisions affecting their care and support.

- People with dementia participate, with the involvement of their carers, in a review of their needs and preferences when their circumstances change.

- People with dementia are enabled, with the involvement of their carers, to take part in leisure activities during their day based on individual interest and choice.

- People with dementia are enabled, with the involvement of their carers, to maintain and develop relationships.

- People with dementia are enabled, with the involvement of their carers, to access services that help maintain their physical and mental health and wellbeing.

- People with dementia live in housing that meets their specific needs.

- People with dementia have opportunities, with the involvement of their carers, to participate in and influence the design, planning, evaluation and delivery of services.

- People with dementia are enabled, with the involvement of their carers, to access independent advocacy services.

- People with dementia are enabled, with the involvement of their carers, to maintain and develop their involvement in and contribution to their community.

(NICE, 2013)

Janicki (2011) describes how a range of mainstream Alzheimer's organisations across the world have published their own recommendations and guidelines for quality care (Alzheimer's Association, 2006; Alzheimer's Australia, 2007). Within services for people with intellectual disabilities and dementia, Janicki (2011) described how care organisations are facing the need to adapt their techniques and methods of care. He proposed that it is useful to have a framework for determining what factors of care services and settings would be the most prominent determinants of quality care. Inherent in this approach is having an understanding of what is meant by quality care.

Many of the principles contained in these documents were already made explicit by *The Edinburgh Principles* (Wilkinson and Janicki, 2002), proposing that governments, organisations, and service providers adopt the list of principles and promote their use. By writing them as inputs rather than outcomes, it is left to local interpretation to determine how compliance with the principles should be measured. Janicki (2011) concluded that the literature on quality care in dementia programmes pointed to four critical components underpinning the provision of quality care, and therefore by extension, enhanced quality of life. These are: clinically relevant, early and periodic assessments; functional modifications in living settings; constructive staff education and functionality for stage-adapted care; and flexible long-term services that recognise and plan for progression of decline and loss of function. Unlike other frameworks and quality standards, Janicki's framework (2011) emphasised the importance of recognising that dementia is a progressive condition and that care needs to be adapted to the stage of dementia. This is a major issue that seems to have been missed in much of the literature on caring and measuring care for people with dementia, where dementia seems to be seen as a 'single condition' rather than a condition which presents ongoing and continuous change in the person, and thus an ongoing and continuous need to change how care is delivered. Janicki (2011) concluded that translating these quality indicators into practice is more challenging.

An accepted approach in mainstream dementia services in the UK is to use Dementia Care Mapping (Bradford Dementia Group, 1997) to observe and evaluate the quality of life of people living with dementia, and to enhance person-centred care. Finnamore and Lord (2007) suggest that Dementia Care Mapping (which was originally adapted from the intellectual disabilities field), may be useful in care planning for people with intellectual disabilities and dementia. In their small study of eight adults with intellectual disabilities and dementia, Dementia Care Mapping highlighted examples of good and poor practice. The process demonstrated positive outcomes after an intervention, however they concluded that the Dementia Care Mapping training and time requirements to achieve this may be beyond the resources of many intellectual disabilities services.

In 2009, the British Psychological Society and the Royal College of Psychiatrists (British Psychological Society, 2009) worked together to publish guidance on the 'assessment, diagnosis, treatment and support for people with intellectual disabilities and dementia'. This included a self-assessment checklist with 15 standards that can be used to evaluate the provision of dementia care across health, social care and voluntary agencies in a geographical area. Many areas are known to be using this as a basis of developing their local dementia strategy for people with intellectual disabilities and to benchmark their services and develop an action plan.

The self-assessment checklist took a similar approach to that in the 'Green Light toolkit' (Cole and Gregory, 2004) and *Challenging Behaviour: A unified approach* (Royal College of Psychiatrists *et al.*, 2007). The checklist reflects the content of the report, and translates the guidance into 'standards you should see if the recommendations are being met'. However, it differs from previous quality standards in that each standard is written as an outcome rather than an input. The list of standards can be seen below. Each standard should be rated using red, amber or green, with clear descriptors given for each of these for every standard.

Standards in British College of Psychiatrists self-assessment checklist

- Legal framework and guidance
- Population
- Multi-agency dementia strategy
- Care pathway
- Multidisciplinary approach to assessment, diagnosis and support
- Assessment and diagnosis
- Person-centred dementia care
- Care management and review
- Interventions
- Dementia friendly environments
- Dying in place
- Choices and rights of people with intellectual disabilities and dementia
- Support to family carers
- Capable workforce
- End of life care.

(BPS, 2009)

The self-assessment checklist can be completed in a variety of ways. Bush (2010) described how it was used within Sheffield Health and Social Care Trust, UK, to rate the care provided, and to develop a local dementia and intellectual disabilities multi-agency strategy and action plan. Bush recommends identifying an appropriate stakeholder group to decide which standards should be included. Different stakeholder groups may be needed for different standards depending on how the local service is configured. At the review meeting, the stakeholders need to be honest in identifying what they are doing well that meets the standard, and when they are not doing what is recommended in the standard. Each standard is then given an overall rating of red, amber or green, and actions identified where improvements are needed. A similar approach has been undertaken in other areas allowing a stocktake of current provision across a geographical area, identification of strengths and gaps.

Outcome measurement for people with intellectual disabilities and dementia

Outcome measurement for people with intellectual disabilities and dementia is still in its infancy. Strydom *et al.* (2009) on behalf of the International Association for the Scientific Study of Intellectual and Developmental Disabilities (IASSIDD), Special Interest Research Group on Ageing and Intellectual Disabilities undertook a systematic literature search from 1997–2008. This review identified no specific literature on measuring outcomes for people with intellectual disabilities and dementia.

Although dementia has been a growing issue in services for people over the last 20 years, the focus was initially on prevalence and epidemiology, together with assessment and diagnostic issues. More lately there has been a greater focus on the management of people with intellectual disabilities and dementia, but there is still very little focus on measuring the outcomes for people with intellectual disabilities and dementia. This means that as practitioners there is a lack of evidence about what makes a difference. The last ten years have seen the development of a number of specific resources to inform family carers, staff and people with intellectual disabilities of ways to support people with dementia (Dodd *et al.*, 2002, 2009; Watchman *et al.*, 2010). Clinicians and professionals working with people with intellectual disabilities are often clear about what works in practice, but this has not resulted in a substantial evidence base. This was highlighted by Jokinen (2005) who concluded that there is a lack of published research on the efficacy of strategies to guide the provision of daily care.

One study by Chaput (2002) found that small group living may provide better opportunities to maintain or enhance quality of life for the person with an intellectual disability and dementia as compared to large group settings, such as nursing homes. Two further studies indicated that specific approaches to measuring quality of life could be undertaken. McCallion and McCarron (2007) proposed nine quality of life indicators that could be used to form a basis for proactive service planning. They wrote that 'Common concepts within a quality of life framework may need to be adapted or modified in dementia care and offer potential for the establishment of a proactive approach' (p. 56). Courtenay *et al.* (2010) in their summary paper looking at caregiving aspects of the review undertaken by Strydom *et al.* (2009) indicated that another avenue of research may be to further investigate quality of life indicators.

Another small stream of the literature has looked at outcomes for specific interventions. Rosewarne (2001) demonstrated that structured psychotherapeutic groups could be used to promote individual quality of life and maintain the person's level of functioning. Kalsy *et al.* (2007) showed that staff training which is focused on behaviour that challenges others can positively influence staff knowledge by changing attributions of the controllability of the behaviour associated with dementia. However, the subsequent outcome for the individual with dementia was not clear. Nichols (2011) demonstrated that using personalised technology made a positive difference to the lives of people with intellectual disabilities and dementia.

Although the intellectual disability literature is very sparse, there has been more of a focus on measuring either specific outcomes or quality of life measures within the mainstream dementia literature. A number of approaches have been utilised. There are an increasing number of studies that have looked at a specific element of a person's life or functioning. These fall into a number of categories. Some studies focus on trying to reduce the changed behaviour of the person with dementia, for example Husebo *et al.* (2011) and Chenoweth *et al.* (2009) demonstrated reduction in agitation. Interestingly, Husebo *et al.* (2011) demonstrated that a systematic approach to the management of pain significantly reduced agitation in residents of nursing homes with dementia. They postulated that improved treatment of pain could help to reduce the unnecessary use of antipsychotics in people with dementia in nursing homes. Other studies have focused on different facets of dementia care. Morgan-Brown *et al.* (2013) showed improvement in social engagement after implementing household environments in two Irish nursing homes. Phillips *et al.* (2013) in a review paper showed that case conferencing provided opportunities to improve care and palliative care outcomes for older people by engaging family and all relevant internal and external health providers in prospective care planning. Similarly, Acton and Kang (2001) have written about the effectiveness of interventions with caregivers or co-residents in the form of education, training and support groups. Peterson *et al.* (2012) found a lack of appropriate evaluation tools when they undertook a review of available quality of life outcome assessments that could be used to assess outcomes of the use of assistive technology for people with dementia.

Other work has focused on developing, evaluating or reviewing quality of life or other specific outcome measures that can be used either with people with mild or moderate dementia or with carers. Brod *et al.* (1999) developed a 29-item instrument designed to assess quality of life by direct interview with people with mild to moderate dementia. They thought that health care professionals might have a better ability to intervene to improve quality of life than to change other aspects of living with dementia. Ready and Ott (2003) reviewed nine measures of quality of life indicators available at that time. They concluded that one important issue was whether quality of life measures are sensitive to change over time, which they thought was critical in evaluating response to treatment and to determine the effects of the progression of dementia on quality of life.

Banerjee *et al.* (2009) reviewed the use of dementia specific measures of health-related quality of life, concluding that little is known about this, or what interventions promote or inhibit health-related quality of life for people with dementia. In a further study, Hurt *et al.* (2010) found that impaired insight is associated with better health-related quality of life in people with moderate dementia. This study has important implications for interventions which focus on increasing the awareness of the person with dementia, as this may not improve their health-related quality of life.

Quirk *et al.* (2012) described the development of the carer wellbeing and support questionnaire, which they hypothesised could be a reliable and valid measure to determine and address areas of support for carers, including assessing the effectiveness of new interventions and approaches. In a review of outcome measures, Moniz-Cook *et al.* (2008) found measures that covered a large number of different areas. For the person with dementia, these included domains of quality of life, mood, global function, behaviour and daily living skills. Family carer domains included mood and burden, which incorporated coping with behaviour and quality of life. The only specific staff domain identified was morale, but this included satisfaction and coping with behaviour. Moniz-Cook *et al.* (2008) concluded that 22 measures across nine domains could be recommended in order to improve the comparability of intervention studies in Europe. Overall, they argued that a more cohesive approach to outcome measurement in dementia care research will lead to a more robust evidence base.

The challenge of outcome measurement in individuals with intellectual disabilities and dementia

Preliminary work was undertaken by Dodd (2010) to see if accepted health-related quality outcome measures, DEMQOL and DEMQOL-Proxy (Smith *et al.* 2005) were appropriate to use with people with Down syndrome and dementia.

Dodd (2010) concluded that in a trial with 30 people, DEMQOL was not an appropriate tool to use with people with intellectual disabilities and dementia because of the complexity of the language and concepts. Similarly, DEMQOL-Proxy is not an appropriate tool to use with carers of people with Down syndrome and dementia because of the way staff perceive or think about people with intellectual disabilities and dementia. What is clear from reviewing the literature is that current measures in place seem to see dementia as a 'stable' condition rather than one which is progressive. It seems vital that any measure is sensitive to the progression (Janicki, 2011), and not just able to be used for people with early or mid stage dementia in line with the thinking of Ready and Ott (2003).

Dodd and Bush (2011) described their thinking about measuring quality outcomes for people with Down syndrome and dementia. From their clinical experience of working with people with Down syndrome and dementia and their caregivers, it had become clear that one of the key components of excellence in dementia care was the ability of the system to continuously adapt their understanding, care and resources as the person's dementia progresses. They had observed that often staff in home and day services for people with intellectual disabilities receive training only when people are identified as having dementia. This allows them to become proficient at meeting the needs of people who are newly diagnosed with dementia. However, as the dementia progresses, they are less able to adapt what they do in line with the person's changing needs. This often leads to staff feeling that they cannot care for the person with the changing needs and that they are always 'lagging behind'. In turn, this can lead to poorer outcomes for the person with mid or late stage dementia.

Other clinicians had also contacted Dodd and Bush (2011) asking for their advice on tools to measure outcomes for people with dementia. These issues led to the development of a measure that is able to look at quality outcomes across the progression of dementia, and which measures quality across the whole of the person's life, rather than specific issues. Dodd and Bush had both been involved in the British Psychological Society and Royal College of Psychiatrists working party to develop the guidance (BPS, 2009) and wanted to build on this work to think about standards and outcomes for individuals with an intellectual disability and dementia. The Quality Outcome Measure for Individuals with Dementia (QOMID) (Dodd and Bush, 2013) is in line with the thinking of Janicki (2011) who also identified the concept of 'stage adapted care' for people with dementia, and other publications (Grieg, 2013; Pickup, 2012) that focus on outcomes for the person, rather than processes.

The aims of the QOMID are that the quality outcome measure:

- could be used with anyone with dementia

- was stage specific (early, mid and late stage dementia)

- reflected the guidance in the British Psychological Society and Royal College of Psychiatrists document for assessment, diagnosis, treatment and support of people with intellectual disabilities and dementia

- was fairly quick to administer

- could be used in any setting

- could be used to help both evaluate quality outcomes and plan to improve them.

The measure needed to be able to distinguish how a quality outcome may change in a particular domain as the dementia progresses. This led to a format that identified common domains from both clinical experience and from a review of the literature, both of which were important in assuring quality outcomes for the individual.

After an initial pilot study, the final tool has 17 domains as shown in Table 16.1. Each domain has a description of the required quality outcome for each of the three main stages of dementia: suspected/ early, mid and late stage.

Table 16.1: Quality outcome measure for individuals with dementia (QOMID)

Area	Suspected/early stage dementia	Mid stage dementia	Late stage dementia

1. Person-centred approaches to support	The person experiences support which is underpinned by planning based on:
	• the person's own wishes,
	• their capacity (maximising their decision making wherever possible)
	• their needs and history as shown in their individualised support plan which includes
	  ○ their person centred plan
	  ○ health care plan
	  ○ communication passport
	  ○ life story book
	  ○ advanced directives, and
	  ○ end of life planning.
		The person experiences support which is underpinned by planning based on:
		• the person's own wishes,
		• their capacity (maximising their decision making wherever possible),
		• their needs and history as shown in their individualised support plan which includes
		  ○ their person centred plan
		  ○ health care plan
		  ○ communication passport
		  ○ life story book
		  ○ advanced directives, and
		  ○ end of life planning.
			The person experiences support which is underpinned by planning based on:
			• the person's own wishes,
			• their capacity (maximising their decision making wherever possible),
			• their needs and history as shown in their individualised support plan which includes
			  ○ their person centred plan
			  ○ health care plan
			  ○ communication passport
			  ○ life story book
			  ○ advanced directives, and
			  ○ end of life planning.

2. Positive risk taking	The person is supported to take appropriate risks that enhance their opportunities to live an independent, fulfilled life.	The person is supported to take appropriate risks that enhance their opportunities to live an independent, fulfilled life.	The person is supported by people who take positive action to ensure that the person still has a range of fulfilling life experiences.

cont.

Table 16.1: Quality outcome measure for individuals with dementia (QOMID) (*cont.*)

Area	Suspected/early stage dementia	Mid stage dementia	Late stage dementia
3. Respect for human rights	The person's human rights are fully respected by ensuring that there is full compliance with: • prescribed medication is in line with NICE guidelines • Mental Capacity Act – choice and decision making. The person is supported to make as many decisions for themselves as is possible • Best Interest Decisions that are made on behalf of the person are fully documented • absence of inappropriate restrictions. If the person tends to wander, this is managed through respectful and positive approaches that do not impact on their human rights.	The person's human rights are fully respected by ensuring that there is full compliance with: • prescribed medication is in line with NICE guidelines • Mental Capacity Act – choice and decision making. The person is supported to make as many decisions for themselves as is possible • Best Interest Decisions that are made on behalf of the person are fully documented • absence of inappropriate restrictions. If there is a need to deprive somebody of their liberty, the appropriate Deprivation of Liberty Safeguards are in place.	The person's human rights are fully respected by ensuring that there is full compliance with: • prescribed medication is in line with NICE guidelines • Mental Capacity Act – choice and decision making. The person is supported to make as many decisions for themselves as is possible • Best Interest Decisions that are made on behalf of the person are fully documented • absence of inappropriate restrictions. If there is a need to deprive somebody of their liberty, the appropriate Deprivation of Liberty Safeguards are in place.

4. Consistency of approach	The person experiences consistency of approach in all settings e.g. <ul><li>They are supported by familiar people.</li><li>Family/Staff fully understand the content of their support plan.</li><li>New staff are properly introduced to the person before they start working with them.</li><li>The use of unfamiliar or agency staff is minimised and staff are well briefed about the person before they start to support them.</li></ul>	The person experiences consistency of approach in all settings e.g. <ul><li>They are supported by familiar people.</li><li>Family/Staff fully understand the content of their support plan.</li><li>New staff are properly introduced to the person before they start working with them.</li><li>The use of unfamiliar or agency staff is minimised and staff are well briefed about the person before they start to support them.</li><li>They are not moved unnecessarily because of funding issues (e.g. need for waking night staff).</li></ul>	The person experiences consistency of approach in all settings e.g. <ul><li>They are supported by familiar people.</li><li>Family/Staff fully understand the content of their support plan.</li><li>New staff are properly introduced to the person before they start working with them.</li><li>The use of unfamiliar or agency staff is minimised and staff are well briefed about the person before they start to support them.</li><li>They are not moved unnecessarily because of funding issues (e.g. need for waking night staff).</li></ul>
5. Interaction with others	The person experiences calm and constructive interaction with family, staff and friends, who adapt the amount of language used and use symbols and pictures as required to ensure the person experiences positive interactions.	The person experiences calm and constructive interaction with family, staff and friends, with no confrontation; no time pressures; and validation of roll back memories. The person experiences positive interactions and is always approached from the front to prevent surprise and panic.	The person experiences calm and constructive interaction with family, staff and friends, with protected 1:1 time each waking hour to ensure that the person experiences positive interactions.

cont.

Table 16.1: Quality outcome measure for individuals with dementia (QOMID) (*cont.*)

Area	Suspected/early stage dementia	Mid stage dementia	Late stage dementia
6. Emotional reassurance	The person receives explanations about their dementia and reassurance about the effects of the disease as appropriate to their wishes and level of ability.	The person is reassured about the changes they are experiencing through both verbal and non-verbal interaction.	The person is reassured about their condition by the way people interact both verbally and through appropriate touch.
7. Orientation	The person is oriented to time and place through approaches that are appropriate to their level of ability. Their support plan describes routines that are likely to be important to the person as the dementia progresses. There is evidence that the team has made plans to ensure that any future changes that are envisaged for the person are properly considered and take account of possible effect on the person's orientation.	The person is able to understand their daily routine through the use of appropriate cues and aids e.g. daily picture timetable, picture menus, picture staff rotas. There is evidence that the team has made plans to ensure that any future changes that are envisaged for the person are properly considered and take account of possible effect on the person's orientation.	The person feels safe in having a consistent and familiar routine.
8. Daily living	The person is able to complete personal care and daily living activities as much as they are able, but without pressure. The person's abilities and additional assistance required to help maintain independence are recognised, and the person is supported appropriately e.g. having increased prompting.	The person is able to complete parts of personal care and daily living tasks that they can do and are assisted as necessary so they do not fail. Their support plan details the additional assistance required to help maintain as much independence as possible in a failure free manner.	The person experiences care that is dignified and respectful of them as a person for all their personal care and daily living activities.

9. Carrying out preferred activities	The person continues to access and enjoy activities which build upon on their lifelong interests and preferences and are appropriate to their level of ability and dementia. Activities are adapted to meet their changing needs.	The person continues to access and enjoy activities which build upon their lifelong interests and preferences and are appropriate to their level of ability and dementia. Activities are adapted to take account of their attention span and memory and ensure that the person is not stressed or experiences failure.	The person continues to access and enjoy activities appropriate to their level of ability and dementia. The person has opportunities to interact with people/objects which give them enjoyment and in ways that take full account of their preferences and attention span.
10. Flexibility of support	The person continues to attend familiar social, leisure, work, respite and recreational activities in their local community, with adjustments made as appropriate to meet their needs.	The person continues to enjoy familiar social, leisure, work, respite and recreational activities in their local community through flexible supports e.g. short days, flexible transport, 1:1 support following the person.	The person continues to access and enjoy the community as much as their dementia allows and as agreed in their support plan.
11. Environment	The person lives and spends their time in environments that are familiar to them and can find their way around easily with depth perception problems minimised, e.g. flooring colour is consistent.	The person lives and spends their time in environments that are familiar to them and have all the necessary aids/adaptations to help them find their way around and meet their needs, and minimises risks of falls, e.g. red toilet doors, red toilet seats, colour contrasts, good signage, handrails, chairs at right height.	The person lives and spends their time in environments that are familiar to them and have all the necessary adaptations to meet their needs. e.g. hoists, adapted bath/shower, special bed, appropriate wheelchair and armchair, changing facilities.

cont.

Table 16.1: Quality outcome measure for individuals with dementia (QOMID) (*cont.*)

Area	Suspected/early stage dementia	Mid stage dementia	Late stage dementia
12. Behaviour	Behavioural issues are minimised by ensuring that the person experiences support that: • understands the context of their behaviour • responds with compassion and avoids confrontation. If the person needs support from services because of their behaviour this is underpinned by: • a comprehensive assessment of the person, their care and the environment • a formulation that enables carers or staff to understand the likely reasons for the behaviour • a proactive support plan that includes triggers to be avoided • reactive strategies that are non-restrictive and the effectiveness of the approach is reviewed regularly.	Behavioural issues are minimised by ensuring that the person experiences support that: • understands the context of their behaviour • responds with compassion and avoids confrontation. If the person needs support from services because of their behaviour this is underpinned by: • a comprehensive assessment of the person, their care and the environment • a formulation that enables carers or staff to understand the likely reasons for the behaviour • a proactive support plan that includes triggers to be avoided • reactive strategies that are non-restrictive and the effectiveness of the approach is reviewed regularly.	Behavioural issues are minimised by ensuring that the person experiences support that: • understands the context of their behaviour • responds with compassion and avoids confrontation. If the person needs support from services because of their behaviour this is underpinned by: • a comprehensive assessment of the person, their care and the environment • a formulation that enables carers or staff to understand the likely reasons for the behaviour • a proactive support plan that includes triggers to be avoided • reactive strategies that are non-restrictive and the effectiveness of the approach is reviewed regularly.

13. Health	The person's physical and mental health needs are met promptly and appropriately including attention to: • pain recognition and management • thyroid function • vision • hearing • blood pressure • diabetes • mental wellbeing Medication is prescribed appropriately and reviewed regularly. The person experiences care with regard to Vitamin D in line with DH guidance.	The person's physical and mental health needs are met promptly and appropriately including attention to: • pain recognition and management • thyroid function • vision • hearing • blood pressure • diabetes • mental wellbeing Medication is prescribed appropriately and reviewed regularly. The person experiences care with regard to Vitamin D in line with DH guidance.	The person's physical and mental health needs are met promptly and appropriately including attention to: • pain recognition and management • thyroid function • vision • hearing • blood pressure • diabetes • mental wellbeing Medication is prescribed appropriately and reviewed regularly. The person has: • no pressure sores • no aspiration • no urinary tract infections The person experiences care with regard to Vitamin D in line with DH guidance.
14. Support from well coordinated agencies	The person's needs are met by people from providers in primary care, secondary care, social services and voluntary sector who have a good understanding of the needs of people with dementia, and who work well together with the person and their families.	The person's needs are met by people from providers in primary care, secondary care, social services and voluntary sector who have a good understanding of the needs of people with dementia, and who work well together with the person and their families. Where necessary good links are made with neurology services re management of epilepsy.	The person's needs are met by people from providers in primary care, secondary care, social services and voluntary sector who have a good understanding of the needs of people with dementia, and who work well together with the person and their families. Good links are made with local palliative care services.

cont.

Table 16.1: Quality outcome measure for individuals with dementia (QOMID) (*cont.*)

Area	Suspected/early stage dementia	Mid stage dementia	Late stage dementia
15. Nutrition	The person enjoys a good and appetising diet and adequate hydration. The person maintains an appropriate weight which is monitored through regular weight checks.	The person enjoys a good and appetising diet and adequate hydration as appropriate to their needs over each 24 hour period. The person maintains an appropriate weight which is monitored through regular weight checks. Any swallowing difficulties are identified and support plans take these into full account.	The person enjoys a good and appetising diet and adequate hydration as appropriate to their needs over each 24 hour period which also prevents dysphagia and aspiration. There is a full assessment of all eating and swallowing problems by an appropriate clinician. Any needs are well documented, a support plan is in place and staff are trained to deliver it safely. The person maintains an appropriate weight which is monitored through regular weight checks.
16. Mobility	The person maintains good mobility. They access regular exercise that is appropriate to their needs and interests.	The person is able to mobilise safely and has appropriate aids and adaptations in place. They access regular exercise that is appropriate to their needs and interests. Risk assessments are in place to prevent falls.	The person is supported to be moved appropriately. They access regular exercise that is appropriate to their needs and interests. Risk assessments are in place to prevent falls.

| 17. Continence | The person maintains their baseline level of continence. | The person maintains their baseline level of continence through environmental changes e.g. clear signage for toilets; regular prompting to use the toilet; and attention to relevant health issues where possible. Continence products are only used when the person needs them. | The person experiences dignified management of incontinence through the use of appropriate aids and continence products. |

Source: Dodd and Bush, 2013

The QOMID should be completed by the professional in discussion with the relevant people for the particular stage of dementia that the person has. Wherever possible, and depending on ability, the person with dementia should be asked how they would rate their experience in each domain. Additional information for the professional to make an inclusive judgement may come from family, support staff, advocates, care managers or anyone else involved with the person and their support, often at a care review meeting.

The person completing QOMID needs to decide which stage of dementia the person currently falls into, based on current assessment and professional opinion. They should then use the column for that stage of dementia and rate each domain using a four-point rating scale, where 1 is 'this is rarely achieved for this person', to 4 where 'this is completely and consistently achieved for this person'. All the domains in the measure must be completed. If the domain is rated less than 4, the person completing the measure should specify what needs to happen to improve the person's quality outcome in that area of their life.

A full QOMID total score is 68, which means that the quality outcomes for the person scored 4 completely and consistently for the person, on all domains. The following categories were assigned for QOMID scores as shown in Table 16.2.

Table 16.2: QOMID category breakdown

Category	Score	Description
Excellent	60–68	On average a 4 is achieved for more than 50 per cent of the domains with 3 on the others
Good	51–59	On average a score of 3 or more is achieved on all domains
Adequate	43–50	On average scores of 2 and 3 are achieved across all domains
Poor	34–41	On average scores of 2 are achieved across all domains
Unacceptable	Under 33	On average scores of 1 and 2 are achieved across all domains

Source: Dodd and Bush, 2013

The aim in supporting the person with intellectual disabilities and dementia is for them to have high quality outcomes throughout the progression of their dementia. As dementia is a progressive condition, it is vital to ensure that the person's changing needs are recognised and met. This means that as the person moves into each stage of dementia, the quality outcome score for each domain may start at 2 or 3, but as people work together to improve the person's quality outcomes, the scores should reach the maximum of 4 in each domain. This may mean that scores may fluctuate during the course of the dementia as support 'catches up' with the person's changing needs.

The QOMID is also designed to help everyone involved in supporting the person to work with the person and their carers to both prevent deterioration in quality outcome and to forward plan effective care. For each domain that is scored at less than 4, the support team is asked to specify what needs to be put in place to improve the person's quality outcome for that domain. These actions can then be included in the person's support plan. In addition, by looking at the descriptions for the next stage of dementia, the professional can begin to help the person and their supporters to think about what needs to be put in place to maintain the person's quality outcome.

Dodd et al. (2013) report on the piloting of the measure across 11 services, ten for people with intellectual disabilities and dementia and one for older people with dementia. Evaluation forms on the use of the tool were received for 73 people across all stages of dementia. Analysis suggested that the QOMID has good reliability and face validity, and that it also had excellent clinical utility as people found it easy to understand, easy to use and effective in practice. Dodd et al. (2013) concluded that it met the initial aims that they had set out for the tool. Moreover, it also meets the requirement of measuring life-related care rather than processes (Greig, 2013) and helping people to 'Live Well with Dementia' (Department of Health, 2009).

Conclusion

Services for people with intellectual disabilities and dementia are at different stages in their development. Whilst person-centred care has been a basis of care for people with intellectual disabilities for many years, the need to focus specifically on dementia adds further layers of complexity. Services appear to progress through a number of stages as they both come to terms with, and learn to offer excellence in care to the person with intellectual disabilities and dementia. These stages start with recognition that people with intellectual disabilities may be vulnerable to dementia, and an understanding of the early signs. This leads services to identify the need for assessment and diagnosis. Once a diagnosis is made, then the next stage is to begin to explore how best to care for the person as the dementia progresses.

However, assurance of quality and outcome measurement for people with intellectual disabilities and dementia is still in its infancy. There needs to be a much greater focus on ensuring that our local services can meet the needs of the increasing numbers of people with intellectual disabilities and dementia, as well as ensuring a quality outcome for each person throughout the course of the condition.

References

Acton, GJ. and Kang, J. (2001) Interventions to reduce the burden of caregiving for an adult with dementia: A meta-analysis. *Research in Nursing and Health 24*, 5, 349–360.

Alzheimer's Association (2006) *Dementia Care Practice Recommendations for Assisted Living Residences and Nursing Homes.* Available at www.alz.org/professionals_and_researchers_dementia_care_practice_recommendations.asp, accessed on 7 December 2013.

Alzheimer's Australia (2007) *Quality Dementia Care Standards: A Guide to Practice for Managers in Residential Aged Care Facilities.* Available at www.fightdementia.org.au/common/files/NAT/20070200_Nat_QDC_QDC2QualDemCareStandards.pdf, accessed on 7 December 2013.

Alzheimer's Society (2013) *Treating Behavioural and Psychological Symptoms of Dementia.* Available at www.alzheimers.org.uk/site/scripts/documents_info.php?documentID=1191&pageNumber=3, accessed on 7 December 2013.

Banerjee, S., Samsi, K., Petrie, CD. *et al.* (2009) What do we know about quality of life in dementia? A review of the emerging evidence on the predictive and explanatory value of disease specific measures of health related quality of life in people with dementia. *International Journal of Geriatric Psychiatry 24*, 1, 15–24.

Bradford Dementia Group (1997) *Evaluating Dementia Care: The DCM Method.* 7th edition. Bradford: University of Bradford.

British Psychological Society and Royal College of Psychiatrists (2009) *Dementia and People with Learning Disabilities: Guidance on the Assessment, Diagnosis, Treatment and Support of People with Learning Disabilities who Develop Dementia.* Leicester: British Psychological Society.

Brod, M., Stewart, AL., Sands, L. and Walton, P. (1999) Conceptualization and measurement of quality of life in dementia: The dementia quality of life instrument (DQoL). *The Gerontologist 39*, 1, 25–35.

Bush, A. (2010) *Assuring Quality Services for Elderly People with Down's Syndrome.* Conference Presentation, 21 October 2010. Rome: International Association for the Scientific Study of Intellectual and Developmental Disability (IASSID).

Care Quality Commission (2013) Time *to Listen in NHS Hospitals. Dignity and Nutrition Inspection Programme 2012.* Available at www.cqc.org.uk/sites/default/files/media/documents/time_to_listen_-_nhs_hospitals_main_report_tag.pdf, accessed on 7 December 2013.

Carnaby, S., Roberts, B., Lang, J. and Nielsen, P. (2011) A flexible response: Person-centred support and social inclusion for people with learning disabilities and challenging behaviour. *British Journal of Learning Disabilities 39*, 1, 39–45.

Chaput, J. (2002) Adults with Down's syndrome and Alzheimer's disease: Comparison of services received in group homes and in special care units. *Journal of Gerontological Social Work 38*, 1/2,197–211.

Chenoweth, L., King, MT., Jeon, Y-H. *et al.* (2009) Caring for Aged Dementia Care Resident Study (CADRES) of person-centred care, dementia-care mapping, and usual care in dementia: A cluster-randomised trial. *Lancet Neurology 8*, 4, 317–325.

Cole, A. and Gregory, M. (2004) *Green Light for Mental Health: A Service Improvement Toolkit.* London: Foundation for People with Learning Disabilities.

Courtenay, K., Jokinen, NS. and Strydom, A. (2010) Caregiving and adults with intellectual disabilities affected by dementia. *Journal of Policy and Practice in Intellectual Disabilities 7*, 1, 26–33.

Department of Health (2009) *Living Well With Dementia: A National Dementia Strategy.* London: The Stationery Office.

Department of Health (2012) *Prime Minister's Challenge on Dementia.* London: The Stationery Office.

Dodd, K. (2010) *Using the DEMQOL to Measure Quality of Life of People with Intellectual Disabilities and Dementia.* Conference presentation, 21 October 2010. Rome: IASSID.

Dodd, K. and Bush, A. (2011) *Measuring Quality of Life for People with Intellectual Disabilities and Dementia.* Manchester: Presentation on 1 September 2011 at EMHID Conference.

Dodd, K. and Bush, A. (2013) *Quality Outcome Measure for Individuals with Dementia (QOMID).* Available at http://dcp-ld.bps.org.uk/dcp-ld/useful-links-and-info/useful-links-and-info_home.cfm, accessed on 7 December 2013.

Dodd, K., Kerr, D. and Fern, S. (2006) *Dementia Workbook for Staff.* Teddington: Down's Syndrome Association.

Dodd, K., Turk, V. and Christmas, M. (2002) *Resource Pack for Carers of Adults with Down's Syndrome and Dementia.* Kidderminster: BILD Publications.

Dodd, K., Turk, V. and Christmas, M. (2009) *Resource Pack for Carers of Adults with Down's Syndrome and Dementia.* 2nd edition. Kidderminster: BILD Publications.

Finnamore, T. and Lord, S. (2007) The use of Dementia Care Mapping in people with a learning disability and dementia. *Journal of Intellectual Disabilities 11*, 2, 157–165.

Francis, R. (2013) *Report of the Mid Staffordshire NHS Foundation Trust Public Inquiry.* Available at www.midstaffspublicinquiry.com, accessed on 24 March 2014.

Grieg, R. (2013) *Dignity, Institutionalisation and the Francis Report.* Available at www.ndti.org. uk/blog/dignity-institutionalisation-and-the-francis-report, accessed on 7 December 2013.

Hurt, CS., Banerjee, S., Tunnard, C. *et al.* (2010) Insight, cognition and quality of life in Alzheimer's disease. *Journal of Neurology, Neurosurgery and Psychiatry 81*, 3, 331–336.

Husebo, BS., Ballard, C., Sandvik, R., Nilsen, OB. and Aarsland, D. (2011) Efficacy of treating pain to reduce behavioural disturbances in residents of nursing homes with dementia: Cluster randomised trial. *British Medical Journal 343*, d4065.

Janicki, M. (2011) Quality outcomes in dementia care review. *Journal of Intellectual Disability Research 55*, 8, 763–776.

Jokinen, N. (2005) The content of available practice literature in dementia and intellectual disability. *Dementia 4*, 3, 327–339.

Jokinen, N., Janicki, MP., Keller SM., McCallion, P., Force, LT. and the National Task Group on Intellectual Disabilities and Dementia Practices (2013) Guidelines for structuring community care and supports for people with intellectual disabilities affected by dementia. *Journal of Policy and Practice in Intellectual Disabilities 10*, 1,1–24.

Kalsy, S., Heath, R., Adams, D. and Oliver, C. (2007) Effects of training on controllability attributions of behavioural excesses and deficits shown by adults with Down's syndrome and dementia. *Journal of Applied Research in Intellectual Disabilities 20*, 1, 64–68.

McCallion, P. and McCarron, M. (2007) Perspective on quality of life in dementia care. *Intellectual and Developmental Disabilities 45*, 1, 56–59.

Moniz-Cook, M., Vernooij-Dassen, M., Woods, R. *et al.* for The Interdem Group (2008) A European consensus on outcome measures for psychosocial intervention research in dementia care. *Aging and Mental Health 12*, 3, 14–29.

Morgan-Brown, M., Newton, R. and Ormerod, M. (2013) Engaging life in two Irish nursing home units for people with dementia: Quantitative comparisons before and after implementing household environments. *Aging and Mental Health 17*, , 57–65.

National Institute for Health and Care Excellence (2010) *Dementia, QS1.* Available at http://guidance.nice.org.uk/QS1, accessed on 7 December 2013.

National Institute for Health and Care Excellence (2013) *Quality Standard for Supporting People to Live Well with Dementia, QS30.* Available at http://publications.nice.org.uk/quality-standard-for-supporting-people-to-live-well-with-dementia-qs30, accessed on 7 December 2013.

Nichols, E. (2011) How personalised technology can play an important role in supporting people with learning disabilities as they age and face the onset of dementia. *Journal of Assistive Technologies 5*, 3, 158–163.

O'Brien, J. (1989) *What's Worth Working For? Leadership for Better Quality Human Services.* Syracuse, NY: The Center on Human Policy, Syracuse University for the Research and Training Center on Community Living of University of Minnesota.

Peterson, CB., Prasad, NR. and Prasad, R. (2012) Assessing assistive technology's quality of life outcomes with dementia. *Gerontechnology 11*, 2, 195–203.

Phillips, J., West, PA., Davidson, PM. and Agar, M. (2013) Does case conferencing for people with advanced dementia living in nursing homes improve care outcomes: Evidence from an integrative review? *International Journal of Nursing Studies 50*, 8, 1122–1135.

Pickup, S. (2012) Improving the lives of people with dementia and their carers: The Prime Minister's challenge and a challenge for us all. *Journal of Care Services Management 6*, 1, 3–9.

Quirk, A., Smith, S., Hamilton, S. *et al.* (2012) Development of the carer well-being and support questionnaire. *Mental Health Review Journal 17*, 3, 128–138.

Ready, RE. and Ott, BR. (2003) Quality of life measures for dementia. *Health and Quality of Life Outcomes 1*, 11 doi: 10.186/1477-7525-1-11.

Robertson, J., Emerson, E., Hatton, C. *et al.* (2005) The *Impact of Person Centred Planning.* Lancaster: Institute for Health Research, Lancaster University.

Rosewarne, M. (2001) Learning disabilities and dementia: A pilot therapy group. *Journal of Dementia Care 9*, 4, 18–20.

Royal College of Psychiatrists, British Psychological Society, Royal College of Speech and Language Therapists (2007) *Challenging Behaviour: A Unified Approach. Clinical and Service Guidelines for Supporting People with Learning Disabilities who are at Risk of Receiving Abusive or Restrictive Practices.* London: Royal College of Psychiatrists.

Smith, SC., Lamping, DL., Banerjee, S. *et al.* (2005) Measurement of health-related quality of life for people with dementia: Development of a new instrument (DEMQOL) and an evaluation of current methodology. *Health Technology Assessment 9*, 10, 1–93, iii–iv.

Strydom, A., Lee, LA., Jokinen, N. *et al.* (2009) *Report on the State of Science on Dementia in People with Intellectual Disabilities.* IASSID: Special Interest Research Group on Ageing and Intellectual Disabilities.

Watchman, K., Kerr, D. and Wilkinson, H. (2010) *Supporting Derek: A Practice Development Guide to Support Staff Working with People who Have a Learning Difficulty and Dementia.* Brighton: Joseph Rowntree Foundation / Pavilion Publishing.

Wilkinson, H. and Janicki, MP. (2002) The Edinburgh Principles with accompanying guidelines and recommendations. *Journal of Intellectual Disability Research 46,* 3, 3, 279–284.

Contributors

Tiina Annus

Tiina is a PhD candidate and research assistant at the Cambridge Intellectual and Developmental Disabilities Research Group at the Department of Psychiatry, University of Cambridge, UK. She has a background in pharmacology and particular interest in the neuropharmacology and neuropathology of Alzheimer's disease. Since 2011, Tiina has been working on a Medical Research Council funded project investigating the role of brain fibrillar beta-amyloid in cognition, cerebral atrophy and Alzheimer's disease in adults with Down syndrome, using 11C-PiB PET and structural MRI techniques.

Susan Mary Benbow

Susan is an old age psychiatrist and family therapist, who has held NHS consultant posts in Manchester and Wolverhampton, UK and is now Director of Older Mind Matters Ltd. She redesigned her working life in 2009, retiring early from NHS consultant work to complete a PhD by published work and pursue a portfolio career involving research, education and consultancy. She joined the primary care memory clinic team at Gnosall Health Centre, Staffordshire, in 2012. Her research interests are broad, including systemic therapy, service development, and user and carer participation. Susan was a member of the Faculties of Old Age Psychiatry and Intellectual Disability Psychiatry Interface Group between 2006 and 2010 and on the working group which wrote a College report on Dementia and Intellectual Disabilities. She was also involved in two interface projects: one, a survey of the views and experiences of old age and intellectual disability psychiatrists, and the second, a local project to set up screening for dementia in adults with Down syndrome.

Christine Bigby

Christine is Research Programme Leader and Deputy Chair Academic Board at La Trobe University, Australia. She has an established national and international reputation for her research on the social inclusion of adults with an intellectual disability. The focus of her work is policy issues, programme effectiveness and frontline practice that supports quality of life outcomes for people with an intellectual disability. Her current ARC and other grants are examining the effectiveness of supported accommodation services, the nature and meaning of social inclusion for people with intellectual disabilities, the history of self-advocacy, and the capacity of disability and mainstream organisations to support active and healthy ageing for people with a lifelong disability. She is a Fellow of the International Association for the Scientific Study of Intellectual and Developmental Disability and Chair of the IASSIDD Special Interest Group on Ageing and Intellectual Disability, Founding Editor of Research and Practice in Intellectual and Developmental Disabilities, and a Fellow of the Australian College of Social Work. She convenes an annual round table on Intellectual Disability Policy at La Trobe University.

Noelle Blackman

Noelle is a registered dramatherapist and is the Chief Executive Officer of Respond, a charity in the UK which specialises in providing psychotherapy to people with intellectual disabilities who have been abused. In 1997, she founded a unique NHS Loss and Bereavement Service for people with intellectual disabilities and after moving to Respond set up the Elder's Project. Noelle is the co-founder of the Palliative Care for People with Learning Disabilities Network. She co-facilitates a user involvement group of older people with intellectual disabilities, which began as part of the GOLD research project in 1997 for The Foundation for People with Learning Disabilities. Her recent work involves supporting the former patients of Winterbourne View and their families. Noelle is an Honorary Fellow at the University of Hertfordshire, UK.

Rachel Carling-Jenkins

Rachel is an independent researcher and trainer. Previously, she held research fellow positions with the Intellectual Disability Research Group at La Trobe University, Australia and with the Centre for Developmental Disability Health, Victoria. Her current research focus is on dementia care, social inclusion and the role of caregivers. She completed her PhD in the School of Social Work and Social Policy at James Cook University with an APA scholarship. Her thesis explored the Disability Rights Movement in Australia. She is a member of the Disability Reference Group at the Victorian Equal Opportunity and Human Rights Commission. In 2011, she was sponsored by Alzheimer's Australia Research to travel to the UK and Ireland, where she studied dementia care for people with an intellectual disability.

Trevor Chan

Trevor is a consultant psychiatrist in intellectual disability at Oxleas NHS Foundation Trust, London, UK. Besides providing inpatient and outpatient psychiatric service to individuals with an intellectual disability in the Royal Borough of Greenwich in South East London, he has also been involved in the development of, and lead for, the local multidisciplinary Memory and Ageing Issues clinic service. He developed his research interest in dementia in the intellectual disability population when working on his dissertation on validity of dementia criteria for his MSc at University College London. He has since contributed to research work in subjects including carer reports of early symptoms, validity of diagnostic criteria, mild cognitive impairment and incidents of dementia in this population.

Antonia M.W. Coppus

As a medical doctor in Dutch intellectual disability care since 1990, and an epidemiologist, Antonia started a longitudinal research project in 1999 on predictors of dementia and mortality in Down syndrome at the Department of Epidemiology of the Erasmus Medical Centre, Rotterdam in the Netherlands which was completed in 2008 with a PhD thesis. The original cohort of 500 people with Down syndrome have been followed since then. In 2007, Antonia developed, and is the Director of a specialised national multidisciplinary outpatient department for adults with Down syndrome. In 2010, she was one of the founders of the Dutch multidisciplinary Down Team Research

Consortium (DOC). The DOC is a joint venture of representatives of the Dutch Down Syndrome Patient Organisation and health care and research professionals. Since January 2012, she has been Head of the Radboud University research pillar 'Down syndrome'. Her research at the Erasmus University Rotterdam, Department of Epidemiology and the Radboud University Nijmegen Medical Centre, Department of Primary and Community Care focuses on dementia and ageing in people with intellectual disabilities.

Ken Courtenay

Ken is a consultant psychiatrist working with adults with intellectual disabilities in a community service in London, UK. His work involves assessing, managing and supporting people who have dementia and their carers. Ken established the 'Dementia in Intellectual Disabilities – Special Interest Group' in 2009 in recognition of the need among clinicians working with people with an intellectual disability who had dementia to belong to a clinical forum that would provide education and support. The group is a multi-professional group that draws on the experience of members to share good practice and to raise standards in services. It has grown in strength since 2009 extending its reach across the UK.

Karen Dodd

Karen is Associate Director, Specialist Therapies: Intellectual Disabilities and Older Peoples Mental Health Services and a consultant clinical psychologist for Surrey and Borders Partnership NHS Foundation Trust, UK. Karen has worked with people with intellectual disabilities for almost 30 years. Her interest in people with Down syndrome and dementia arose out of her clinical work, and has included an ongoing longitudinal study of adults with Down syndrome; developing work with peers of people with Down syndrome and dementia. She is invited to speak at regional, national and international conferences and workshops on the needs of people with Down syndrome and dementia. Karen co-chaired the joint group between the British Psychological Society and Royal College of the Psychiatrists Intellectual Disability Faculties to write national guidance on the assessment, diagnosis, treatment and support of people with intellectual disabilities and dementia.

Nicole Eady

Nicole is a higher trainee in intellectual disability psychiatry. She is currently completing a MSc in Psychiatric Research at University College London, UK in the Faculty of Brain Sciences (Mental Health Sciences Unit). Her current research is focused on the treatment outcomes of dementia in adults with an intellectual disability.

Andrew Griffiths

Andrew works as a consultant in older adult psychiatry with the Black Country Partnership NHS Foundation Trust in Wolverhampton, UK where he runs a Young Onset Dementia Service. He is dual trained in older adult and intellectual disability psychiatry.

Moni Grizzell

Moni is an advanced nurse practitioner/research sister and visiting lecturer at Wolverhampton University, UK. She works in Wolverhampton Memory Clinic with the Black Country Partnership NHS Foundation Trust, and is actively involved with her local church. Other interests include raising Alzheimer's awareness via roadshows, services for people with an intellectual disability and dementia, and assisting in developing the Journal of Geriatric Care and Research.

Anthony J. Holland

Anthony holds the Health Foundation Chair in the Psychiatry of Learning Disabilities in the Department of Psychiatry at the University of Cambridge, UK and leads the Cambridge Intellectual and Developmental Disabilities Research Group. He is also an honorary consultant psychiatrist with Cambridgeshire and Peterborough Foundation Trust and the Cambridgeshire Learning Disabilities Partnership.

Teresa Iacono

Teresa is Professor of Rural and Regional Allied Health at La Trobe Rural Health School, La Trobe University, Australia. In her role as Head of the Department of Allied Health in the Rural Health School, Teresa oversees the delivery of undergraduate programmes in exercise physiology, physiotherapy, podiatry, occupational therapy and speech pathology. With a background in speech pathology, her clinical and academic interests have been in severe communication impairment in people with intellectual disabilities, as well as health and mental health issues faced by this group. Teresa is a member of the Faculty of Health Sciences Living with Disability research programme. Current projects address services for ageing people with an intellectual disability and those who care for them, Down syndrome and Alzheimer's disease assessment and caring needs, active support for people with an intellectual disability living in group homes, promoting positive relationships for people with an intellectual disability and predicting success in augmentative and alternative communication intervention for young children with autism.

Nancy S. Jokinen

Nancy is a faculty member of the School of Social Work at the University of Northern British Columbia, Canada. Her interests include: aging, aging with intellectual disabilities, dementia care, health and quality of life. She has over 20 years of experience in services and supports to adults with an intellectual disability and their families. Prior to attending doctoral studies, she was the manager of a special care unit for persons with Alzheimer's disease and other dementias. In Canada, Nancy co-chairs a local group on aging and intellectual disabilities, serves as co-president on the British Columbia Psychogeriatric Association, and is a member of Community Living British Columbia's Advisory Committee on Aging. She is also an active member on the Ontario Seniors Health Knowledge Network's Community of Practice on Aging and Developmental Disabilities. At an international level, she was elected president of the AAIDD's Gerontology Division (2009–2014) and is a member of the executive committee of IASSIDD's Aging and Intellectual Disabilities Special Interest Research Group (International Association for the Scientific Study of Intellectual and Developmental Disabilities). Nancy is actively involved with the US National Task Group on Intellectual Disabilities and Dementia Practices.

Sunny Kalsy-Lillico

Sunny is a consultant clinical psychologist with over 20 years of experience in working with people with intellectual disabilities in the UK. She currently specialises in working with older people with intellectual disabilities and early onset dementia. As a qualified systemic family therapist she also works extensively with families and care teams supporting people with intellectual disabilities. As a result of her work with people with Down syndrome and dementia, she was presented with the British Psychological Society's May Davidson award, for her contribution to British clinical psychology.

Philip McCallion

Philip is Professor in the School of Social Welfare at New York State's University at Albany, a Hartford Geriatric Social Work Faculty Scholar and Mentor and co-Director of the Centre for Excellence in Aging and Community Wellness. He holds an appointment as a Visiting Professor at the School of Nursing and Midwifery at Trinity College Dublin, Ireland where he is co-principal investigator for the Intellectual Disability Supplement to the Irish Longitudinal Study of Ageing (TILDA). Philip's research has included system design work on creating ageing and disability prepared communities and on embedding evidence-based health promotion, care transitions strategies and participant-directed practices in ageing and in disability services delivery. He has been responsible for the evaluation of non-pharmacological interventions for persons with dementia, psycho-educational interventions for family caregivers, and of quality of life maintenance and enhancement strategies. Philip has developed innovative demonstration projects designed to maintain ageing persons with intellectual disabilities in the community and has adapted palliative care principles for end of life care for people with intellectual disabilities.

Mary McCarron

Mary is Dean of the Faculty of Health Sciences, at Trinity College, Dublin, Ireland and an internationally recognised researcher on quality of life and care in the areas of intellectual disabilities, ageing, chronic illness, dementia and palliative care. Mary is the principal investigator of the longitudinal study on Ageing in Persons with Intellectual Disabilities, a landmark study with comparative data to compare the ageing process in people with an intellectual disability with other population groups. Mary is a Policy and Service Advisor on Dementia to the Daughters of Charity Service and a consultant to services providers and advocacy groups, advising on dementia diagnosis, person-centred care and service redesign for people with an intellectual disability. She acts as spokesperson on ageing-related issues for key organisations both nationally and internationally.

Niamh Mulryan

Niamh is a medical graduate of Trinity College Dublin, Ireland and is currently the acting Clinical Director of the Daughters of Charity Intellectual Disability Services, Dublin, Ireland. She has trained both in general psychiatry and the psychiatry of intellectual disabilities and has developed special interests in ageing and mental health issues in those with an intellectual disability.

Liam Reese Wilson

Liam is a research assistant and PhD student at the Cambridge Intellectual and Developmental Disabilities Research Group (CIDDRG), Department of Psychiatry, University of Cambridge, UK. He is working on a MRC funded study investigating the role of cerebral beta-amyloid in Alzheimer's disease in Down syndrome using MRI, [11C] PiB PET and several neuropsychological measures of memory and executive functioning.

Evelyn Reilly

Evelyn has had a particular interest in ageing and dementia in people with Down syndrome for the past 15 years. As one of the first qualified clinical nurse specialists in intellectual disabilities and dementia, Evelyn manages the day-to-day operations of a service-wide memory clinic for the Daughters of Charity Service in Dublin. She is involved in the ongoing service development for people with an intellectual disability and dementia including cognitive screening and assessment, non-pharmacological psychosocial approaches to care and promoting best practice at end of life. She offers comprehensive training in dementia care to all levels of staff, to peers and family. Currently, lecturing on the MSc in Specialist Nursing (Dementia and Intellectual Disabilities) in Trinity College Dublin, Evelyn was key in the planning and design of a new Special Dementia Home Setting for people with an intellectual disability. This specially tailored environment was designed to compensate for the losses and challenges associated with dementia, and to enable the people living there to experience the highest possible quality of life.

Amanda Sinai

Amanda is a clinical research associate at University College London, UK in the Faculty of Brain Sciences (Mental Health Sciences Unit) and is currently working towards an MD (Res). She has recently completed her training in the psychiatry of intellectual disability. Her research interests include behavioural phenotypes and dementia in people with Down syndrome.

Andre Strydom

Andre is a senior lecturer at University College London, UK in the Faculty of Brain Sciences (Mental Health Sciences Unit) and a consultant psychiatrist in intellectual disabilities. His research is focused on the epidemiology and aetiology of mental disorders in adults with neurodevelopmental conditions, and the development and evaluation of interventions to reduce associated morbidity. He is particularly interested in ageing-related conditions such as dementia in adults with an intellectual disability and Down syndrome.

David Thompson

David is a specialist nurse safeguarding adults at Hounslow and Richmond Community Healthcare NHS Trust, UK. He brought together the Growing Older with Learning Disabilities (GOLD) group when he was managing a project on ageing at the Foundation for People with Learning Disabilities, UK in 1998. He has a wide experience of direct work with people with intellectual disabilities, including as a teacher, sex educator and advocate. He has also had national roles relating to support for family carers, the Mental Capacity Act 2005 and adult safeguarding; including being vice chair of the Ann Craft Trust. David works as a Court of Protection Visitor having completed his training as a mental health nurse.

Christine Towers

Christine is Research and Service Development Manager at the Foundation for People with Learning Disabilities, UK where she has worked since 2005. Christine's areas of interest include planning with families, supporting people with intellectual disabilities as they grow older, people with intellectual disabilities with caring roles and the development of social and community networks. Her research interests include the experiences of fathers of children with intellectual disabilities and supporting families to plan for the future. Her research projects have led to the development of practical resources for family carers and practitioners. Prior to working at the Foundation for People with Learning Disabilities, Christine worked on national research projects on direct payments and the impact of person-centred planning. Over the past 30 years, she has worked in a variety of roles developing opportunities for people with intellectual disabilities and their families in health services, social services and non-governmental organisations. Christine has also managed and developed services and organisations supporting people with mental health problems.

Irene Tuffrey-Wijne

Irene qualified as a nurse in the Netherlands in 1985. She has worked as a residential care assistant and home manager in the L'Arche London Community for people with intellectual disabilities and as a palliative care nurse at Trinity Hospice, London, before changing to an academic career in 2001. She is a Senior Research Fellow at St George's University of London and Kingston University, UK and at Maastricht University in the Netherlands. Irene has carried out a range of research projects around intellectual disabilities, cancer and palliative care. Her research includes studies of the care and safety of patients with intellectual disabilities in hospitals, the personal experiences of people with intellectual disabilities who have cancer and the development of a new model for breaking bad news to people with intellectual disabilities. Inclusion of people with intellectual disabilities as study participants and as salaried co-researchers is a key part of her work. Irene chairs the Palliative Care for People with Learning Disabilities Network and the Taskforce on Intellectual Disabilities of the European Association of Palliative Care.

Leslie Udell

Leslie is the Interim Executive Director, Winniserv Inc., Canada, an agency that provides residential supports to adults with an intellectual disability. She has been with the organisation for over 20 years, first as a Programme Coordinator, then as the Coming of Age Project Coordinator and currently as the Interim Executive Director. Leslie's primary areas of focus are on the issues of ageing, supporting people with dementia and person-centred care. She has contributed to publications on intellectual disabilities and dementia through the US National Task Group on Intellectual Disabilities and Dementia Practices.

Karen Watchman

Karen is Alzheimer Scotland Lecturer in Dementia at the Alzheimer Scotland Centre for Policy and Practice, University of the West of Scotland, UK. With experience of supporting people within both dementia care and intellectual disability services, Karen's research and teaching stems from her practice and academic background. This includes her role as Director of Down's Syndrome Scotland and subsequent development and delivery of online undergraduate and postgraduate programmes on intellectual disabilities and dementia in Scotland. Karen developed the internationally recognised Intellectual Disabilities and Dementia: Train the Trainer course to cascade information through organisations and services. Karen is a committee member of the Down Syndrome Special Interest Research Group, IASSIDD and is actively involved in the work of the Palliative Care for People with Learning Disabilities Network.

Heather Wilkinson

Heather has been based at the University of Edinburgh, UK since 2001. She is co-Director at the Centre for Research on Families and Relationships, Director of Research and Knowledge Exchange and Head of Interdisciplinary Social Science in Health at the School of Health in Social Science. Her research intersects across several key areas, within an overall focus on the experience of people with dementia and people with an intellectual disability and dementia, and improving their care experience. She has linked this work into knowledge exchange and public engagement. Much of Heather's work has been methodologically ground-breaking to ensure that the research participants with dementia and/or intellectual disabilities are included in research and dissemination. Heather was a founder member of the Scottish Dementia Working Group.

Shahid H. Zaman

Shahid is a consultant psychiatrist for the Cambridgeshire and Peterborough NHS Foundation Trust and affiliated lecturer at the Department of Psychiatry, University of Cambridge, UK. Shahid has undertaken research in the synaptic pathophysiology of Alzheimer's disease using rodent transgenic models and is working on understanding the pathogenesis of dementia in people with Down syndrome.

Subject Index

Author Index